PACIFIC NORTHWEST MEDICINAL PLANTS

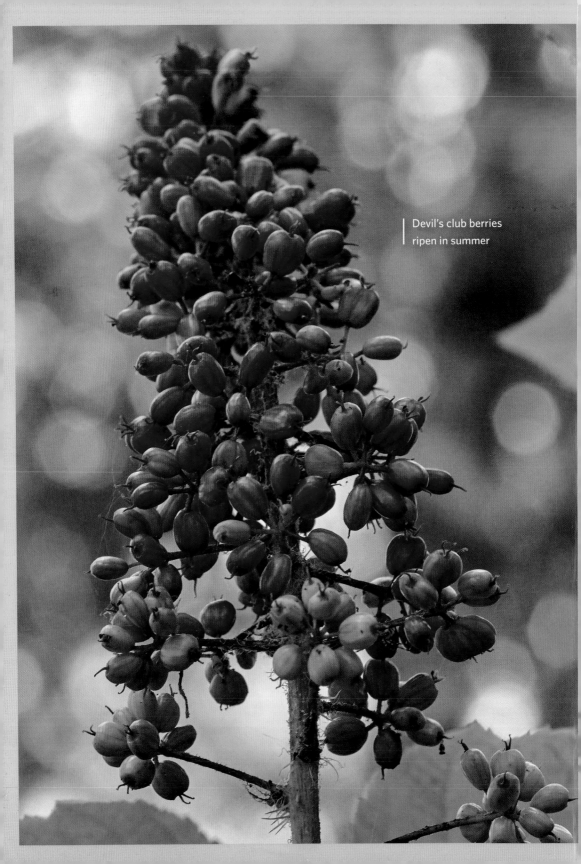

Devil's club berries
ripen in summer

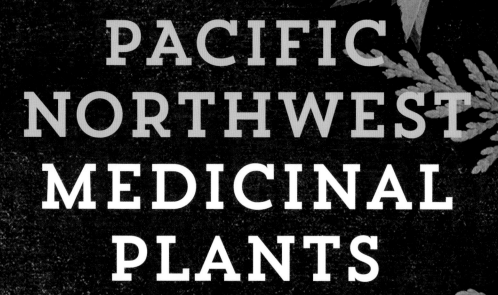

PACIFIC NORTHWEST MEDICINAL PLANTS

IDENTIFY, HARVEST, AND USE
⚜ 120 WILD HERBS ⚜
FOR HEALTH AND WELLNESS

SCOTT KLOOS

The information in this book is true and complete to the best
of our knowledge. All recommendations are made without guarantee
on the part of the author or Timber Press. The author and publisher
disclaim any liability in connection with the use of this information.
In particular, ingesting wild plants and fungi is inherently risky.
Plants can be easily mistaken and individuals vary in their physiological
reactions to plants that are touched or consumed. Please do not
attempt self-treatment of a medical problem without
consulting a qualified health practitioner.

Published in 2017 by Timber Press, Inc.
The Haseltine Building
133 S.W. Second Avenue, Suite 450
Portland, Oregon 97204-3527
timberpress.com

Printed in China
Second printing 2017
Text and cover design by Adrianna Sutton

Library of Congress Cataloging-in-Publication Data
Names: Kloos, Scott, author.
Title: Pacific Northwest medicinal plants: identify, harvest, and use 120 wild
    herbs for health and wellness / Scott Kloos.
Description: Portland, Oregon: Timber Press, 2017. | Includes bibliographical
    references and index.
Identifiers: LCCN 2016036947 | ISBN 9781604696578 (pbk.)
Subjects: LCSH: Medicinal plants—Northwest, Pacific. | Herbs—Northwest,
    Pacific.
Classification: LCC QK99.A1 K67 2017 | DDC 581.6/3409795—dc23 LC record
    available at https://lccn.loc.gov/2016036947

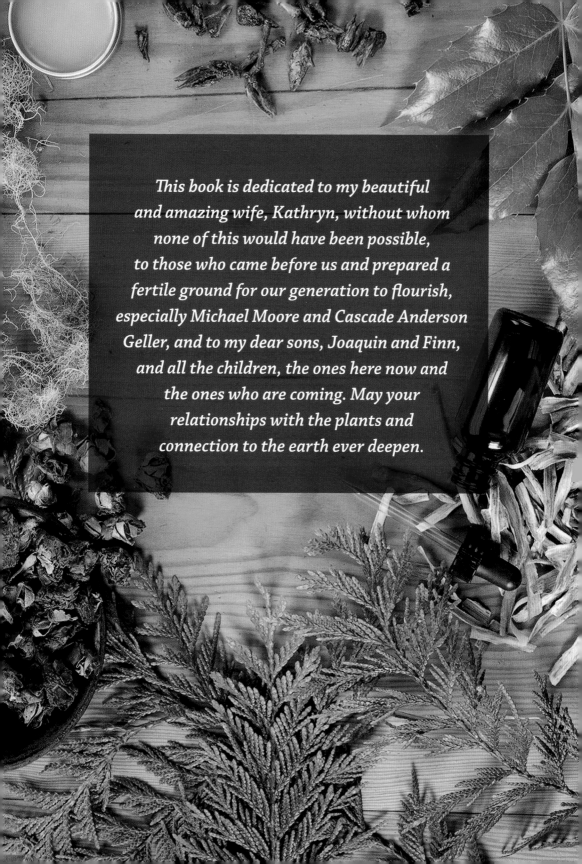

This book is dedicated to my beautiful and amazing wife, Kathryn, without whom none of this would have been possible, to those who came before us and prepared a fertile ground for our generation to flourish, especially Michael Moore and Cascade Anderson Geller, and to my dear sons, Joaquin and Finn, and all the children, the ones here now and the ones who are coming. May your relationships with the plants and connection to the earth ever deepen.

CONTENTS

Preface • 9

WILD MEDICINAL PLANTS OF THE PACIFIC NORTHWEST • 85

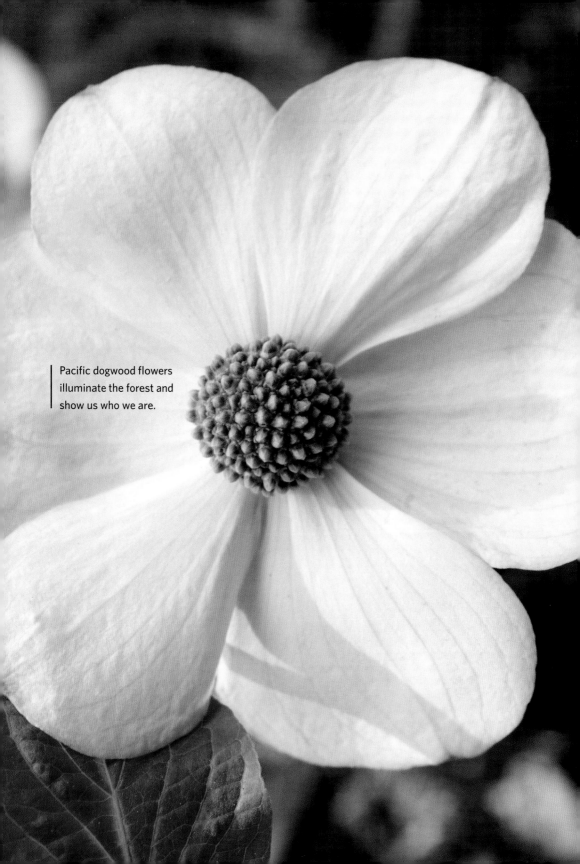

Pacific dogwood flowers illuminate the forest and show us who we are.

PREFACE

My first field-guides still sit on a bookshelf in my office at home. Each crease, dirt smudge, dried plant specimen, and dog-eared page in those books is a testament to days of adventure pregnant with the promise of meeting new plant friends and allies in the forests, mountains, valleys, and deserts of my cherished Pacific Northwest home. I used those books so much that the information they contained became a part of me, but one day I knew it was time for me to take off the training wheels and leave the field guides at home.

I very clearly remember that day. It was a day tinged with sadness because knowing the plants well enough to leave the books behind also meant saying goodbye to the thrill of discovery and the wonderment that propelled me on many epic quests. At the time I knew there would always be new things to discover, relationships to deepen, and aspects of nature to wonder upon, but it would never be like it was in those early days.

If you are just beginning your journey on this green path, I envy you. Out in the wild, many new friends and allies await. Amid the earth's myriad flowering colors and the infinite shades of green knowledge within her

whispering leaves, you will experience the excitement, joy, and awe that comes when you finally discover and meet a new plant that's been calling to you. Instead of just gazing longingly at the pictures in this book, you will have the opportunity to smell the sweet scent of the flowers, stroke the subtle fuzz on the underside of the leaves, and watch how the plants sway in the wind to greet you as you enter the forest.

Getting to know plants is like meeting a lifelong friend. You will need to give as much or more than you receive. It takes dedication to develop these relationships, but you will never be alone again. Wherever you go you will be surrounded by friends. Like the books that inspired me, I hope that this book helps you find, remember, and renew your connection to the wild. You will meet plants that grow along your favorite hiking trails and in your neighborhood park, plants that grow way out in the mountains and absolutely won't grow in anybody's garden, and others that will happily grow in your garden or that thrive in ground disturbed by the presence of humans. The thing that unites these plants is that they grow without our aid and sometimes despite our attempts to eradicate them. They embody the forces of nature and possess a spirit that renews and invigorates our own wildness. By connecting with and using these plants as medicine, we can retune our physical bodies in relationship to the land. By connecting with the wild places within ourselves and by harvesting and making medicine from these wild plants, we remember how to be in harmony with nature.

How did I get started on this path? After watching my grandparents die without dignity in the hospital, I was unable to go near a hospital for years without having a panic attack. These and other mainstream health care experiences affected me deeply. I knew that I never wanted to end up in the hospital. Even as a teenager, I knew that the hospital was not a suitable environment for healing. It was a place to die, not a place to get well.

In my early twenties, I started learning about herbs and wanted to make my own medicine because I was sure that civilization had no interest in my well-being and, in any case, it was headed for a collapse. I knew that if I wanted to survive the downfall, I would have to take matters into my own hands. As I've cultivated this rebellious spirit of self-reliance over the years, my views on how to bring about societal change have shifted.

Rather than hunker down and wait for the end of civilization, I've spent the majority of my adult life making medicines to share with my community, empowering others to do the same, and teaching classes that allow people to experience the magic and power of plant medicine so that we ourselves can shape the world in which we want to live.

The wild plants have become my friends and teachers. Harvesting them to make medicine has brought health and happiness to my life on so many levels. While I understand that wild plants will never be the main supply of medicine for the modern world, they will always have their place.

Health care is a right all humans ought to share equally. As people continue to become disillusioned with a system increasingly dependent on developing new drugs to increase profits for shareholders, it becomes more important that we have access to medicines that grow in the backyards, fields, meadows, and wild areas near our homes. It is refreshing to return to the roots of healing and find natural remedies that support our own health and well-being as well as that of our families and friends.

Wild medicinal plants carry a different medicine than herbs cultivated in gardens. They not only create the conditions for physical health and inspire harmony within our bodies, but they remind us of the wild places within ourselves and connect us to nature. Can we truly be healthy without a connection to the foundations of all life here on Earth? I say no, and in my experience it is this disconnect that is at the root of so much of our current dis-ease as a society.

Retaining and developing a connection to the wild through making medicine from and ingesting wild medicinal plants can enliven and invigorate our lives in a very special way. It can lead us to the remembrance of a

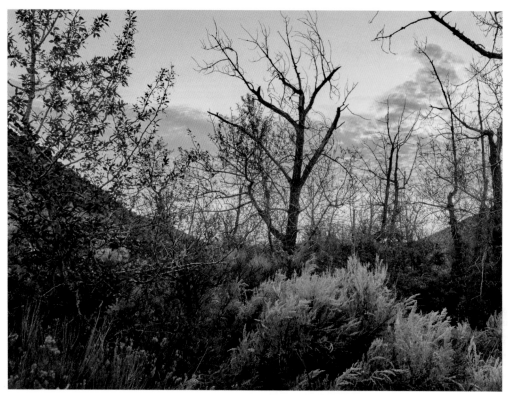

Dawn breaks over a high desert creek lined with sagebrush and cottonwood.

culture that respects the land and all creatures of the earth, one that is guided by the very same principles that the natural world uses to organize itself.

So now I take another step on my path as I write this book for you. I am honored to share the knowledge that I've gathered in more than two decades of wildcrafting, medicine making, and working with plant medicine. Connecting with these plants has helped me connect with parts of myself that have been marginalized, pushed aside, and forgotten. By studying these plants and the places where they grow, I remember who I am. I see their dignity, power, and beauty reflected in me. I remember my indigenous self as the presence of the ancestors who lived intimately with these lands—digging roots, gathering leaves, and making medicine by the cycles of the moon—reverberates through my being.

Without my first field guides, I would never have experienced these things. To their authors I am deeply indebted and forever grateful. I can only hope that you will find similar inspiration in the pages that follow and wish you the best on adventures of your own.

May these chapters inspire you to seek out your own philosophy of health, and may the plants be agents of healing, teaching, and guidance for you in the same way that they've been for me.

Open yourself to the wild. The plants await.

Take a moment to listen.

They are calling.

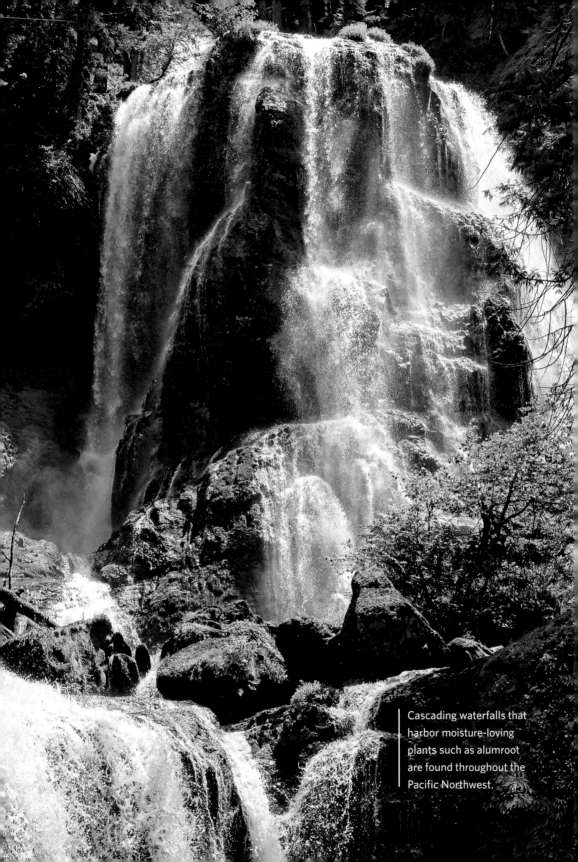

Cascading waterfalls that harbor moisture-loving plants such as alumroot are found throughout the Pacific Northwest.

HOW TO USE THIS BOOK

This book describes 120 of the most important medicinal plants growing in this region. The geographical area covered includes Alaska, British Columbia, Oregon, Washington, and northern California, ranging from temperate rain forests to rich-soiled river valleys, from rugged coastal bluffs to glacier-topped mountains, and from urban wilderness and green spaces to high desert landscapes.

The introductory chapters include detailed information to inspire confidence in and deepen your relationship with the natural world and the plants that you will find growing there. Therein I describe basic botanical concepts, herbal energetics, an overview of tools for harvesting and making medicine, ethical and sustainable wildcrafting practices, how to use plants for medicine, herbal safety, and a breakdown of the harvesting season. In the section "Making Herbal Medicines," I describe the detailed steps involved in preparing infusions, decoctions, tinctures, herb-infused oils, salves, syrups, compresses, and poultices. These are the general recipes to be used when making the herbal preparations presented in the 120 plant profiles.

Each plant profile is accompanied by photographs showing the growth habit and important parts of the plant and includes a description of the plant's identifying characteristics. I list the geographical distribution and habitats where you will most likely find each plant, the best time of year to harvest, and harvesting instructions. I discuss the plant's medicinal uses and methods for preparing each part as medicine. Finally, I highlight cautions and contraindications relating to each plant, if warranted, and offer tips for sustainable harvesting and propagation. Be sure to read the whole entry for each plant thoroughly before harvesting or using it for medicine so that you are aware of any pertinent wildcrafting information or important cautions.

It is my sincerest hope that this book will empower you to trust in your own senses and experience. In the pages that follow, I present you with all of the tools necessary to begin harvesting wild plants in an ethical and sustainable way and offer simple, clear, and concise directions for processing these plants into medicine for personal use or to share with family, friends, and community.

Plant Names

Plants have two types of names: a scientific name and common names. The scientific name, also known as a Latin binomial, comprises two words written in italics, such as *Oplopanax horridus* (the name for devil's club). *Oplopanax* refers to the genus, a grouping of closely related plants that share similar physical characteristics and common genetics. This part of the name is capitalized. The second part of the name, *horridus*, known as the specific epithet refers to the species and is written lowercase. As a rule, plants that look very similar and are able to produce fertile offspring together are considered to be of the same species.

Some people may feel intimidated by scientific names, but they often help us understand various morphological, geographical, or historical aspects of the plant. For example, both the genus and species names of Saint John's wort, *Hypericum perforatum*, have stories to tell. *Hypericum* comes from the Greek words *hyper* (meaning "over or above") and *icon* ("image"). It was understood that when people worked with Saint John's wort, the image or spirit of the plant watched over them. In ancient times it was hung above doorways to keep negative spirits away. Today we ingest the tincture to relieve depression that may be caused by negative thought forms. The specific epithet, *perforatum*, reminds us that the leaves have holes or perforations in them.

As you familiarize yourself with botanical terminology, you will find many useful hints about plants based on the words used to name them. For example, the word *glabra* means "smooth" or "without hairs," *glauca* means "covered in a whitish or bluish waxy coating or bloom," and *trifolium* means "three-leaved." The specific epithets *officinale* or *officinalis* are used to denote species within a genus that are preferred for use as medicine, such as *Taraxacum officinale* (dandelion) and *Melissa officinalis* (lemon balm).

The scientific names have other things to tell us as well. The species name of *Umbellularia californica* tells us that California bay is primarily found in California, although an alternate common name, Oregon myrtle, tells us something else. The suffix *-ensis* added to the end of a species name means "of that place," as in *Solidago canadensis* (Canada goldenrod). The suffix *-oides* is used to denote a morphological relation to another species. For example, the name *Scutellaria antirrhinoides* tells us that the flowers of this species of skullcap look like those of the genus *Antirrhinum*, the snapdragons, and indeed one of the common names of *S. antirrhinoides* is snapdragon skullcap.

Plants may also be named after the botanist who first described them or as a way for this person to honor someone else. California poppy (*Eschscholzia californica*) was named after the German botanist Johann Friedrich von Eschscholtz who accompanied Adelbert von Chamisso, the man who named the plant, on a Russian scientific expedition to the west coast of North America in the early 1800s.

With the arrival of DNA sequencing to more accurately determine the genetic relationships between plants, the scientific names, which were intended to remove

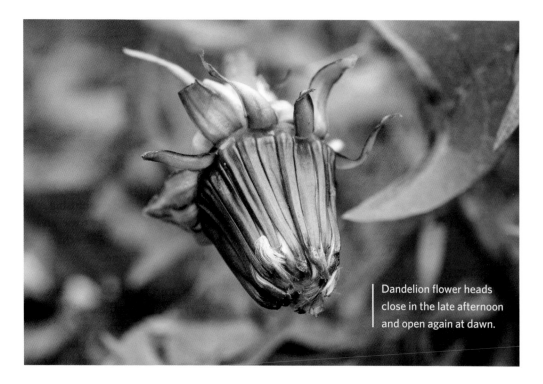

Dandelion flower heads close in the late afternoon and open again at dawn.

confusion in nomenclature, are currently undergoing a lot of change and creating some measure of confusion. Although truly understanding the evolutionary links between plants is a useful endeavor, the current upheaval is creating difficulty for those of us who just want to be able to align ourselves with others regarding plant names.

This is of particular concern to herbalists who, like me, develop a fondness for the names of plants. For two centuries Oregon grape was known as *Mahonia nervosa*, but it is now considered a member of the genus *Berberis*. It's as if someone told you that your grandmother, whom you've known all of your life as Molly, should now be called Gertrude. It's just weird. However, in this book I use the currently accepted scientific names and note the previously used names. We can only hope that the rapidly changing botanical name game will subside soon so we can all be on the same page regarding plant names.

Common names are the names most often used for plants, but their use alone may cause confusion, because the same plant may have many different common names. In addition, completely unrelated plants may share the same common name. There are many plants around the world, for example, that go by the name woundwort, but there is only one *Stachys chamissonis* var. *cooleyae*.

Herbalists often use common names that refer to the medicinal properties of plants. I've opted to use the common name given by the USDA Plants database (plants.usda. gov) unless this name severely conflicts with the name commonly used by herbalists in western North America. I've included other common names used to describe each plant when applicable.

Photographs

Photographing plants is one of my passions. When possible, I've included several

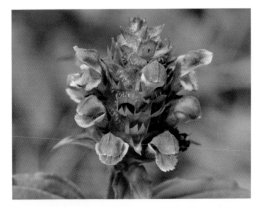
Selfheal's two-lipped flowers are a common feature in the mint family.

How to Identify

In an effort to bring the plants to life on the page, in this section of each plant profile I describe the morphological characteristics of plants as they grow throughout the seasons and across the span of their lives. I've used language accessible to the lay person but have included common botanical terms that you will encounter as you delve more deeply into your study of plants. Under this heading, I also mention potentially confusing look-a-likes, especially if they are toxic, and make note of closely related species that may be used similarly for medicine.

Where, When, and How to Wildcraft

Based on the range maps in the USDA Plants database, I present the geographical regions where you can expect to find each plant. While there may be stands or individuals that fall outside of these areas, the information ought to give you a pretty good idea of any given plant's distribution.

photographs to help you correctly identify each plant, highlighting identifying characteristics, important features, and the overall growth habit of the plant in question. Refer to the photographs as you read the text descriptions of the plants, but realize that even within species plants can exhibit a wide morphological range.

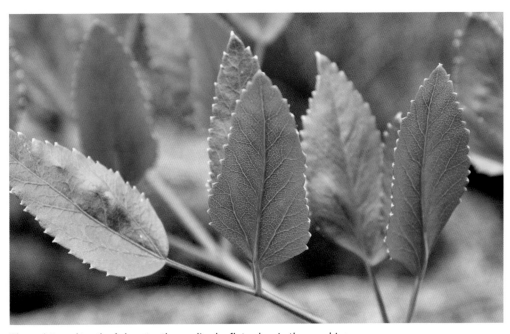
The red-tipped teeth of sharptooth angelica leaflets glow in the sunshine.

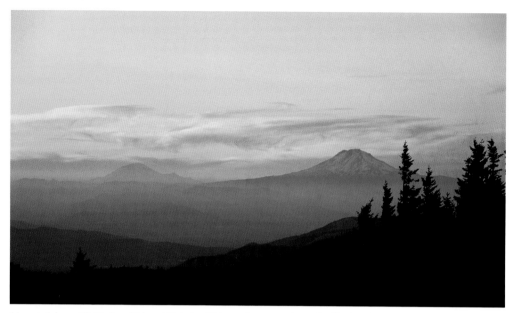

Mount Adams (Pahto) and Mount Rainier (Tahoma) as seen from the flanks of Mount Hood (Wy'east), where you will find high-elevation plants like western pasqueflower.

Elevation Ranges

- Low elevation: sea level to 2000 feet
- Middle elevation: 2000 to 5000 feet
- High elevation: above 5000 feet

Because the geographically diverse Pacific Northwest extends across many degrees of latitude and includes wide spans of elevation—from sea level to more than 14,000 feet at the top of this region's highest peak, Mount Rainier in Washington—it is difficult to pinpoint exact harvest times that will apply equally in all places. For example, Saint John's wort usually starts blooming in the lowlands around Portland, Oregon, in early to mid June, but at higher elevations on the flanks of Mount Hood, it may not start blooming until early August. At the northern extent of this region plants may bloom later than they do in the southern portions of this region. I've presented a wide harvesting range to accommodate for this and used seasonal names rather than months.

Some plants have very specific requirements for growth, whereas others can thrive in widely varying environmental conditions. Based on my own experience and through extensive research, I've endeavored to present the most likely types of habitat that the plant will occupy and listed the ranges of elevation within which you are most likely to encounter these plants. In this section I also offer harvesting and drying tips specific to each plant that go beyond the techniques laid out in the "Ethical and Sustainable Wildcrafting" section.

Medicinal Uses

In this section I have combined information from my own experience with the work of authors whom I deeply trust and respect, including Michael Moore, Matthew Wood, Robin Rose Bennet, Peter Holmes, Deborah Frances, and the Eclectic physicians who in the text are referred to as early American botanical doctors. When writing about the properties of plants beyond their first aid uses, I've tried to avoid the "What is this good for?" mentality when referring to the medicine of the plants. Instead I start with the question "What can the human body, psyche, and/or spirit learn from this plant, and how can it restore harmony and balance within the system as a whole?" Where applicable, I've included psycho-spiritual indications, and when possible I've tied these subtler forms of healing potential directly to the physical ailments to which they are so often related.

Herbal Preparations

This section lists various ways to prepare each plant for use as medicine and provides safe and effective dosages. I've listed the most common modes of preparation, but there may be other ways to make medicine from a plant. If it seems to you that a plant might make a good infused oil but it's not listed in the text, try it and see how it goes.

In describing tincture-making formulas, I list the ratio of plant material by weight to the amount of menstruum by volume, whether the medicine is made with fresh or dry plant material, and the percentage of alcohol (ethanol), distilled water, and in some cases vegetable glycerin (to stabilize the tannins). When I present two versions of the formula, the first is the preferred method.

For infused oils, I have simply listed the ratio of plant material by weight to the amount of oil by volume and whether to make the oil from fresh or dried plant material. I prefer to use olive oil, but there are many different types of oil, each with its own virtue,

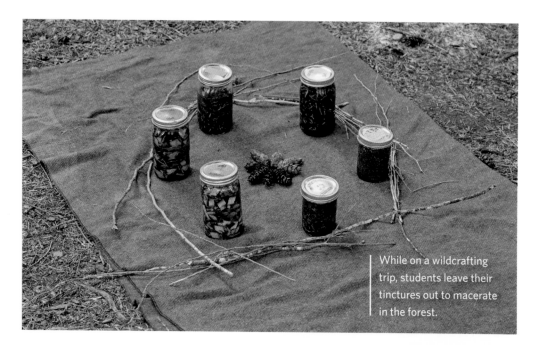

While on a wildcrafting trip, students leave their tinctures out to macerate in the forest.

suitable for making medicine. All salves, which are made by adding beeswax to an infused oil, are prepared using the same formula.

⚠ Caution

Although ingesting most medicinal plants is very safe, there are some instances where it is important or even imperative to consider the potentially harmful effects of an herb. When applicable, this section describes the toxicity, undesirable effects, dosage precautions, and contraindications for each plant.

Future Harvests

It is important to ensure that the stands of medicinal plants that we harvest from remain healthy and viable for many generations to come. In this section I describe various harvesting techniques and methods of propagation. Use the latter methods to propagate plants directly in the wild, to grow them in your garden, or to start them at home to transplant back into the wild.

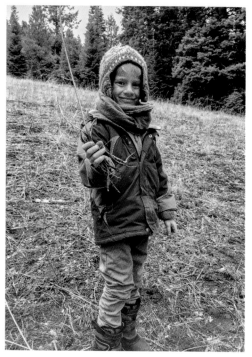

My son harvests Gray's lovage in the Ochoco Mountains.

WILDCRAFTING BASICS

Wildcrafting is the craft of harvesting medicinal plants from the wild. Humans have been wildcrafting since the dawn of time, but today when medicines are so easily procured, one might question the effort and time required to gather your own. I can assure you that the benefits of harvesting and making medicine from wild plants are many. It is not only more sustainable to use the medicinal plants that grow in the regions where we live, but the herbs we gather will be fresher and more potent. Also, because they are born of the same forces that give shape to our own physical and spiritual beings, local plants are more likely to offer deep healing benefits for our bodies, minds, and souls. In the sections that follow, I share with you the many elements wildcrafters ought to consider in order to safely and sustainably practice this age-old craft.

SPEAKING THE LANGUAGE OF PLANTS

If we are to work with wild plants for medicine, we must first study their external forms so we can learn to correctly identify them. Once a plant has been positively identified, it can be harvested and made into medicine. After we've made the medicine, we need to understand the medicinal activity of the plant so we can correctly administer it for the ailments we wish to heal.

Early in my wildcrafting career, I was on a backpacking trip with a couple of my classmates in mid autumn. We were walking the Timberline Trail on Oregon's Mount Hood in search of medicinal plants. As we made our

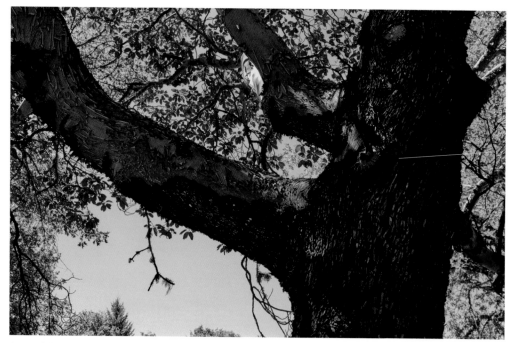

A careful and deep study of the natural world and its energetic patterns reveals many hidden secrets. Madrone teaches us to shed our old skin so that our new selves can emerge.

way around the mountain, I saw the familiar leaves of red baneberry. I excitedly showed the plant to my friends and explained how I had identified it.

We decided that there were enough plants here to make a harvest. We sat with the plants, prayed, made offerings, and then began to dig up the roots. After a little while of digging, I noticed that the plant I was digging up had small seed pods on it. "Something is not right here," I thought. Red baneberry, of course, has bright red berries. "If this isn't red baneberry then it must be black cohosh!" I had been searching for our native black cohosh for years.

I pulled out Michael Moore's *Medicinal Plants of the Pacific West* and read: "*Cimicifuga laciniata*, a sparser plant, with shorter and less elaborately divided basal leaves, is found only around the base of Mt. Hood in Oregon and across the Columbia River Gorge in Washington. It is found at much higher elevations, and

with decades of extensive logging, has been reduced to a few stands in wilderness areas. It is a threatened plant and should *not* be picked." Upon further examination I noticed that only a few of the plants in the stand had flowered and set seed.

I was horrified and embarrassed. Not only had I harvested the wrong plant, but I had harvested an endangered plant. From that day forward I paid closer attention, making absolutely sure of the identity of any plant I was going to harvest.

Picking the wrong plant can have serious consequences and be potentially life threatening. Before you venture off in search of plants to harvest, it is important to have a fundamental understanding of plant identification and an awareness of both toxic and threatened, endangered, and sensitive plant species of the area. Don't let your excitement get in the way of careful observation.

Basic Botany

Botany is western civilization's science of studying plants. It is a wide-ranging field that covers all aspects of plant life from the cell biology of plants to the roles they play in ecosystems. Here we will focus on the way that botany describes the structure of plants, known as plant morphology, so that we can correctly and positively identify plants that we encounter in the wild. The specific tool designed by botanists for this task is known as a botanical key.

Understanding how to use a botanical key, also called a dichotomous (that is, divided into two parts) key, is a must for any wildcrafter. In these books, sequences of two choices are presented that help guide the reader to a plant's specific identity. The most commonly used keys in this region are Leo Hitchcock and Arthur Cronquist's *Flora of the Pacific Northwest*, Helen Gilkey's *Handbook of Northwestern Plants*, and Eugene Kozloff's *Plants of Western Oregon, Washington, and British Columbia*.

Through careful observation and by reading the plant descriptions in this book and viewing the photographs, you ought to be able to identify many of the important medicinal plants of the Pacific Northwest. But when it comes to the parsley family (Apiaceae), which contains several very toxic plants that can be confused with plants commonly used for medicine, it is essential that you absolutely and correctly identify the plant in question using a botanical key.

If you are just starting out, find an experienced plant person who has an understanding of basic botany or sign up for a field botany course. As you are introduced to new plants, ask to be walked through the process of identification. Be sure to ask how the plant is positively identified. Learn the defining characteristics of the plants: the thing(s) that distinguish a plant from others that look

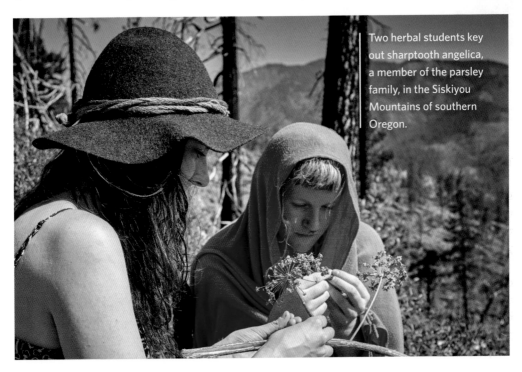

Two herbal students key out sharptooth angelica, a member of the parsley family, in the Siskiyou Mountains of southern Oregon.

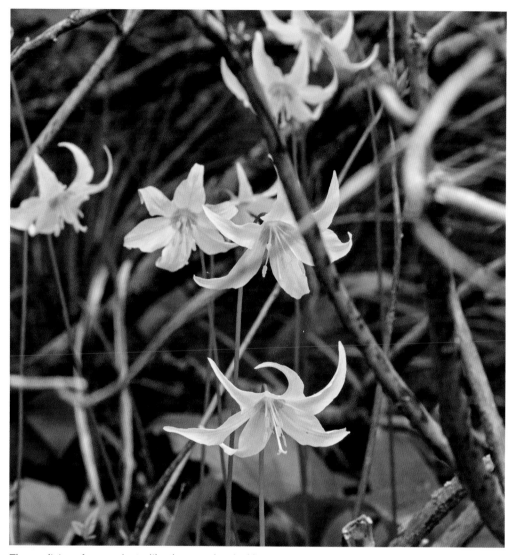

The medicine of some plants, like these avalanche lilies, is in their beauty alone.

similar. After you familiarize yourself with the process of identification, spend days in the field working through botanical keys on your own.

Studying botany and the morphological characteristics of plants helps hone the skills of perception and observation, but botanical keys have limitations. For example, it can be frustrating to key out a plant in April, which requires you to know the shape of the seed that doesn't ripen until August. So in addition to botany, study the tastes, smells, and other sense impressions of the plants. Observe the way the plants hold themselves and look for commonly occurring or strangely formed patterns. Using all of these tools in conjunction will aid you greatly as you learn to identify plants and will help minimize the risk of mistaken identity.

Steps to Identifying a Plant

Before you start reading the plant descriptions in this book or open a botanical key, make note of these important characteristics.

Growth habit Is it a tree, shrub, vine, or herb? Does is grow thin and tall, or does it spread itself wide?

Habitat Where is the plant growing? Is it sunny or shady? What type of soil is it growing in?

Trunks, stalks, and branches Is the bark smooth or furrowed? Are hairs or spines present? Do trunks, stalks, and branches grow straight, or do they twist and turn?

Leaves What shape are the leaves? What is their texture? Are they hairy, smooth, thick, or thin? Are they arranged alternately, oppositely, or in whorls along the stem? If present, how long are the leaf stalks? Are the leaves entire or are they divided into segments, lobes, or compound leaflets?

Flowers What color is the flower or flowers? How are they arranged on the plant? Are they solitary or in clusters? If present, how many petals or sepals are there? Are they fused or separate? Examine the reproductive parts for further clues.

Fruits and seeds What shape and form do fruits and seeds take? Are they fleshy, woody, or hard-skinned? Do they have a crown of hairs? For some plants the seeds are the most reliable means of identification, but unfortunately they are not always present.

PLANT MORPHOLOGY

These are the most important parts of a plant that every beginning wildcrafter ought to know.

LEAF SHAPES

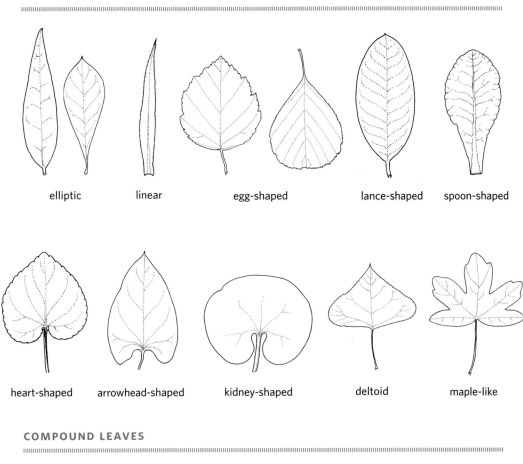

elliptic

linear

egg-shaped

lance-shaped

spoon-shaped

heart-shaped

arrowhead-shaped

kidney-shaped

deltoid

maple-like

COMPOUND LEAVES

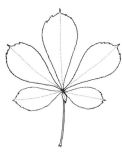

palmate compound

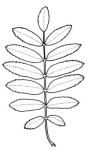

pinnate compound

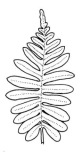

pinnate lobed

LEAF MARGINS

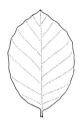 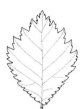 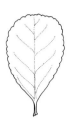 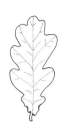 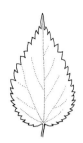

smooth-edged   double-toothed   scalloped   lobed   toothed

LEAF ARRANGEMENTS

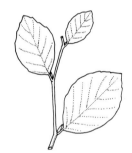

alternate

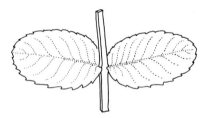

opposite

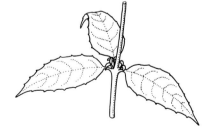

whorled

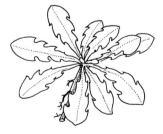

basal

CONIFER LEAVES

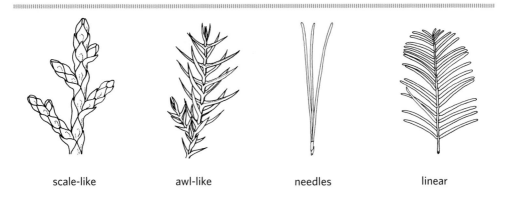

scale-like   awl-like   needles   linear

LEAF PARTS

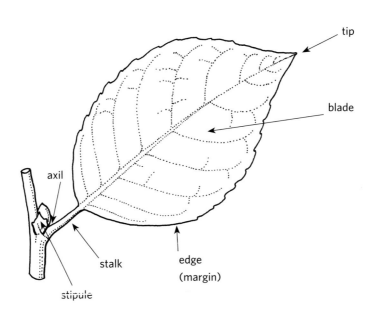

tip

blade

axil

stalk

stipule

edge
(margin)

FLOWER PARTS

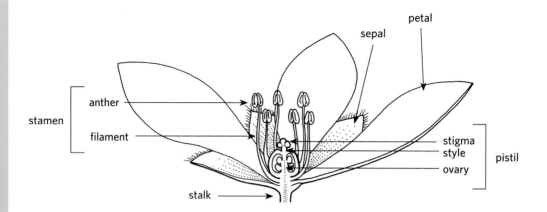

stamen

anther

filament

sepal

petal

stigma
style
ovary

pistil

stalk

COMPOSITE FLOWER PARTS

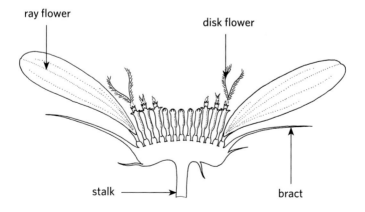

ray flower

disk flower

stalk

bract

The Doctrine of Signatures

After first learning about the Doctrine of Signatures, I sat in front of a goldenrod plant in the garden where I was working. At the time I knew nothing about the medicine of goldenrod. I carefully observed the plant's form for a few minutes and then closed my eyes. In my mind a saw a golden fountain of urine. I opened my eyes and saw the resemblance between my vision and the yellow flower clusters at the ends of the stalks. When I got home, I looked goldenrod up in a book and found that it was useful for healing infections and other conditions of the urinary tract. I was so excited!

If one believes that there is an underlying force or energy that gives shape and form to the universe, it is easy to see that there would be correlations between things that have been shaped by similar permutations of this universal force. This force creates patterns that are found throughout nature in forms that include the golden ratio, the golden rectangle, Fibonacci sequence patterns, Overbeck jets, and toroids.

In order to see these patterns, we must perceive on an intuitive level where connections can be made, freely and without inhibition. Here we can tap into deeper levels of experience and bring back symbols that bridge the gap between the conscious and unconscious minds as well as the spiritual and material dimensions. This is the magic place that we seek when working with the Doctrine of Signatures.

A careful and deep study of the natural world and its energetic patterns reveals many hidden secrets. Information is all around us waiting to be received. Working with the Doctrine of Signatures allows us to penetrate to deeper levels of understanding. It is the overall feel of a plant and its energetic essence that gives us clues to its medicinal and psycho-spiritual properties. If we are able

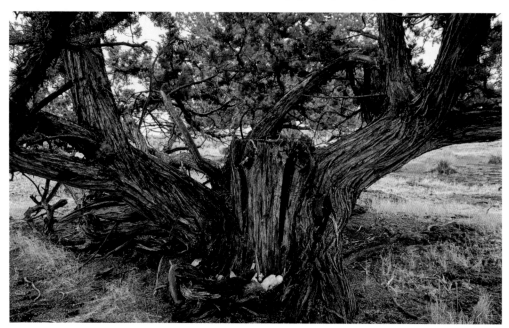

Western juniper twists and turns in response to environmental stresses. The tree teaches us about how the traumas we experience shape our lives.

to experience plants in their totality, patterns based on their habitat, their form including shape, color, and texture, and their energetic qualities including temperature, taste, and elemental associations may begin to emerge.

Some Useful Signatures

Cascade Oregon grape's yellow roots relate to the liver. Think of the way jaundice, a liver disorder, causes a yellowing of the skin.

Devil's club's spines are protective. Developing a relationship with this plant creates a layer of spiritual protection and beats the devils or negative thought forms away with its club.

Mullein's hairy leaves relate to cilia of the lungs. Mullein leaves help clean the lungs.

Pacific dogwood flower heads remind us of the third eye chakra. Pacific dogwood opens one's capacity for visions.

Red alder and red root have nitrogen-fixing nodes on their roots that look like lymph nodes. Both plants clear waste products from the lymphatic system. Both have red bark and have an effect on the blood.

Western pasqueflower's wild-haired seed head looks like the head of a person who just stuck a finger in an electrical socket. Western pasqueflower is an excellent remedy for a person with a fried, overstimulated nervous system.

Yerba santa's taste changes from bitter to sweet. It shows us how to find the value in the bitter experiences of life.

TOXIC PLANTS

Learning to correctly identify toxic plants can save you and others from serious harm. I don't want to instill fear of the wild in you, but there are some toxic plants in this region that can be confused with commonly used medicinal plants. Here is an overview of the toxic plants you may encounter in the Pacific Northwest. Please do your own research. Find a book that deals specifically with poisonous plants and study it well. Pay close attention to the buttercup (Ranunculaceae) and the parsley (Apiaceae) families. They contain some of this region's most beneficial and most poisonous plants.

First, let's define toxic. Plants considered toxic or poisonous have one or more parts that cause a harmful reaction when people consume, inhale, or come into contact with them. There are degrees of toxicity to consider as well. We've all probably consumed foods that when eaten in moderation give us no trouble, but when consumed in larger quantities the same food may make us sick to our stomachs, such as foods high in fats or sugars.

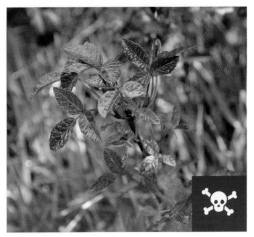

The irritating oil urushiol, present in all parts of the poison oak plant, can cause severe rashes in some people.

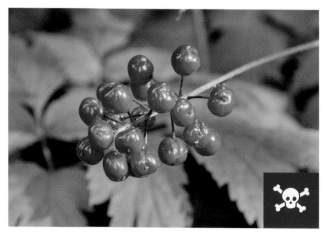

Baneberry's enticing but toxic berries live up to their name, but the roots and leaves are safe to consume.

or vomiting if ingested, but the berries (minus the seeds) and flowers when ingested cause no adverse reaction.

There is also a common misconception that if birds or other animals can safely consume a plant, it must be edible for humans to eat as well. This not true. The digestive systems of other animals differ from those of humans and correspondences do not apply. This goes the other way as well. If an animal consumes a plant and it causes a toxic reaction, it doesn't mean that the same plant will cause an adverse reaction in humans.

If one part of a plant is edible, that doesn't mean that all parts of it are edible. Conversely if one part of a plant is toxic, that doesn't mean that all parts of it are toxic as well. The leaves, bark, roots, and seeds of blue elder, for example, contain the toxic compound hydrocyanic acid that can cause nausea and/

Unfortunately, much of the information we rely on for determining which plants are toxic to humans comes from animal studies or cases of livestock poisoning. For example, despite the fact that Saint John's wort

What to Do If Someone Consumes a Toxic Plant

- Stay calm.
- If the person has stopped breathing or doesn't respond to being touched or shaken, call 911 immediately. Otherwise, call the local poison control center. In the United States, dialing 1-800-222-1222 will connect you with the nearest poison control center. In British Columbia, the local poison control center can be reached at 1-800-567-8911. As best as you can, describe the plant responsible for the poisoning, the symptoms of the poisoning, and the amount of plant material the person ingested.
- Wait for professional help, and do not administer syrup of ipecac or attempt to force the person to vomit by any other means. Inducing the poisoning victim to vomit can make the problem worse.
- If you are in the field and far from medical attention, administer activated charcoal. The recommended dosage for adults is 25–100 grams of powder mixed with water. For children 1–12 years old, it is 25–50 grams mixed with water. For children less than 1 year old, give 10–25 grams mixed with water. Then seek emergency medical help as quickly as possible.

has a reputation for causing photosensitive reactions in humans, there have been few documented cases of such reactions occurring. In *Poisonous Plants of the United States and Canada*, the most referenced book when it comes to toxicity, John M. Kingsbury cites a 1920s study showing that in order for sheep to exhibit symptoms of Saint John's wort photosensitization, they need to eat 5 percent of their body weight of dry Saint John's wort herb. For cattle it is 1 percent. If we take the average human body weight at 150 pounds and assume that our digestive systems are similar, this would mean that a human would have to eat 1½ pounds of dry Saint John's wort to have a reaction. We know that our systems are quite different, but it would be hard for a human to even come close to this amount. In moderate doses the vast majority of people are fine consuming medicinal preparations of Saint John's wort.

Take Care with the Parsley Family (Apiaceae)

Because several toxic plants in this family grow in the Pacific Northwest and may be confused with common medicinal plants, it is vitally important to accurately and positively identify the plants you intend to harvest. Two of these poisonous plants, water hemlock and poison hemlock, look similar to medicinal plants described in this book, and both are deadly toxic even when consumed in small quantities. Do not ingest any part of wild carrot, angelica, or any other member of the parsley family unless you are 100 percent confident in your ability to correctly identify the plant in question. Your life or the lives of others depend on it.

Wild carrot and poison hemlock both grow in dry, disturbed soils. To avoid inadvertently gathering poison hemlock (*Conium maculatum*) when you are seeking to harvest wild carrot (*Daucus carota*) roots or seeds, pay close attention to these distinguishing characteristics. Wild carrot's hairy stems are usually not purple-spotted, and its white, carrot-like roots are pleasant smelling. Wild carrot's nest-like seed head is made up of bristly haired seeds. Poison hemlock's usually purple-spotted stems are hairless, and the roots usually exude a disagreeable aroma. The seed heads, made up of hairless seeds, remain open as the seeds mature.

The angelicas and water hemlocks both prefer wet soils and have compound leaves with

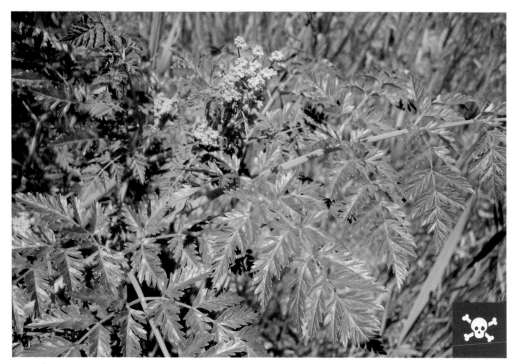

Poison hemlock

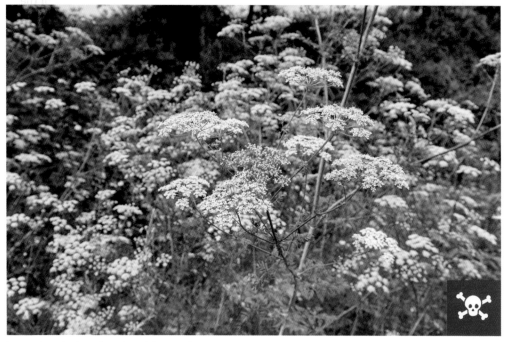

Poison hemlock, with its lacy foliage, white, small-flowered umbels, and purple-spotted stalks, may look similar to other members of the parsley family.

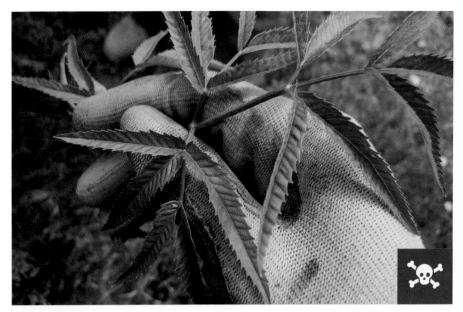

Water hemlock

large leaflets. To avoid inadvertently gathering water hemlock (*Cicuta douglasii*) when you are seeking to harvest angelica (*Angelica* species) roots or seeds, pay close attention to these distinguishing characteristics. Angelica roots have a very specific perfumey, soap-like smell and a usually unchambered, solid root. Angelica's leaf veins usually terminate at the tips of the teeth. In contrast, water hemlock usually has chambered roots, and its leaf veins usually terminate at the cut between the teeth.

You may have noticed that I used the word *usually* several times in the previous two paragraphs. I did this because the form of individual plants of the same species can sometimes differ greatly. Do not rely exclusively on any one of the traits described here to make a positive identification, and keep in mind that the most reliable way to accurately differentiate plants in this family is to identify them by the form and structure of their seeds. Before attempting a harvest, identify the plants while in seed using a botanical key, and get to know the differences intimately.

Toxic Plant Quiz

To prepare my students for wildcrafting, I hand out a toxic plant quiz that we go over together in class. Here, I've included what I consider the most important part of that quiz. These are seven of the most deadly toxic plants of this region. Know how to identify these plants because they can kill you if you ingest them.

List the Latin name, defining characteristics, look-a-likes, and symptoms of poisoning for the following plants:

1. water hemlock
2. poison hemlock
3. monkshood
4. false hellebore
5. foxglove
6. death camas
7. wild cucumber

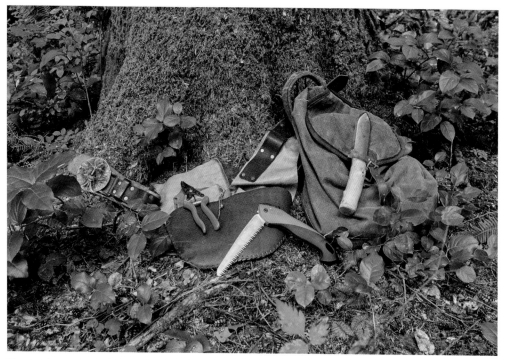

You can harvest just about anything with a pair of pruning shears, a hori hori knife, and a saw. Add the custom-made tool belt and the backpack and you're ready to go in style.

TOOLS OF THE TRADE: AN HERBALIST'S FIELD AND PANTRY KIT

Certain items are indispensable for wildcrafting and medicine making. You won't need every item on these lists right away, and, in fact, you probably already own or can borrow many of them.

If you are starting from scratch, I'd recommend getting a few key things: a pair of pruning shears, a digging tool, and some paper or cloth bags for wildcrafting and some mason jars, an inexpensive kitchen scale, a measuring cup, and a pair of scissors or a knife and cutting board for medicine making. If you choose to use the folk method for making medicine, you can skip the scale and measuring cup.

Resist the urge to buy cheap harvesting tools. It's better to buy a couple of good tools than to get a bunch of inexpensive, poorly made tools. Well-made, high-end tools last years longer, operate more smoothly, and most have replaceable parts, which means less waste in the end. My current pair of pruning shears is 15 years old, and it works as well now as the day I bought it. I've watched frustrated students give up on harvesting jobs because they were using inadequately made or poorly maintained tools. High-quality, well-maintained tools allow for more work with less effort.

Harvesting Tools

Clippers and pruners I prefer smaller pruning shears, because they are more versatile and can do finer work. Find a pair that feels good in your hand. Consider a pair of long-handled pruners, also known as loppers, for cutting thicker branches.

Saws A high-quality saw makes for easier work. Don't allow the saw blade to come in contact with dirt or rocks, as this will quickly dull the cutting teeth. Replace the blade if the teeth become dull. Consider a second saw for cutting large woody roots. Whenever I replace the blade on my branch cutting saw, I switch the old blade to the root cutter.

Knives A good pocket or fixed-blade knife comes in handy for stripping bark and many other things.

Hori hori digging knife The hori hori knife, with its heavy and dense blade, might be the single most useful tool I own. It digs, cuts, saws, and pounds, and its blade will never break. Hand trowels, on the other hand, are meant for digging in fluffy garden soil. They are lighter, offer little leverage, and break easily when subjected to the rigors of digging roots in the wild.

Shovels and digging forks Shovels are effective tools for many applications, but I prefer digging forks because they do less damage to roots. The tines of the fork loosen the soil around the root without slashing through the flesh or bark of the root. This isn't a tool for leveraging out large rocks, but neither is a shovel. Applying too much force will bend the tines or break the blade of the shovel. Consider a digging or wrecking bar for working in very rocky soil.

Brushes, bags, backpacks, and belts Vegetable brushes are helpful for cleaning dirty roots. Stay away from plastic bags, because they encourage molding. Instead use paper or cloth shopping bags to carry your harvest. For larger harvests, use a mesh feed bag or a sheet that can be tied at the corners. You'll also need a backpack or bag to carry this book and others, tools, maps, snacks, water, offerings, and anything else you might need for a day of harvesting in the wild. Carrying tools in a tool belt or in pocket holsters makes them more accessible while you are harvesting.

Tool Care Tips

Always use the proper tool for the job.

Keep blades sharp with a sharpening stone or a carbide sharpener.

Keep moving parts well oiled with a natural, nontoxic oil.

Account for all of your tools before filling in holes or leaving a site.

Clean and dry tools after each day of harvesting.

Oil wooden handles at the end of the harvest season.

Medicine-Making Supplies

Teas
tea pot or jar
tea ball
pot with a lid
strainers
tea cup

Tinctures
alcohol (ethanol)
distilled water
vegetable glycerin
mason jars
kitchen scale
measuring cup or graduated cylinder
scissors
knife and cutting board
grinder
labels or masking tape
small herb press or cheesecloth
funnels
bottles of various sizes for storing
    and administering medicine

Salves and Oils
oil
beeswax
double boiler

ETHICAL AND SUSTAINABLE WILDCRAFTING

I remember with fondness the first time I found and harvested arnica flowers. My knees were in agony as I came near the end of a 20-mile day of backpacking in the mountains of Washington. I'd been searching for arnica for months, inspecting every medium-sized, yellow-flowered aster family plant I came across. None of the plants I'd encountered was the one. I continued my search while on this trip, and at the end of that long day of hiking, I came across a patch of flowering arnica. Rubbing the crushed flowers, pungent and rich with aromatic oils, onto my knees brought almost instant relief and invigorated my spirit. Finding this plant that I was so eagerly seeking made every torturous minute of that hike worth it.

Harvesting plants in the wild is one of my favorite things to do. From the season's first harvest of black cottonwood buds in winter to the root harvests of autumn, each moment in the field for me is pure joy. Knowing when the plants are ready for harvesting connects me with the seasonal cycles, and I often lose myself in the work of wildcrafting and forget to eat or even notice that I am hungry or tired.

With the joy comes responsibility. For me, the craft part of wildcrafting is all about employing harvesting practices that maintain the abundance of wild populations of plants and the integrity of the ecosystems in which they live. As the numbers of people relocating to the Pacific Northwest increases and foraging and wildcrafting become more

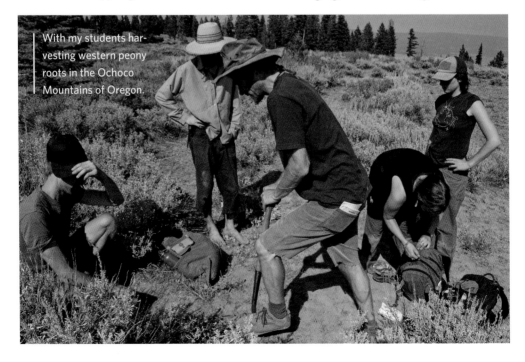

With my students harvesting western peony roots in the Ochoco Mountains of Oregon.

popular in this region, it is becoming even more crucial that we pay close attention to the effect that we humans have on the natural landscape.

When you first start harvesting plants, exercise caution. Be conservative and careful. As your confidence and discernment increase, your understanding of ethical and sustainable harvesting will grow. But no matter how experienced you are, I urge you to continue critically examining the effects of your wildcrafting. If you realize that you've adversely affected the ecosystem or a stand of plants, try to make reparations if possible, learn from your mistakes, and alter your practices.

Even while practicing the craft with a heightened sense of awareness, it is possible to cultivate a healthy respect for the wild without becoming overly cautious and fearful. In my experience, an excessive fear of

doing harm arises from the same place that leads some to clear cut forests and dump toxins into the rivers: a place of separation from self and nature. For me, wildcrafting is a sacred act. It helps me connect with forces beyond myself that invigorate my body, mind, and soul.

I encourage you to approach plants with respect and humility as a way of strengthening your relationship with the physical and energetic ecosystems of the wild. To be conscious and sustainable wildcrafters, we must try to understand how life organizes itself in the forests, meadows, fields, and high desert landscapes where we will be harvesting. It should be the goal of everyone gathering wild plants to have as little impact as possible. Our presence in nature is not inherently negative. If we immerse ourselves in a deep study of the natural world and examine the physical characteristics of

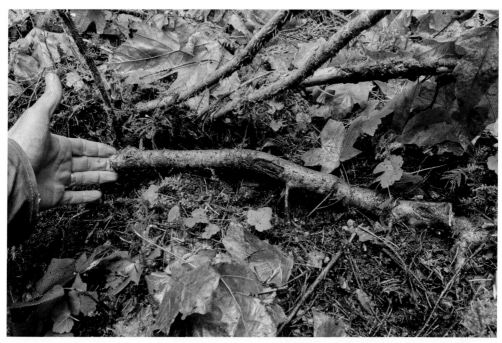

Removing a chunk of devil's club root from between two well-rooted nodes allows the aboveground portions of the plant to continue to grow.

different ecosystems, our actions may even have a positive impact on the places we visit. To determine whether harvesting is appropriate and to ensure that the places where we harvest medicinal plants remain healthy and viable for many generations to come, I encourage you to gain as much understanding as possible of the intricate web of interrelations that keep ecosystems functioning in a healthy way. We each have a role to play in this process, and as we each gather and share this information, we will increase our collective appreciation for the import of these relationships. So how do we do this?

Start by learning about the places you visit most often. As you become comfortable in these places, expand your reach and visit as many different types of habitat as you can. Spend time in natural areas without a thought of harvesting. Just be. Go there to give and receive on other levels. Open your heart to the forces of nature. Develop relationships with the plants you are intending to harvest for medicine. Not only will you learn a lot, but the medicine you make will be more effective.

Study different ecosystems. Each has differing requirements to sustain itself. The needs of a coastal wetland community vary greatly from those of a high desert scrubland community. Visit natural areas that have been impacted by human activity. Sit or walk silently in an old-growth forest or in wild remote places where the impacts of human contact are barely detectable. What are the components of a healthy ecosystem? What happens when these requirements are not met? What differences do you notice in the way plants grow? Are there plants or animals you find in one place but not the other? What are some of the effects of increased human presence?

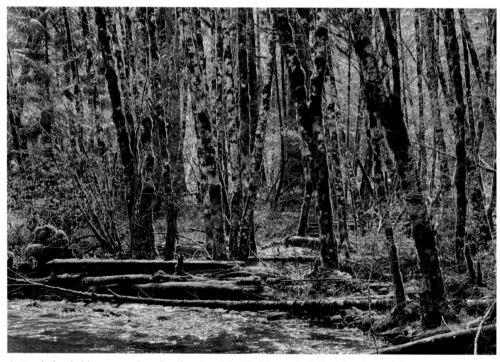

A stand of red alder grows along Panther Creek in Washington's Gifford Pinchot Wilderness.

Topics to Stimulate Your Inquiry

How do the weather and changing climatic conditions affect different ecosystems and the plants in which they grow? For example, in dry years I've noticed that some plants like sharptooth angelica or western peony choose to conserve energy by not ripening their seeds. Others like yerba santa produce bountiful seed crops. Consider this factor in your harvesting assessment. Don't do anything that will unduly stress the plants in drier years.

How do variations based on elevation or local geography affect the ecosystem? A plant that grows abundantly at lower elevations or in sunny conditions may grow more sparsely at higher elevations or in the shade. Does the wind affect growth or the orientation of the slope on which a plant grows? Some plants prefer growing on south-facing slopes that receive full sun all day long. Is a plant thriving in a small area because of a particular microclimate? Perhaps this is the only thriving community in the area. If so, find somewhere else to harvest.

How does the type of soil in which a plant lives affect its growth? Plants are highly adaptable. A plant species may prefer to grow in rich soil. If it grows in a less than optimal dry, rocky soil, it can survive but its rate of growth may be severely stunted. This ought to be considered when you decide whether to harvest a plant.

What are the effects of fire or other disturbances on the landscape and what species come in after fire? Understand the life cycle of different ecosystems. In dry areas *Ceanothus* species and yerba santa often sprout up after a fire. *Ceanothus* adds nourishment to the soil by fixing nitrogen in nodules on its roots, and yerba santa creates an extensive lateral root system that prevents erosion. In wetter areas affected by fire or flooding, fast-growing alders also fix nitrogen and drop lots of leaf matter to build the soil. Slow-growing conifers arrive when the conditions are right and eventually shade out the alders, which die off once their job is done. Trees in an old clear cut where I'd been harvesting red root (*Ceanothus velutinus*) started growing tall enough that they were shading out the red root. The red root had done its job, building the soil and depositing seed to wait for the next forest disturbance or fire. It became a prime harvesting spot before the red root completely died out.

What animals make their home in the ecosystem, what role do the animals play in the ecosystem, and which plants or animals do they rely on for food? For example, if we remove too many plants upon which an insect deposits its eggs, how will this affect other insects or animals who feed on that insect?

How have humans affected the landscape? Clear cuts, road cuts, and power lines all have detrimental effects on ecosystems. How can we navigate around these and not create more disturbances? Can we take advantage of some of these disturbances while we work to prevent them in the future?

This is a brief introduction to the topic, and the questions that can be asked are endless. We can't possibly know all of the factors involved in maintaining a healthy ecosystem, but as we continue to ask these questions, we, as a community of wildcrafters, will eventually come to a place where we can have little negative impact on the ecosystems where we harvest medicinal plants. Thank you for your contribution to this very important effort.

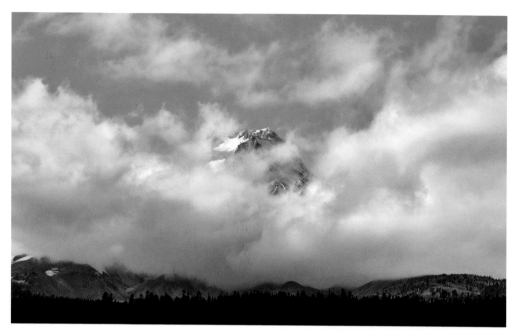

Wy'east, also known as Mount Hood, peeks through clouds that hide fields of medicinal plants.

A Short Meditation to Deepen Your Connection with the Wild

Feel your feet on the ground. As you breathe in, feel the energy of the earth rise up through your feet and into your body. With each exhale, send roots deeper and deeper into the earth. Let this energy fill your body. As you continue to inhale and exhale, the energy will reach the top of your head and burst forth into the sky. Now, as you breathe in, draw energy up from the earth and into the sky above. As you breathe out, pull energy in from the sky and send it down into the earth. You are now a conduit between the sky and the earth. From this place radiate awareness from your heart in all directions. Tune into the life energies that surround you. Listen to the sounds of the birds and insects. Feel the wind as it moves across your skin. Experience the subtle movements of the plants and trees. Do you feel more connected now?

Asking Permission and Making Offerings

Once while on a search for cascara sagrada, I found a tree with many inward growing branches that was perfect for harvesting. I asked permission and the tree said "no." I was baffled, but as I continued up the trail just a bit, I found a tree with a large broken branch that was still full of life and ripe for harvest.

Another time, I sat in front of wild ginger in early October completely exhausted after an incredibly busy year of harvesting and teaching. When I asked permission to harvest, I was told that I was too tired to harvest and was instructed to go lie under a tree and take a nap.

Always ask the plants for permission to harvest. Develop your listening skills. The answers come differently to each person.

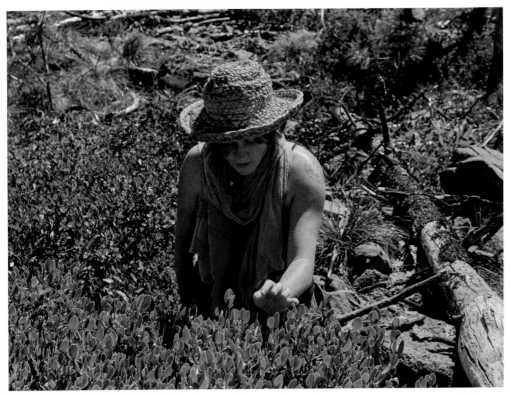

As you find your connection with nature and to the spirits of the plants, you will find that more often than not they happily and willingly offer up their gifts of healing. They know that we really need their help.

For me a "yes" may be a feeling of openness in my heart or a vision of arms reaching out to hand me a bunch of plants. A "no" will feel like a shrinking of my energetic being or my head will begin to nod from side to side. At first you might hear "yes" a lot and may doubt yourself, but when you hear the first "no," you will begin to trust your ability to hear the plants.

Reverence and gratitude open the pathways for us to receive. Offer tobacco, cornmeal, beads, shells, some kind words, a song, or some of your hair to express your gratitude to the plants. As I make offerings to the plants, I thank them for all of the healing that they have brought to me and my community and very clearly describe the help that I and others will need from them.

Endangered, Threatened, and Sensitive Species

The history of the expansion of human communities across the globe is filled with stories of plants that we can no longer harvest from the wild in good conscience. As the final frontier of American migration, the western part of North America has fewer chapters to contribute to this sad tale, but we still need to be acutely aware of plants that grow very slowly, plants whose habitat is diminished by human development, or plants whose popularity is leading to more harvesting than the land can support. Getting to know these plants and the ways we can sustainably work with them will ensure that these medicines will not be harvested out of existence.

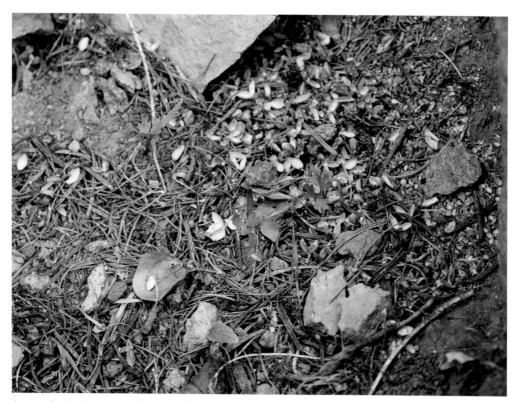

A year after being sown in the hole where a root was dug, these Gray's lovage seedlings start their slow growth to maturity.

We should look at the effects of our harvesting with a long-term vision, but with humans' current state of disconnect from the land and the loss of traditional knowledge, we don't have much to go on in terms of longer harvesting cycles. While some plants may thrive from our continued picking, other slow-growing, long-lived species may need long spaces of rest between harvests. We may find locally abundant stands of desert parsley, Gray's lovage, or western trillium that contain hundreds of plants, but we must ask ourselves how long it took for those stands to establish themselves. Desert parsley, for example, may only sustain a few years of even minimal harvesting before needing 50 years or more to rest and regenerate. In some instances it may take only one day of overzealous harvesting to seriously harm a stand of slow-growing plants. If our harvesting leads to a decline in a stand of plants or in the health of an ecosystem, we need to find other wildcrafting sites so the places that we've been harvesting from can rejuvenate themselves.

We should also consider the collateral damage we may cause when harvesting plants in the wild. For example, sundew (*Drosera rotundifolia*), various orchid species, and other rare plants grow in the meadows where I find king's gentian. A misplaced footstep can damage or kill these delicate plants and leave a long-lasting impression in the soft soil. Be mindful of your impact, and stay on trails to avoid damaging meadows or other sensitive ecosystems.

With a continuing and careful study of the natural cycles of life in the wild, including the consequences of our wildcrafting, we can reestablish an understanding of the needs of ecosystems and the plants that inhabit them. We can then pass this vital information on to our children, grandchildren, and those who will follow for many generations to come.

Be Cautious of Your Impact on These Plants

These plants live in fragile ecosystems, have limited distribution, and/or they (cascara sagrada) or their relatives in other places (arnica, gentian, western aralia, and western trillium) have been subject to unsustainable harvesting practices that have threatened their existence in the wild.

arnica (*Arnica* species)
cascara sagrada (*Frangula purshiana*)
gentian leaf (*Gentiana* species)
goldthread (*Coptis* species)
pipsissewa (*Chimaphila umbellata*)
western aralia (*Aralia californica*)
western trillium leaf (*Trillium ovatum*)

Harvest These Plants with Great Care

The roots of these slow-growing plants take a long time to reach a suitable harvesting size, so the effects of their removal from the ecosystem and the amount of time it takes for their stands to regenerate post-harvest should be monitored closely.

desert parsley (*Lomatium dissectum*)
Gray's lovage (*Ligusticum grayi*)

Never Harvest These Plants from the Wild

Whether due to their slow rate of growth, the loss of their preferred habitat (it is illegal to harvest California pitcherplant for this reason), and/or the pressures of over-harvesting, these once-popular medicinal plants are at risk of extinction. Please enjoy the beauty of these plants if you encounter them, but do not harvest them under any circumstances.

California pitcherplant (*Darlingtonia californica*)
coralroot (*Corallorhiza* species)
lady's slipper (*Cypripedium* species)
Mount Hood bugbane (*Actaea laciniata*)
roundleaf sundew (*Drosera rotundifolia*)
spleenwort-leaved goldthread (*Coptis aspleniifolia*)
tall bugbane (*Actaea elata*)

The Legality of Wildcrafting

Research the rules and regulations in the area. Generally, if you are harvesting for personal use, you won't need a permit. If you are harvesting on privately owned land, always get permission from the land owner. On public land, permits are necessary for commercial wildcrafting. Some governmental agencies will give out permits, usually for a small fee, whereas others, despite having a permitting process in place, will never give out permits. When attempting to obtain a permit from one such agency in my area, I was told that they didn't have enough employees to do a survey of the area. You'll have to decide for yourself how to proceed in such cases of moral ambiguity.

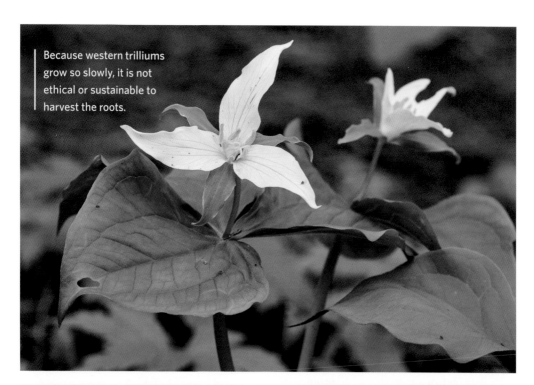

Because western trilliums grow so slowly, it is not ethical or sustainable to harvest the roots.

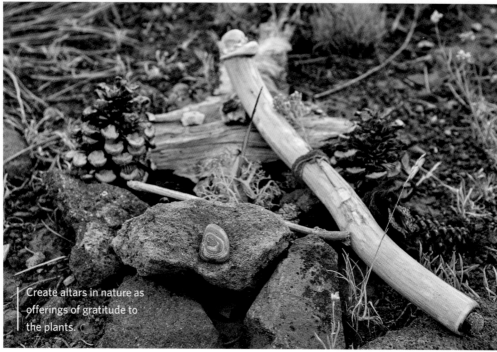

Create altars in nature as offerings of gratitude to the plants.

Rare and Endangered Plant Resources

United Plant Savers is an organization started by Rosemary Gladstar and other herbalists to bring awareness to ethical and sustainable wildcrafting practices. They publish a list of "at-risk" and "to-watch" plants. For more information, visit their website at unitedplantsavers.org.

The U.S. Forest Service and **Bureau of Land Management** work together to put out a list of threatened, endangered, or sensitive species for the states of Washington and Oregon. For more information, visit fs.fed.us/r6/sfpnw/issssp/.

The British Columbia Ministry of Environment publishes a red list that includes any ecological community and indigenous species and subspecies that is extirpated, endangered, or threatened and a blue list that includes any ecological community and indigenous species and subspecies considered to be of special concern for the province. For more information, visit env.gov.bc.ca/atrisk/faq3.html.

Determining Whether a Harvest Is Ethical and Sustainable

Imagine you are out in the field sitting in a stand of wild plants. You have positively identified the plant and are sure that it is not endangered or toxic. To determine whether it is sustainable and ethical to harvest this plant, clear your mind and ground yourself. Tune in to your surroundings. Open your heart and use all of your senses. Very carefully observe the area around you with an unattached mind and ask yourself these questions.

- Am I in the proper emotional state to make a harvest?
- Am I prepared to be honest with myself in regards to making decisions about my impact on this stand of plants and the ecosystem in which they live?
- How much of this medicine can or will I realistically process and use?
- If the plant is rare, can I use a more widely available plant in its place?
- Is this stand of plants healthy? Are the individual plants healthy?

- Are there other plants like this in the area, or is this an isolated stand? Is there a larger stand around the bend?
- How old are the plants?
- Will my harvest result in the death of the plants? Is there some way to mitigate this? If not, how long will it take for other plants of this species to take their place?
- If my harvest won't require taking the plant's life, how long will it take the harvested part(s) to grow back?
- Will my impact be noticeable?
- Is there evidence of others harvesting here?
- Will my harvest adversely affect the ecological balance of the stand or the intricate web of interrelations that ensure its continued existence?
- Are there animals or insects that depend on this plant for food or other uses? How will my harvesting impact these relationships?
- What is the terrain like? Will my harvest, including the path I take to arrive there, adversely impact the integrity of a river bank or cause erosion on a slope?

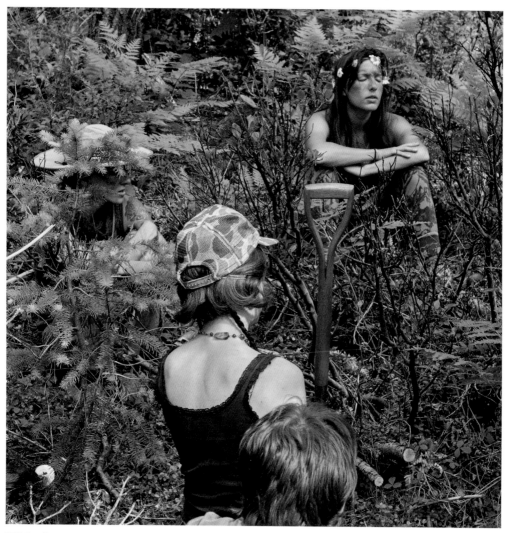
Wildcrafters contemplate a potential red root harvest.

Only after thoroughly contemplating and answering these questions will you be able to determine whether harvesting is acceptable in this place. If the answer is "yes" and you feel confident in proceeding with the harvest, you can now ask the plant for permission, make offerings, and state your intention to the plant. At this point, based on the more objective information you've gathered from the questions above and the more subjective response you've gotten from the plant, you should be able to determine how many plants you can safely harvest from the stand. There is no formula for this. You must make an informed decision based on the life cycle of the plant in question, the variables listed above, and any other information that seems pertinent. Ultimately your goal should be to increase life in the forest rather than diminish it. Please err on the side of caution.

Guidelines for Ethical Wildcrafting

- Know the rare and endangered plants of the area and don't harvest them.
- Determine whether a harvest is ethical and sustainable.
- Exercise caution when harvesting at the outer limits of a plant's geographical range.
- Pick from different stands or spots in a stand to minimize impact.
- Care for and develop a relationship with the stand.
- Don't harvest the Grandmothers and Grandfathers. The oldest and largest plants in a stand are the most successful survivors with the strongest genes. Let them continue to reproduce.
- Leave any area you harvest from in the same or better condition than you found it. Fill in holes after harvesting roots. Don't leave discarded leaves or other plant parts lying around where others can see them. Whenever possible replant root crowns or scatter seeds.
- Observe the stand over time so that you can continue to refine your personal assessments. Be aware of the impact of your harvesting and/or any natural environmental changes that have affected the health of the stand. Based on this information, be prepared to alter your wildcrafting practices or stop harvesting altogether from this spot.

Mutually Beneficial Wildcrafting

Developing harvesting techniques that benefit the growth of plants will ensure that we have access to these medicines for many generations to come. For example, when working with shrubby plants, cutting above a leaf node that is facing out from the center of the plant will promote a more bushy growth habit, resulting in plants that are bigger and lusher than those that haven't been harvested. Cut the stem or branch at a 45 degree angle about ¼ inch above the leaf node. For plants with opposite leaves, cut straight across. Observing the correct cutting angle and distance from the node prevents unnecessary damage to the plant.

Replant root crowns whenever possible, leaving a portion of the root with some visible root hairs. Dig only the back end of roots or rhizomes of herbaceous perennials and leave the front end with next year's bud to sprout the following spring. If you dig the whole plant up, snip off the back end and replant the front end.

Dig roots in summer or autumn after the seeds mature, the leaves begin to die back, and the plant's energy descends downward into the roots. At this point in a plant's growth cycle, the roots are full of the life force and medicinal constituents that the plants have accumulated during the growing season. The timing is more important for fleshy roots like those of sharptooth angelica or Gray's lovage than for woody perennials with dense, hard roots, like red root or California bayberry. Roots are generally more sweet and tonic when dug in spring and have a gentler effect than autumn-dug roots.

Rather than harvesting roots, consider using other parts of the plant such as the leaves. We traditionally use only the roots of some plants, not because this is the only part that is medicinal, but because the roots are more easily transported and retain their freshness and viability for longer periods of time, making them better for commerce and trade. Western aralia is a great example of

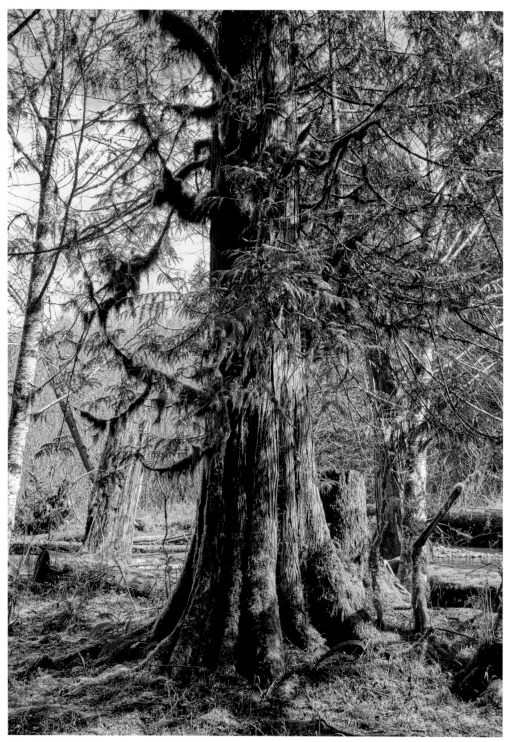
Western redcedar, the tree of life, stands tall and straight.

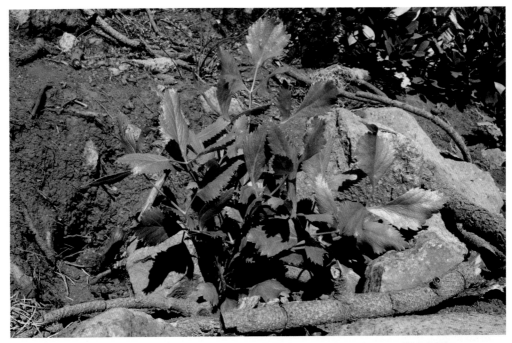

After its root was harvested the previous year, the replanted crown of this sharptooth angelica is sprouting new leaves.

this. Not long ago it was thought that only the roots and berries were useful as medicine, but at some point someone started making medicine from the leaves and found it to be quite useful. Harvesting and using the leaves for medicine is becoming common practice.

For years, almost all of the bark I've harvested has come from already-downed trees that are still alive. If the fallen tree is still rooted and it is not a conifer species, I cut the tree at the base so it will resprout from the crown. If left alone, the tree usually sprouts many new potential trunks along the length of the original trunk. In the end the tree is unable to sustain all of this new growth and the original trunk dies. Cutting it and using the bark for medicine is a win–win situation. The tree can more rapidly create its new sustainable trunk, and my community and I are blessed with lots of good medicine.

I also look to harvest broken branches that are still attached to a tree and alive or to cut branches that are growing into the center of a tree, both of which will ultimately die. Branches that cross and rub against other branches may open wounds in the tree that invite infection or disease. I cut these branches for medicine, and trim away and discard dead branches as I harvest. When practicing any of these techniques, I often feel a sense of relief from the trees.

Harvest bark from standing trees when the sap is running; sap generally begins to run when the leaves emerge. When the sap is running the bark easily separates from the heartwood.

Make clean cuts when removing branches. Using a sharp saw and proper technique minimizes damage and reduces the risk of infection for the tree. If you don't end up with a straight cut through the branch, cut a

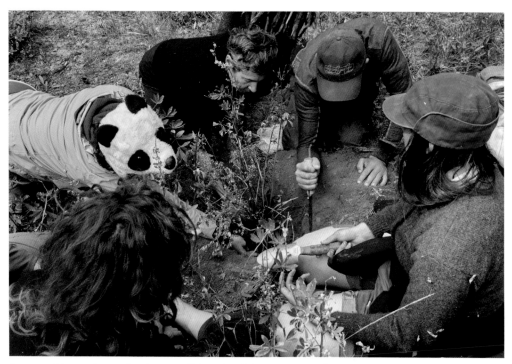

A group of harvesters gather bear medicine, Gray's lovage root, in the mountains of central Oregon.

little more off so that you leave a flat-surfaced stub.

When cutting larger branches, first make a 1-inch-deep cut under the branch before sawing in the same plane from above. By doing this, the bark on the bottom part of the branch won't strip past the cut you've made as the branch falls of its own weight.

Strictly observe the guidelines that relate to sustaining the health of the plant, while doing your best to follow the guidelines dealing with the timing of harvests given in each plant profile. With so many factors to consider, from seasonal variability to the demands of our own personal schedules, it's not always possible to be at the right place at the exact right time. My personal goal is always to harvest plants for medicine at the peak of their energetic potency, but I've learned to strive for perfection without attachment.

Processing Herbs

Process herbs promptly, and never leave freshly harvested herbs in the sun. Cover them with a white sheet when transporting them home in your vehicle. If possible, prepare tinctures in the field for the freshest, most vibrant medicine.

If you've harvested branches when the sap is running and if they have few secondary branch scars, you can make a slice lengthwise on either side of the branch and pry a knife up under the bark to peel it away in nice long strips that are easy to hang or lay out to dry. If this doesn't work, run the knife perpendicular to the already removed branch, and cut into the bark until the knife hits the woody part of the branch. Use a light touch so it doesn't get caught up in the sapwood. Peel the bark off promptly or the job will rapidly increase in difficulty.

Cleaning and Culling Roots

1. After digging a clump of roots, shake and gently beat the root mass against the handle of the digging fork or other digging tool to remove as much of the dirt as possible without damaging the roots.
2. Disentangle the root mass and remove the roots of the other plants that are intertwined with those you are harvesting. Be sure to leave the aboveground parts attached to aid in positive identification. This is especially important when harvesting Sitka valerian because it grows with other plants that have white roots of similar thickness. (You might think that it would be easy to separate the Sitka valerian roots from the others by smelling them, but the roots are so strongly aromatic that the other roots sometimes take on their scent.)
3. After all of the digging is done, clean the roots more thoroughly in a nearby stream or with a hose back home. Break clumps apart to ease this process, and remove any suspect roots that aren't attached to the aboveground parts of the plant from which you are intending to make medicine.
4. As you weigh the roots to make medicine, do a final inspection to make sure that no imposters have snuck in.

Drying and Storing Herbs

Good airflow is the most important factor when drying herbs. Use racks, screens, or bags, or hang bundles upside down. I generally use a dehydrator only for very moist plant parts like berries. Keep the drying herbs out of direct sunlight. You'll know bark is dry when you can hear an audible "snap" when you break it.

To kill insect eggs or larvae that will eat up the harvest when they mature, place fully dried and well-contained seeds or berries in the freezer for 2 weeks.

After they dry, some leaves need to be stripped from stalks and broken into smaller pieces for storage. I use this process, known as garbling, as another opportunity to remove discolored leaves and to discard foreign plant material. If you leave the plant material somewhat whole rather than cutting and sifting, there will be less oxidation and the herbs will last longer.

Store dried herbs in glass jars or in airtight plastic bags in a cool dry place out of direct sunlight. Check for condensation a day or two after placing freshly dried herbs in a container. Condensation indicates that the herbs were not fully dried. Remove the plant material and completely dry it before putting it back into the jar or bag. If left contained, it will mold.

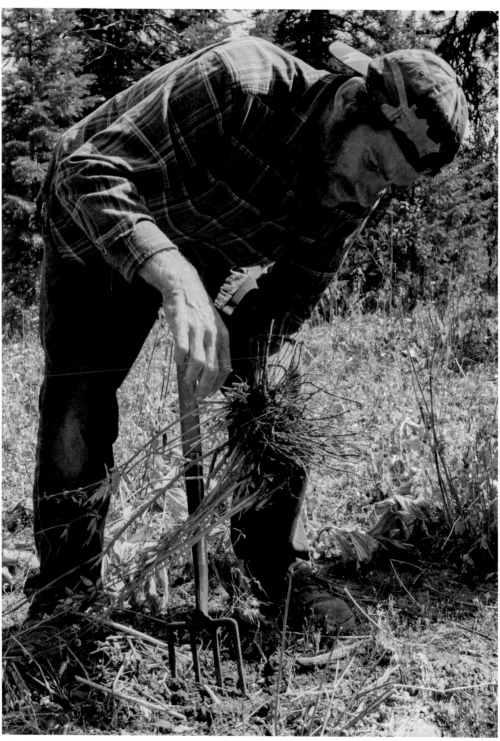

Here I am cleaning a clump of sweetroot.

HERBAL ✤ MEDICINE ✤ PRIMER

I remember the awe that I felt the first time I added alcohol to a jar filled with Saint John's wort flowering tops and watched the liquid instantly begin to turn blood red. I still get a thrill every time I add alcohol and water to a jar of ground up, dried plant material and watch as the liquid churns on its own as it begins to incorporate the medicinal and energetic properties lying hidden in the plant's material body. Making your own medicine is not only rewarding, it is fascinating and fun.

Making good medicine is an alchemical process that calls us to enter into a relationship with the elemental forces of fire, water, earth, and air. Participating in this age-old ritual reconnects us to our ancient wise woman and cunning man healing traditions. Without doubt, an herbal medicine maker exists in every person's family tree. Maybe that herbalist and medicine maker was a mother who knew which tea to give to her feverish children when they were ill, or perhaps he was a grandfather who knew how to make poultices to relieve the pain of sprains or bruises. As a child, you may even have collected sticks and grasses to make your own potions. I urge you to tap into this forgotten part of yourself and remember that making medicine from plants is the birthright of all. It's in our bones, and for the vast majority of human history we as a species have known no other way. As you begin to make medicine, trust and embrace the wise and innate medicine maker within. Don't worry if you are doing it right. Have fun, let your inner child come out to play, and let your imagination run wild.

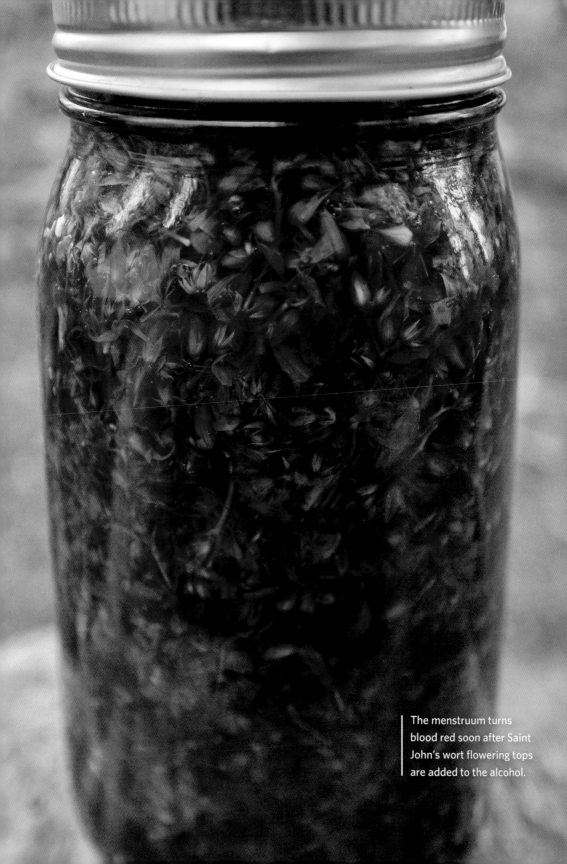

The menstruum turns blood red soon after Saint John's wort flowering tops are added to the alcohol.

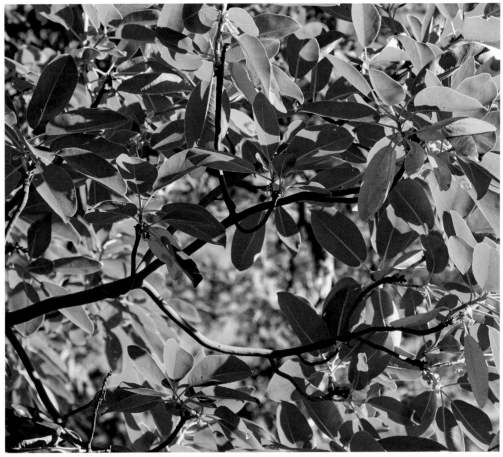

Develop relationships over time to access the special force that resides within each plant. Pacific madrone, for example, evokes the cleansing and healing power of water.

MAKING HERBAL MEDICINES

But before we get started, I'd like to present you with a few practical words of advice. There are two components to making good medicine. First, you'll have to start with high-quality plant material. For me this means harvesting or growing the plants myself. If you are unable to procure plant material directly, you'll have to get your herb material from others. Taste and smell the herb to make sure that it has retained its vitality. Fresh herbs should not be wilted or discolored. Recently dried and well-stored herb material will be vibrantly colored,

have retained its flavor, and, if aromatic, be strongly scented.

The second factor that affects the outcome of making medicine is less tangible. It's a special faculty that develops over time. As you establish relationships with the plants you are using to make medicine, you will gain an energetic understanding of each plant's medicine. This will enable you to make medicine that is more effective and that works on deeper levels of the human body and psyche.

Making Teas

Teas are best prepared in stainless steel, glass, enamel, or clay vessels. You can make teas by adding a handful of herbs to some water, but to make a medicinal strength tea that will be active at the dosages given under the "Herbal Preparations" section in each plant profile, it is best to weigh and measure. For those who scoff at this type of behavior, I'll say this: I weighed and measured my teas until I felt comfortable in my ability to reliably estimate the correct quantity of herb and amount of water to use. I highly recommend that you weigh and measure at least a few times so you will have a baseline idea of what it takes to make therapeutically effective tea.

INFUSIONS

Hot infusions are used to make water extracts of less dense plant parts such as leaves and flowers. It is best to prepare plants high in mucilage, like common mallow, as cold infusions because hot water alters the quality of the mucilage and renders it less effective. Because there is no heat used when making a cold infusion, it is essential that the plant material is held near the top of the infusing vessel to encourage circulatory displacement. This ensures that the medicinal constituents are fully extracted. Suspending the herb at the top of the infusing vessel is recommended but not essential when making a hot infusion.

Hot Infusion

1. Place 1 part by weight of dried plant material (or 2 parts by weight of fresh plant material) in an appropriate vessel, and pour 32 parts by volume of boiling water over the herb.
2. Let sit covered for 15 minutes.
3. Strain, drink the appropriate amount, and store the unused portion in the refrigerator for use within the next 24 hours.

Cold Infusion

1. Place 1 part by weight of dried plant material (or 2 parts by weight of fresh plant material) in a small muslin bag or a piece of cheesecloth, and suspend it in 32 parts by volume of cold water.
2. Let sit covered overnight.
3. Squeeze the retained liquid from the tea bag into the vessel, drink the appropriate amount, and store the unused portion in the refrigerator for use within the next 24 hours.

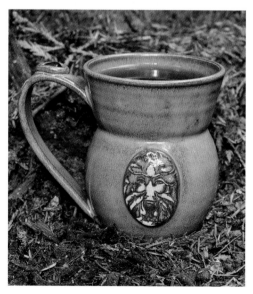

Get ready to enjoy a warm mug of tea in the forest.

DECOCTIONS

For denser parts of a plant such as roots, barks, and seeds, the extra heat of a decoction results in a better extraction of the medicinal constituents. It is helpful but not necessary to soak the herbs in the cooking water for at least 30 minutes before preparing. To make a strong decoction, use twice as much plant material or half as much water.

Standard Decoction

1. In an appropriate cooking vessel, combine 1 part by weight of dried plant material (or 2 parts by weight of fresh plant material) with 32 parts by volume of cold water.
2. Bring the water to a boil, cover the pot, and simmer on low heat for 15 minutes.
3. Strain, drink the appropriate amount, and store the unused portion in the refrigerator for use within the next 24 hours.

Making Tinctures

Tincturing is my favorite way to prepare plants for medicine. Making medicine this way retains the plant's physical and energetic essence, and a plant made into a tincture tastes more like the fresh plant than when the same plant is prepared as a tea because the constituents are not altered by the heat needed to extract them when using water as the primary solvent.

When I make a tincture, it's my goal to make the medicine taste just like the fresh plant because to my mind the taste of the plant reflects the plant's medicinal effect. I've spent years experimenting with alcohol-to-water ratios in an attempt to retain as much of the original flavor of the fresh plant as possible. In the "Herbal Preparations" section of each plant profile, I've explained the ratios that I use for the menstruum, but don't be afraid to experiment and find what works best for you.

In general, the more succulent a plant, the shorter the time needed for maceration. For example, chickweed and cleavers taste much more like the fresh plant if macerated for 1 week. If you let them or other delicate plants macerate for too long, their taste profile changes, which to me indicates a diminishment of the herb's effectiveness. Macerate barks and woody roots longer so the menstruum has a chance to extract all of the constituents.

Tincture making is a very simple process that's easy to follow. Please don't let the fancy words or the math intimidate you. Once you've gone through the steps a few times on your own, it will all make sense. I'll start with a brief introduction to the process of tincture making before I list the steps for using both the folk and scientific methods of making tinctures.

Fresh or Dry Plant Material?

Whenever possible, I prefer making tinctures from fresh plant material. However, I've found that resinous plants, such as balsamroot, extract better when I dry and grind the plant material before tincturing. Also, when tincturing dense plant materials like bark or woody roots, I get a better extraction by drying and grinding. This creates more surface area for extraction so the menstruum can absorb more of the medicinal constituents. Also, because it is difficult to squeeze the retained fluid out of bark and woody roots when they are prepared as fresh plant tinctures, the volume of the final product after pressing is greater when you dry and grind the plant material first.

WHAT IS A TINCTURE?

A tincture is an extract made by macerating or steeping an herb in a menstruum. The menstruum—most often a mixture of pure grain alcohol and distilled water—is the solvent or liquid used to extract the medicinal constituents from the plant material. Alcohol is used most often as menstruum because it is a good all-around solvent and because it is an excellent preservative. I use pure, 190 proof alcohol and add distilled water, if necessary, so that I can create the optimal conditions to extract the full spectrum of a plant's medicine. Sometimes other solvents are added to the menstruum, such as glycerin, to bind tannins and prevent precipitation of the medicinal constituents, or vinegar, to enhance the extraction of alkaloids.

The Benefits of Tinctures

Most alcohol-based tinctures remain stable for many years.

You can carry tinctures in little bottles everywhere you go without need of refrigeration. Dosages can be carefully measured, so you can fine tune your herbal protocols.

Easily assimilated tinctures rapidly disperse their medicine throughout the body, making them especially useful for acute cases.

GOOD MENSTRUUM MAKES GOOD MEDICINE

To get the best extraction, you want the menstruum to be as clear and pure as possible. Solvents have a limited capacity to hold constituents in solution; therefore, using a solvent free of substances like minerals, flavorings, or added coloring allows more of the plant's constituents to be extracted. Imagine that the menstruum is a sponge and the plant constituents are water. If the sponge has some water in it, its capacity to absorb more water is reduced. For this reason, using colorless alcohols with a neutral flavor and distilled water results in more potent and higher quality medicine.

Tinctures made with plants containing high concentrations of tannins tend to clump up and go bad after a few years. Add 10 percent glycerin to tinctures of high-tannin plants such as red root or Oregon white oak bark to slow the rate at which the tannins bind with other constituents and precipitate them out of solution. Not only will the tinctures last longer, but if you ever mix one of these high-tannin plants into a formula with a plant rich in alkaloids you will avoid, for a time, rendering the alkaloids ineffective.

THE FOLK METHOD OF TINCTURING

This is the simplest way to make a tincture. You basically fill a jar with fresh plant material or a quarter to half with dried plant material and cover it with alcohol (most people use 100 proof vodka). If done with care and attention, the folk method yields good-quality medicine, but there are a few disadvantages with this method. First, if you don't tightly pack enough fresh plant material into the jar, you may end up with a weak extract that has only a hint of the plant's taste and medicinal properties, and the medicine may be less effective. Also, if you don't weigh the plant material or measure the menstruum, the tinctures you make won't have a consistent potency from year to year. This makes dosing challenging, especially if you are administering low-dose tinctures.

If you plan to use the folk method, I recommend that you try the scientific method of weighing and measuring a few times to get a sense of how much herb you need to squeeze into a jar when making a full-strength tincture. Try it, you might be surprised.

Making a Tincture Using the Folk Method

1. Cut the fresh herb with scissors or with a knife and cutting board and tightly pack it in a glass jar. Grind dried plant material to the consistency of corn meal with a coffee grinder or other device. If using leaves or flowers, fill the jar about half way; for roots, barks, or berries, fill the jar about a quarter of the way.

2. Add vodka or other alcohol to cover the herb. To prevent spoilage, the menstruum must be at least 40 percent (80 proof) alcohol for a fresh herb extract or 22 percent (44 proof) alcohol for a dry herb extract.

3. Tightly seal and label the jar with the date and the plant's common and Latin names.

4. Shake dry herb preparations once or twice daily. Distributing the plant material throughout the menstruum allows for a better extraction because the solvents can pull more constituents out when they have access to the increased surface area created by the grinding of the herb. (Shaking a fresh plant preparation is not necessary because the alcohol breaks the cell walls to extract the medicinal constituents.)

5. After macerating in a cool dark place for 2–4 weeks, the tincture will be ready to be strained and pressed. Pressing is the act of separating the liquids from the solids by applying pressure. Wrap the herb material in cheesecloth or place it in a tight-mesh muslin bag and squeeze. Using a dedicated mechanical herb press will increase the final yield.

6. Tinctures will last longer and be more visually appealing if you filter out the sediment. Let the tincture sit overnight so any sediments can settle to the bottom, and pour through a coffee filter into a clean, dry jar.

7. Store in a cool dark place.

THE SCIENTIFIC METHOD OF TINCTURING

This method uses commonly agreed upon ratios developed at a world conference of pharmacists and medicine makers held in Brussels, Belgium, in 1902. Standard herb to menstruum ratios are generally 1:2 for fresh herb or 1:5 for dried herb, which is the ratio of the weight of the herb material to the volume of menstruum.

For each plant, I've listed the percentage of alcohol used to get the best extraction. Depending on the constituents you wish to extract from the plant material, you will use more or less alcohol. Neither resins nor balsams are soluble in water, so we use a higher percentage of alcohol to make tinctures from plants with high concentrations of these constituents. Because mucilages, polysaccharides, saponins, and tannins are not soluble in alcohol, we use a lower percentage of alcohol when tincturing plants that contain them.

Before you start, determine the appropriate container size. When making a fresh plant tincture 300 grams of plant material and the resulting 600 milliliters of menstruum will always fit in and nearly or completely fill a standard 1-quart mason jar. (I prefer working with grams and milliliters because it makes the math much easier.) If you get close to the end of the process and it seems like not all of the plant material will fit in the jar, cut the herb more finely. Trust me, it always works. For a dry plant tincture, 140 grams of plant material and the resulting 700 milliliters of menstruum will always fit in and nearly or completely fill a standard 1-quart mason jar. Divide in half for pint jars.

Fresh herb material can be chopped with scissors or clippers into the menstruum, or you can use a knife and cutting board and add it to the jar as you chop. I prefer the former method, because I can't bear to see the leaves oxidizing and the plant's juices oozing out onto the cutting board. I want all of that goodness in my tincture. It is a more difficult process, but for me it is worth the extra work. When processing woodier plants like Oregon grape root, I chop the roots into a bowl with my hand pruners and periodically put the chopped pieces into the jar. With larger roots like those of skunk cabbage or yellow pond-lily, using scissors or clippers doesn't work, so I use a knife and cutting board and practice acceptance.

Fresh Herb Tincture

RATIO OF FRESH HERB TO MENSTRUUM 1:2

1. Weigh the fresh herb material in grams. This gives you the 1 part of the 1:2 weight to volume ratio.
2. Multiply the weight of the herb by 2 to get the liquid part of the 1:2 weight to volume ratio.
3. Determine the amount of alcohol, water, and/or other solvents needed based on the percentage(s) listed in the "Herbal Preparations" section of each plant profile. For example, if you have 300 grams of plant material, you will need 600 milliliters of menstruum. If the formula calls for 75 percent alcohol, multiply 600 by 0.75 to get 450 milliliters of alcohol. The remaining 25 percent or 150 milliliters of the menstruum will be distilled water. Measure out the solvents and pour them into the jar. Reserve one-quarter of the menstruum so you can top off the jar at the end to ensure the herb material is fully submerged.
4. Chop the herb material with scissors or clippers into the menstruum or use a knife and cutting board and add to the jar as you chop.
5. Tightly seal and label with the date, the plant's common and Latin names, the herb to menstruum ratio, whether you used fresh or dry plant material, the percentage of alcohol used, and the total volume of the menstruum.
6. After macerating in a cool dark place for 2–4 weeks, the tincture will be ready to be strained and pressed. Wrap the herb material in cheesecloth or place it in a tight-mesh muslin bag and squeeze. Using a dedicated mechanical herb press will increase the final yield.
7. Tinctures will last longer and be more visually appealing if you filter out the sediment. Let the tincture sit overnight so any sediments can settle to the bottom, and pour through a coffee filter into a clean dry jar.
8. Store in a cool dark place.

Dry Herb Tincture

RATIO OF DRIED HERB TO MENSTRUUM 1:5

1. Weigh the dried herb material in grams. This gives you the 1 part of the 1:5 weight to volume ratio.
2. Multiply the weight of the herb by 5 to get the liquid part of the 1:5 weight to volume ratio.
3. Determine the amount of alcohol, water, and/or other solvents needed based on the percentage listed in the "Herbal Preparations" section in each plant profile. For example, if you have 140 grams of plant material, you will need 700 milliliters of menstruum. If the formula calls for 50 percent alcohol, multiply 700 by 0.50 to get 350 milliliters of alcohol. The remaining 50 percent or 350 milliliters of the menstruum will be distilled water.
4. Grind the herb material to the consistency of corn meal with a coffee grinder or other device and add it to the jar. Grinding it too fine will cause clumping and lead to a less efficient extraction.
5. Measure out and pour the menstruum into the jar.
6. Label with the date, the plant's common and Latin names, the herb to menstruum ratio, whether you used fresh or dry plant material, the percentage of alcohol used, and the total volume of the menstruum.
7. Shake dry herb preparations once or twice daily. Distributing the plant material throughout the menstruum allows for a better extraction because the solvents can pull more constituents out when they have access to the increased surface area created by the grinding of the herb.
8. After macerating in a cool, dark place for 2–4 weeks, the tincture will be ready to be strained and pressed. Wrap the herb material in cheesecloth or place it in a tight-mesh muslin bag and squeeze. Using a dedicated mechanical herb press will increase the final yield.
9. Tinctures will last longer and be more visually appealing if you filter out the sediment. Let the tincture sit overnight so any sediments can settle to the bottom, and pour through a coffee filter into a clean dry jar.
10. Store in a cool dark place.

Making Infused Oils

The alcohol used in tincture making has the ability to extract the medicinal constituents from plant material, but oils do not have this same capacity, so heat must be applied to get a proper extraction. The simplest way to achieve this is to add oil to a jar of herbs, put the jar of infusing oil into a heavy paper bag to prevent exposure to light, and leave it outside in the sunniest, warmest spot you can find. If you use this method to infuse fresh plant material in oil, don't put a lid on the jar for the first few days. Instead cover the top with cheesecloth so the evaporating water can escape.

If the sky is cloudy or you don't want to take any chances with the oil going bad, employ another method to apply heat, like using a yogurt maker or placing the jar next to a woodstove. Ideally you want to keep an even heat of between 100 and 120°F for about a week. Crockpots, even on the warm setting, are too hot for this purpose.

It is preferable to make infused oils with dried plant material, because water from the plant can cause the oil to ferment or develop mold. This process is easy, but there are certain infused oils that need to be made with fresh plant material. Saint John's wort oil, for example, absolutely needs to be made using the fresh flowering tops. Preparations of Saint John's wort made with dried plant material lack the medicinal properties found in the fresh plant preparations.

Standard herb to oil ratios are 1:3 for fresh herb or 1:5 for dried herb, which is the ratio of the weight of the herb material to the volume of oil.

Fresh Herb Infused Oil

RATIO OF FRESH HERB TO OIL 1:3

1. Weigh the fresh herb material in grams. This gives you the 1 part of the 1:3 weight to volume ratio.
2. Multiply the weight of herb by 3 to get the volume of oil. For example, if you have 200 grams of plant material, you will need 600 milliliters of oil.
3. Wilt the plant material by spreading it thinly on a screen or a piece of cardboard overnight. This minimizes the possibility of spoilage before combining with the oil.
4. Place the wilted and chopped fresh herb in the macerating vessel of choice and cover with the oil.
5. Heat evenly at 100–120°F for about a week, stirring several times daily. Leave the lid slightly ajar for the first couple of days and wipe away any condensation that accumulates on the underside of the lid.
6. Place a few layers of cheesecloth in a large funnel, and pour the warm oil through the cheesecloth and into a clean dry jar.
7. Squeeze the collected herb to remove as much oil as possible, but don't use an herb press. It will add too much water to the oil without significantly increasing the amount of oil you get back.
8. Let the oil stand overnight to allow any water or plant debris to settle to the bottom of the jar. Carefully decant by pouring the clear oil into another clean dry jar. Once you begin to see globs of water or streams of sediment nearing the lip of the jar, stop pouring and discard the remaining sludge. Repeat until the oil is completely free of water and sediment.
9. Store out of the light in a cool place. Oils infused with fresh plant material generally last for about 1 year.

Dry Herb Infused Oil

RATIO OF DRIED HERB TO OIL 1:5

1. Weigh the dried herb material in grams. This gives you the 1 part of the 1:5 weight to volume ratio.
2. Multiply the weight of the herb by 5 to get the volume of oil. For example, if you have 140 grams of plant material, you will need 700 milliliters of oil.
3. Grind the herb material to the consistency of corn meal with a coffee grinder or other device. Grinding it too fine will cause clumping and lead to a less efficient extraction. Add it to the macerating vessel of choice, and cover with the oil.
4. Heat evenly at 100–120°F for 3–7 days, stirring regularly.
5. Place a few layers of cheesecloth in a large funnel, and pour the warm oil through the cheesecloth and into a clean dry jar.
6. Squeeze or use an herb press to get back as much oil as possible from the dried herb material.
7. Let the oil stand overnight to allow any plant debris to settle to the bottom of the jar. Carefully decant by pouring the clear oil into another clean dry jar. Once you begin to see streams of sediment nearing the lip of the jar, stop pouring and discard the remaining sludge.
8. Store out of the light in a cool place. Oils infused with dry herb generally last for 1 to 2 years.

Alternative Oil Method

RATIO OF DRIED HERB TO OIL 1:7

This method can be used to make oils in a few hours. It also works well for plant material that is not readily soluble in oil, such as roots, barks, or tough leaves. I generally use this method to make oils that will be processed into salves because it is easier, and I know that a good portion of the alcohol will evaporate during the salve-making process.

1. Weigh the dried herb material in grams. This gives you the 1 part of the 1:7 weight to volume ratio.
2. Multiply the weight of the herb by 7 to get the volume of oil. For example, if you have 100 grams of plant material, you will need 700 milliliters of oil.
3. Grind the herb material to the consistency of corn meal with a coffee grinder or other device and put it in a clean dry jar.
4. Mix 1 part by volume of 90 percent rubbing alcohol (isopropyl alcohol)—for example, if you have 100 grams of plant material, you will need 100 milliliters of rubbing alcohol—into the dried herb material until the alcohol is evenly distributed. Cover and let it sit for 2–3 hours.
5. Put the dried herb and alcohol mixture in a blender, and cover it with the oil. Blend until the whole blender jar gets warm.
6. Place a few layers of cheesecloth in a large funnel and pour the warm oil through the cheesecloth and into a clean dry jar.
7. Squeeze or use an herb press to get back as much oil as possible from the dried herb material.
8. Let the oil stand overnight to allow any plant debris to settle to the bottom of the jar. Carefully decant by pouring the clear oil into another clean dry jar. Once you begin to see streams of sediment nearing the lip of the jar, stop pouring and discard the remaining sludge.
9. Store out of the light in a cool place.

Adapted from Michael Moore

Making Salves

A salve is made by adding beeswax to an infused oil. Whereas oils penetrate into the tissues, salves are indicated when you'd like the plant's medicine to stay at the surface of the skin. They are especially helpful for speeding the healing and preventing the infection of wounds.

Salve

RATIO OF PLANT-INFUSED OIL TO BEESWAX 5:1

1. Heat 5 parts by volume of infused oil to approximately 150°F in a double boiler.
2. Cut 1 part by weight of beeswax into small chunks and add it to the oil. Stir frequently until the beeswax is fully melted.
3. Scoop a small amount of the oil and beeswax mixture into a spoon and place it in the freezer for about a minute until it hardens. Test the consistency. If it is too soft, add more beeswax. If it is too hard, add more oil. Retest until you've obtained the desired consistency.
4. Pour the warm oil and beeswax mixture into jars. Allow the salve to cool and harden before capping and labelling accordingly.

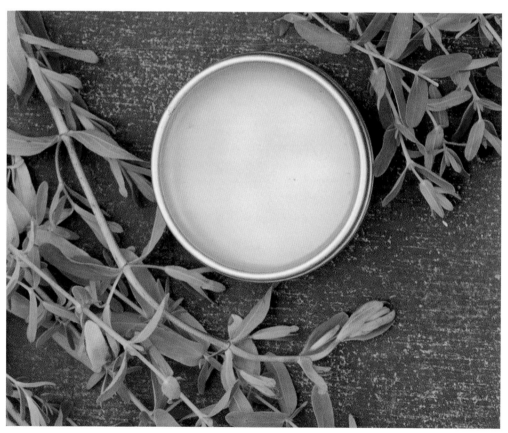

Salve made from St. John's wort flowering tops effectively speeds the healing of wounds.

Making Medicinal Syrups

There are at least two methods for making honey syrups: one uses water to extract the plant's medicine and the other uses the honey itself. The second method works best for succulent roots like Gray's lovage or western aralia.

I often add a few squirts of various tinctures of other plants to the honey to increase the medicinal benefit. If you want to be more technical about it, add 1 part tincture to 20 parts syrup.

The standard dosage for honey syrups is 1 tablespoon up to 5 times per day. Give children 1 teaspoon of syrup up to 5 times per day.

Honey Syrup
THE STANDARD METHOD

1. In a double boiler, combine 1 part by volume of a double-strength infusion or decoction with 3 parts by volume of pure honey. For example, to make horehound syrup, decoct 30 grams of herb in 480 milliliters of water. Combine the resulting volume of tea, let's say 400 milliliters, with 3 times the amount or 1200 milliliters of honey.
2. Simmer at a very low heat, stirring frequently, until the tea is thoroughly assimilated into the honey.
3. Pour the syrup into a completely dry and clean jar.
4. Label with the date, the plant's common and Latin names, the herb to honey ratio, and whether you used fresh or dry plant material for the tea.
5. This preparation is best stored in the refrigerator.

Honey Syrup
THE ROOTSY METHOD

1. In a double boiler, add 1 part by volume of chopped, fresh roots to 4 parts by volume of pure honey. Measure the honey carefully, because in the final stages of the process, you'll need to know the exact volume you started with.
2. Using a double boiler, simmer at a very low heat for 4 hours, while stirring occasionally. (If you heat the honey too high, it will foam up and create a small herbal eruption that will create a huge mess and ruin the medicine.)
3. Place a few layers of cheesecloth in a large funnel and pour the warm honey concoction through the cheesecloth and into a dry clean jar. If the volume of honey is greater than that with which you started, gently heat the honey again to evaporate any water the honey extracted from the plant material. Remove from heat when the honey is back to its original volume. Excess water in the honey may lead to spoilage. Save the honey-infused root chunks; they are like little medicinal candies.
4. Label with the date and the plant's common and Latin names.
5. Store in a cool dry place.
   Adapted from Michael Moore

Making Compresses and Poultices

A compress, also known as a fomentation, is a method of applying an herbal extract in the form of a tea, infused oil, or diluted tincture to soothe conditions such as sprains, strains, bruises, sore muscles, and headaches. To make a compress, simply soak a clean piece of cotton or wool cloth in one of these preparations and apply it to the affected area. For most purposes, the compress is best applied hot and should be refreshed once it loses its heat. Placing a hot water bottle over the compress will aid in the absorption of the medicine. Cold (that is, room temperature) compresses can be used to speed the healing and reduce the pain of wounds or to soothe hot, inflamed tissues.

A poultice, also known as a cataplasm, is a method of applying plant material directly to the skin to speed the healing of external conditions such as abscesses, boils, inflammations, and bruises. Because the plant's medicine can also be absorbed into the tissues under the skin, these preparations are also helpful for clearing swollen or blocked lymph glands or to promote the healing of broken bones or damaged connective tissue. Poultices can generally be left in place for 1–8 hours before they need to be refreshed.

Fresh Herb Poultice

1. Gather enough fresh plant material so you can cover the affected area about ½ to 1 inch thick with herb.
2. Chop and simmer the fresh herb in a pot for a few minutes, or in a blender combine the herb with just enough hot water to make a thick slurry.
3. Completely cover the affected area with the herb material and cover with a clean piece of cotton or wool cloth.
4. Leave it on for several hours or overnight. Reapply with newly prepared plant material as needed.

Dried Herb Poultice

1. In a bowl or blender, mix finely ground herb with hot water. Use enough plant material to make a thick paste that will cover the affected area about ½ to 1 inch thick.
2. Completely cover the affected area with the herb material and cover with a clean piece of cotton or a small towel.
3. Leave it on for several hours or overnight. Reapply with newly prepared plant material as needed.

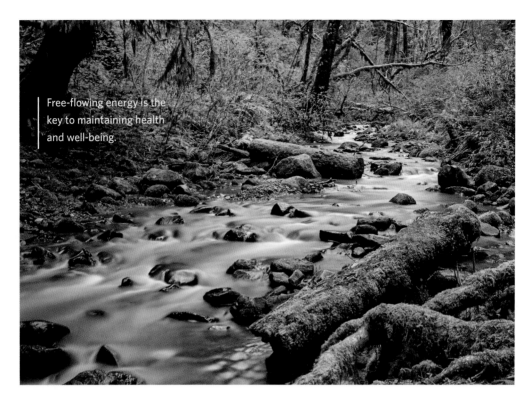

Free-flowing energy is the key to maintaining health and well-being.

WORKING WITH WILD MEDICINAL PLANTS

The body is a holistic system endowed with an innate healing wisdom. Plants remove impediments to health and teach or remind the body how to function in a healthy way. For example, when I say that a plant speeds the healing of chronic intestinal infections, I am implying not only that it kills microbes but that it alters the internal ecology of the body in such a way that the intestines become a less hospitable environment for bacteria or viruses to thrive.

It is easier to maintain health than to correct imbalances. Don't turn to your plant allies only when you are sick. Call upon them to support your physical and emotional well-being and to inspire greater balance and harmony both from within and without your body. If your torso tends to be cold and damp, leaving you susceptible

to lung infections as the weather turns cold and damp in autumn, you can prepare your body for the change in season by taking preparations of sharptooth angelica root to stimulate the warming and drying of your digestive and respiratory systems. A regular course of dandelion root, Oregon grape root, buckbean leaf, or other bitter herbs will keep your liver functioning well. Flavonoid-rich berries help prevent coronary disease by lessening inflammation in the heart and blood vessels and may reduce the risk of cancer by protecting cells from free radical damage.

We often focus only on how a plant or other medicine can get us out of our current state of dis-ease, but plants are intelligent and operate in conjunction with the human body to support a full spectrum of healing. If the plant's medicine is suited to your constitution, it will not only bring you back into a state of balance, but it will teach you how to embody the positive aspects of yourself that run along the same axis as the disease process itself.

Our greatest gifts come from our places of greatest vulnerability and wounding. Western pasqueflower relieves anxiety and worry that result from an overactive mind filled with chaotic thoughts, but it can also show people prone to this way of being how to sharpen their minds and help them organize their thoughts in a meaningful and creative way.

Remember also that working with medicinal plants is only one part of living a healthy life. Diet, exercise, emotional health, the environment in which you live, and how and with whom you choose to spend your time all play an important role in creating and maintaining a state of health.

An Energetic System of Healing

All folk medicine traditions have a language or way of describing energetic patterns that can be observed in the universe. The underlying and animating force that gives shape to and guides these patterns is, by different cultures, variously called qi, prana, pneuma, holy spirit, or the vital force. Some of the patterns this force creates are visible with the naked eye, whereas others may be seen only tangentially or in altered states of consciousness.

All folk medicine traditions also acknowledge that the body is a network of energetic pathways. In Chinese medicine, these are described as meridians that run throughout the body. When any part of this system becomes blocked, whether from physical, mental, emotional, or spiritual reasons, disease occurs. Clearing the blockages in these channels and allowing the body to resume its free flowing state is an essential part of the healing process.

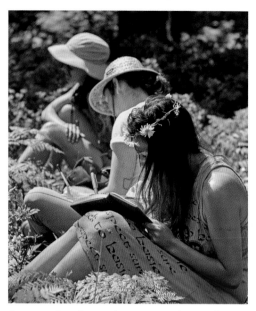

A group of students takes notes as they study plant medicine in the forest.

Traditional Chinese, Ayurvedic, Native American, and Greek medicine, which forms the foundation of our own western herbal tradition, all teach that there is an intelligence that guides and directs the movement and ordering of all the elements of nature, including the lives of humans. Our own culture has abandoned this notion and consequently our system of medicine has evolved without a solid foundation anchoring it to the world around us.

Instead of recognizing patterns of imbalance and harmony, the currently accepted western system of medicine, also known as allopathic medicine, looks for agents of disease—viruses, bacteria, and other microbes—and eradicates them without considering the deeper constitutional factors that lead to states of illness. Folk medicine traditions, on the other hand, view the human body in a holistic way and seek to support the body's innate ability to heal itself. A cure is achieved not by "fixing" one

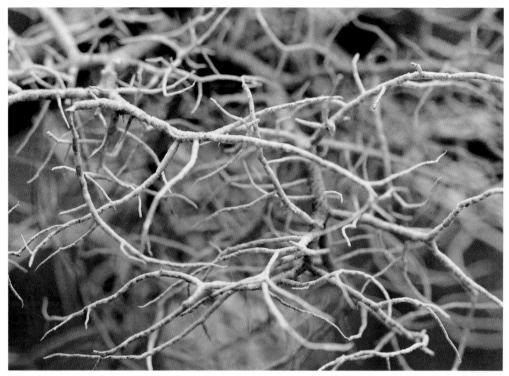

Usnea's branching tufts create intricate patterns that look similar to the paths upon which I imagine the vital force traversing the human body.

part, but by returning harmony and balance to the whole system.

To work with plants in this way, we need to understand how imbalances manifest and how to restore harmony to the human organism. If we can read the energetic patterns visible in the human body, we can select the correct herb or herbs that match the imbalance in the body that needs healing and bring the body back to a state of health.

The most commonly used energetic system in western herbalism comes to us from the Greeks. It is represented by hot, cold, dry, and damp. At the most basic level, it can generally be said that if there is a condition of heat in the body, administer cooling herbs. If there is dampness in the body, give drying herbs. As you progress in your study of plants and the human body, you may find that there

are more subtle interactions that take place, but for our purposes this simple system will serve us well.

The flavor, smell, and taste impressions of herbs can also tell us a lot about their medicine. The human tongue and nose are very sensitive to even the slightest variations in taste and smell. When first learning about a plant's medicine, I highly recommend tasting the plant in a very intentional way and paying close attention to its flavors and how it feels in the mouth. You can do this with the fresh or dried plant, a tincture, or a tea. While doing this type of research, avoid eating spicy or greasy foods, avoid perfumes or strongly scented shampoos and soaps, and keep your palate as clear as possible. It may be difficult to discern the different flavors and impressions at first, but everyone has

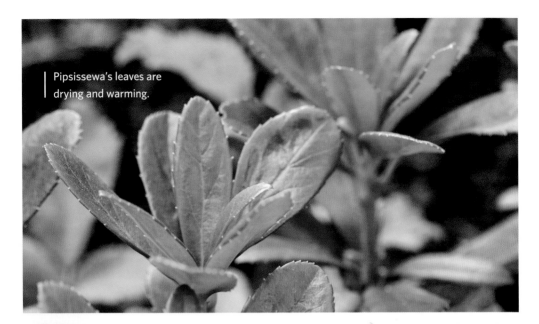

Pipsissewa's leaves are drying and warming.

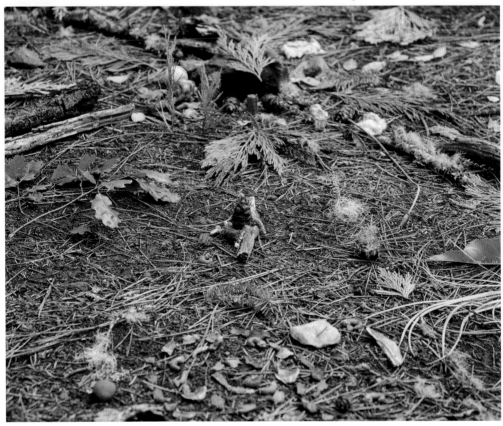

This medicine circle celebrates our connection to the four elements and directions.

the ability to perceive in this way. Keep practicing: the understanding you will gain is well worth the effort.

The Five Flavors

Bitter cools, clears, and stimulates

Pungent warms, stimulates, and disperses

Sweet nourishes, cools, and moistens

Sour tightens and cools

Salty drains, dissolves, moistens, and indicates the presence of minerals

Some Common Taste Impressions

Drying tightens and tones tissues, resolves dampness

Expansive opening, clearing, and clarifying

Saponaceous soapy and slightly irritating; indicates the presence of saponins

Slimy coating, soothing, moistening; indicates the presence of mucilage

Sticky indicates presence of gums and resins; often clears mucus

Tingly points to an effect on the nerves or immune system

Determining Dosages

Many factors alter and affect the body's response to a plant's medicinal and energetic constituents. Considering the fact that each person's body is a uniquely operating biological system, listing exact dosages is all but impossible. A 5-drop dose of Fremont's silktassel leaf may be just right to relieve one woman's menstrual cramps, but another woman may need 30 drops to achieve the same result. A 5-drop dose may work today, but tomorrow the same dose may have little effect or may cause an adverse reaction. This is an extreme example. Most herbs work in a generally reliable manner within certain parameters, but when administering herbs it is important to be mindful of the various factors that come into play when trying to determine an effective and safe dosage.

When trying to find the correct dosage for an individual, the questions to ask are "how much?" and "how often?" For acute conditions, smaller more frequent doses work best. For chronic conditions, larger doses just a few times a day for longer periods of time are preferred. Always start with smaller dosages and work your way up until you find the sweet spot, and remember that what works for one person won't always work for another.

Some Factors Affecting Dosage

Weight Generally the heavier the person, the more medicine needed, but this is not always true.

Age Children and the elderly generally need less medicine than the average adult.

Temperament Sensitive, quiet people may need less medicine than those who are outgoing and more active.

Current state Those weakened by illness are more apt to need less medicine than those in a hearty state of health.

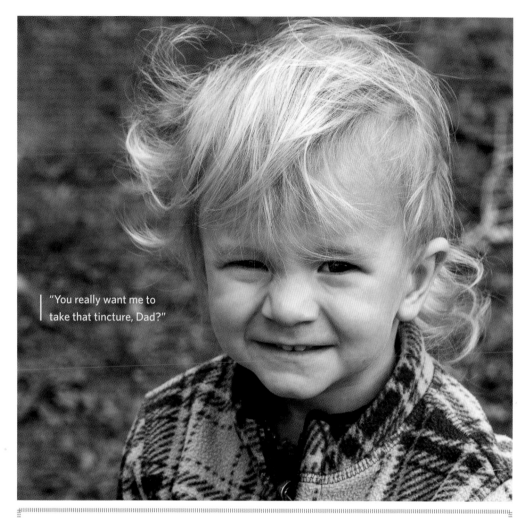

"You really want me to take that tincture, Dad?"

Dosages for Children

Use Clark's rule to determine the appropriate dosage for children between the ages of 2 and 17. Divide the child's weight in pounds by 150. Thus, for a 30-pound child, divide 30 by 150 to get ⅕ or 20 percent. If the normal dose for an adult is listed as 15–30 drops, this child's dose would be 3–6 drops.

HERBAL SAFETY

The possibility of being seriously harmed from taking herbal medicines is pretty slim. Some have estimated that the chance of dying from ingesting an herbal remedy is one in a million. However, some herbs can produce adverse reactions or interact with pharmaceutical medications. If you use medicinal plants according to the recommendations given in this book and don't use ultra-concentrated forms of these medicines, you run very little risk of injury or discomfort.

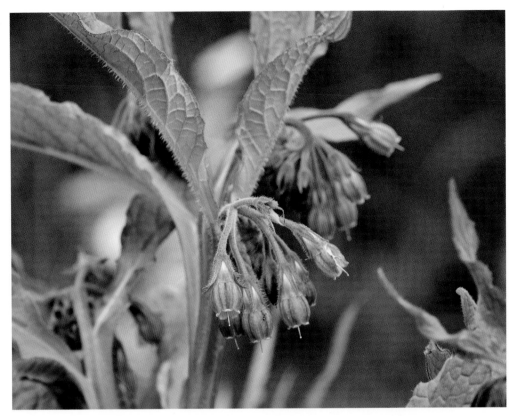

Comfrey leaves and roots contain toxic pyrrolizidine alkaloids that are known to cause a severe and life-threatening disorder known as hepatic veno-occlusive disease.

Guidelines for the Safe Usage of Herbs

Consult with a qualified health practitioner before using herbs to treat serious medical conditions.

Follow the dosage recommendations given in the text. If you notice any adverse reactions, cut back on the dosage or stop taking the herb.

Carefully read the cautions listed for each plant, and pay close attention if you are pregnant or nursing.

Herb–Drug Interactions

As the practice of combining herbs with pharmaceutical medications becomes more common, our understanding of possible adverse interactions increases. Always speak with a qualified health practitioner if you are planning to take herbs along with over-the-counter or prescription drugs. Some herbs may increase or decrease the rate at which your body processes and absorbs medications, which may lead to an unwanted potentiation or decrease in the effect of the drugs. Saint John's wort, for example, increases the liver's ability to process and break down certain medications. Studies have shown taking Saint John's wort in conjunction with cyclosporine, a drug used to prevent the body from rejecting transplanted organs, decreases the concentrations of that medicine in the blood to sub-therapeutic levels. Pay particular attention to combining herbs with MAO-inhibiting or SSRI antidepressants, medications that thin the blood, or drugs that raise or lower blood pressure.

Using Herbs while Pregnant or Nursing

Even though many herbs are safe and pose less risk than over-the-counter or prescription pharmaceuticals, always exercise caution and consult with a midwife, naturopathic doctor, or other health care practitioner if you plan to use herbs while pregnant. Pregnant women should avoid taking most herbs during the first trimester of pregnancy, when the developing fetus is most at risk. Nettle herb and raspberry or thimbleberry leaf, all of which are recommended throughout pregnancy, are exceptions to this rule.

Herbs that stimulate the uterus, have a strong laxative effect, or contain potentially dangerous alkaloids or other compounds are all contraindicated during pregnancy. When applicable, a warning is listed under the "Caution" heading for each plant with these attributes.

The medicine of some herbs can be transferred to a child through the mother's milk. This can be a useful and gentle way to administer medicine to infants. Some stronger acting plants should be avoided to prevent their medicine being passed through the breast milk. Other plants, such as garden sage, can also decrease milk supply. These herbs may be useful if you wish to wean your child, but not so great if you would like to continue nursing.

Low-Dose Plants

Some plants that are safe to use in smaller doses may have toxic effects in larger doses. Use these plants with extreme care, and pay close attention to the cautions and recommended dosages.

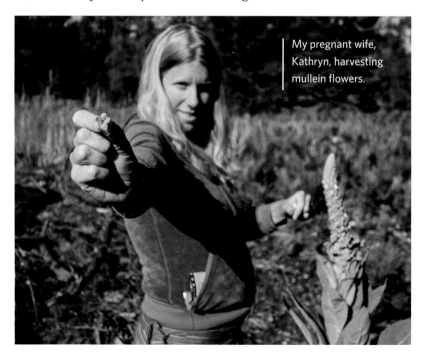

My pregnant wife, Kathryn, harvesting mullein flowers.

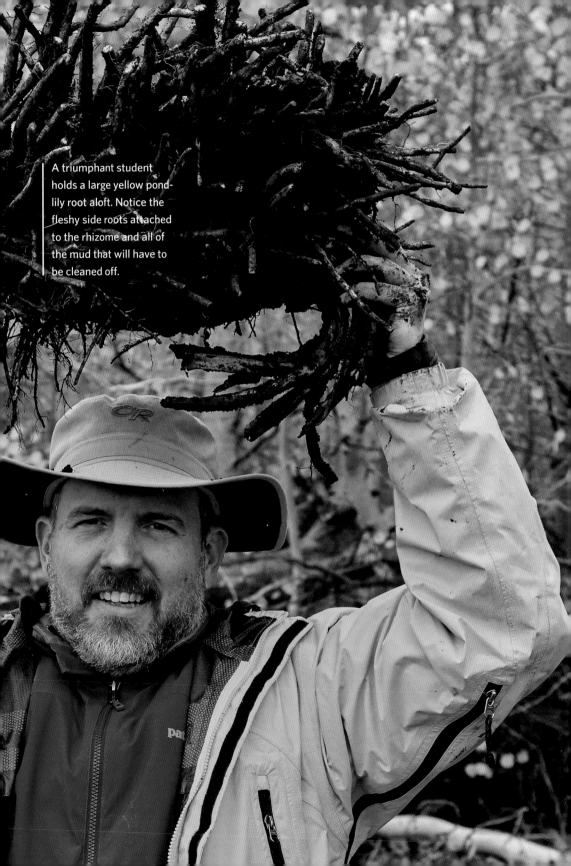

A triumphant student holds a large yellow pond-lily root aloft. Notice the fleshy side roots attached to the rhizome and all of the mud that will have to be cleaned off.

WILDCRAFTING SEASON BY SEASON

highly recommend that you spend lots of time out in the field to attune yourself to the rhythm of the harvest season, and use these lists only as guidelines. Climatic conditions often vary wildly from year to year, and depending on the weather, the leaves will emerge to herald the beginning of bark harvesting season, the plants will bloom, or the plants will pass through their period of prime medicinal activity earlier or later in the season. You learn to flow with it. Also, with some plants there is a very narrow window of opportunity for harvesting. Don't worry: if you miss out on a harvest this year, you can look forward to next year's wildcrafting season.

To account for the wide range of elevation at which some of these plants grow, you will have to make adjustments. Individual plants of the same species growing at lower elevations bloom earlier than those at higher elevations. Yarrow, for example, grows from sea level, where it begins blooming in mid spring, to timberline, where it may not finish flowering until mid autumn. Each plant is listed under the season during which it is first ready to be harvested.

WINTER
Walking among the trees during late winter as you and the life around you prepares to awaken from the darkness of winter, the smell

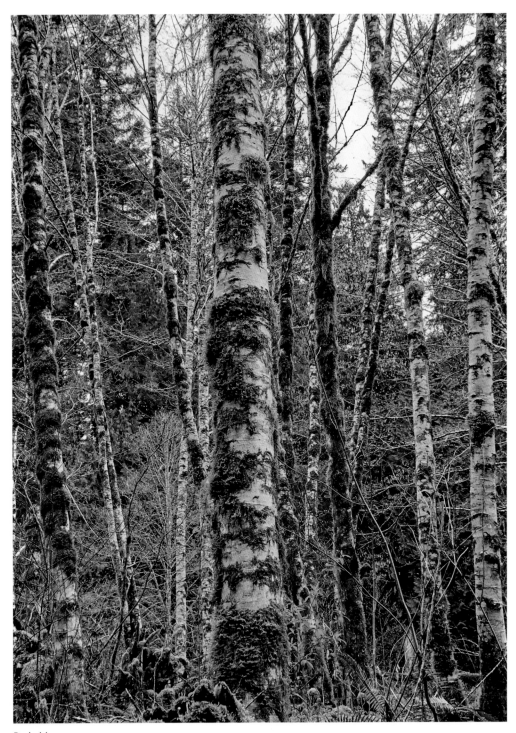

Red alder

of the wet, fecund earth rises to your nostrils. Cutting through this rich, heavy aroma, the faintest hint of a familiar sweet, spicy, and resinous fragrance brings a smile to your face. The black cottonwood buds are swelling, and spring is just around the corner. The nettles start to poke their heads above the ground. The yearly harvest cycle begins once again.

Mid Winter

Woodlands and Partially Shaded Places

black cottonwood bud (until early spring)

Late Winter

Open Meadows, Disturbed Soils, Sunny Areas, and the Edges of Sunny Areas

burdock root (until early spring)
Fuller's teasel root (until early spring)
mullein root (until early spring)
wild carrot root (until early spring)

Woodlands and Partially Shaded Places

nettle herb (until mid spring)

SPRING

As the earth awakens from its winter dormancy, fresh green herbs, nutritive and/or lymphatic cleansing, arrive to help our bodies prepare for the seasonal changes to come. Our forebears who lived through the winter months without the benefit of fresh fruits and vegetables welcomed them with glee because these plants helped them adapt to a different type of diet and cleared the accumulated waste products from the winter diet.

Later in the season the sap begins to run through the bark of the trees, the buds burst open, and the leaves unfurl. Keep an eye out for mutually beneficial bark-harvesting opportunities.

As the season progresses the rate of flowering and leafing out increases to feed the awakening insects and other wildlife.

Early Spring

Open Meadows, Disturbed Soils, Sunny Areas, and the Edges of Sunny Areas

chickweed herb (year-round)
dandelion leaf (until early summer)
dandelion root (until late spring)
Fremont's silktassel leaf (until late summer)
Himalayan blackberry root (year-round)
narrow-leaved plantain leaf (until early autumn)
western juniper leaf (year-round)

Woodlands and Partially Shaded Places

hookedspur violet herb (until late spring)
lungwort thallus (until early summer)
Pacific bleeding heart whole plant (until late spring)
pitch from Douglas-fir, ponderosa pine, western hemlock (year-round)
Scouler's corydalis whole plant (until late spring)
usnea thallus (until mid summer)
western redcedar leaf (year-round)

Wetlands, Riverbanks, Lakesides, Bogs

horsetail stalk (until early summer)
western coltsfoot root (until late spring)

Mid Spring

Open Meadows, Disturbed Soils, Sunny Areas, and the Edges of Sunny Areas

arrowleaf balsamroot root (until mid autumn)
California bay leaf (until early autumn)
chokecherry bark (until mid summer)
cleavers herb (until mid summer)
comfrey leaf or root (until early autumn)

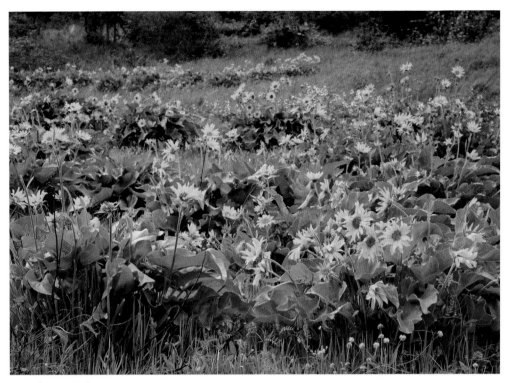

Arrowleaf balsamroot

curl-leaf mountain mahogany leaf or twigs (until early autumn)

Himalayan blackberry leaf (until early summer)

manzanita leaf (until mid autumn)

Oregon white oak bark (until mid summer)

Pacific madrone leaf (until mid autumn)

ponderosa pine bark (until mid summer)

ponderosa pine needle (until mid summer)

ponderosa pine pollen cones (until late spring)

shepherd's purse whole plant (until late summer)

smooth sumac bark or leaf (until mid summer)

uva ursi leaf (until mid autumn)

western white clematis leaf and stem (until late summer)

yarrow leaf and flower (until mid autumn)

Woodlands and Partially Shaded Places

baldhip rose flower (until early summer)

Cascade Oregon grape root (until mid autumn)

cascara sagrada bark (until mid summer)

devil's club root or stem bark (until late spring)

Douglas-fir bark (until mid summer)

Douglas-fir leaves (until late spring)

oceanspray leaf or bark (until early autumn)

oneseed hawthorn leaf and flower (until early summer)

Pacific dogwood flower (until early summer)

Pacific dogwood bark (until mid summer)

quaking aspen bark (until mid summer)

red alder bark (until mid summer)

western hemlock bark (until mid summer)

western hemlock leaf (until late spring)

woodland strawberry leaf (until early autumn)

Wetlands, Riverbanks, Lakesides, Bogs

highbush cranberry bark (until mid summer)

sweet gale leaf (until late summer)

willow bark (until mid summer)

Late Spring

Open Meadows, Disturbed Soils, Sunny Areas, and the Edges of Sunny Areas

arrowleaf balsamroot leaf (until mid summer)

California poppy whole plant (until early autumn)

common mallow whole plant or individual parts (until early autumn)

desert parsley root (until early autumn)

gumweed flower (until early autumn)

Menzies' larkspur seed (until late summer)

mountain monardella leaf and flower (until late summer)

nettleleaf giant hyssop leaf (until late summer)

Oregon figwort leaf and flower (until early summer)

oxeye daisy herb (until mid autumn)

selfheal herb (until early autumn)

sheep sorrel whole plant (until late summer)

yerba buena leaf (until mid summer)

Woodlands and Partially Shaded Places

pipsissewa leaf (until early autumn)

salal leaf (until mid autumn)

thimbleberry leaf (until early summer)

SUMMER

As spring turns to summer, the earth expresses herself in a long procession of flowering and exuberant growth. In response to longer days and increased solar intensity, aromatic oils become more concentrated in the leaves of some of this region's most important medicinal plants. A multi-colored wave of flowers leads you from the lowlands up into the mountains as the pollinated flowers of summer leave a trail of ripening fruits and maturing seeds in their wake.

Early Summer

Open Meadows, Disturbed Soils, Sunny Areas, and the Edges of Sunny Areas

barestem biscuitroot seed (until late summer)

coastal hedgenettle herb (until late summer)

feverfew leaf and flower (until late summer)

fireweed leaf (until early autumn)

hairy arnica flower (until late summer)

herb Robert root (until late autumn)

horehound leaf (until mid autumn)

king's gentian herb (until late summer)

lemon balm leaf (until late summer)

mullein flower (until early autumn)

red clover flowering top (until late summer)

Saint John's wort flowering tops (until late summer)

snapdragon skullcap leaf (until mid summer)

western mugwort leaf and flower (until mid autumn)

western pasqueflower leaf (until late summer)

yerba santa leaf (until late summer)

Woodlands and Partially Shaded Places

ghost pipe flowering stalks (until late summer)

parrot's beak herb (until early autumn)

thimbleberry berry (until mid summer)

thinleaf huckleberry leaf (until early autumn)

western bunchberry whole plant (until early autumn)

Wetlands, Riverbanks, Lakesides, Bogs

buckbean leaf (until late summer)

western aralia leaf (until mid summer)

western coltsfoot leaf (until late summer)

Seashore and Coastal Areas

bladderwrack thallus (until mid summer)

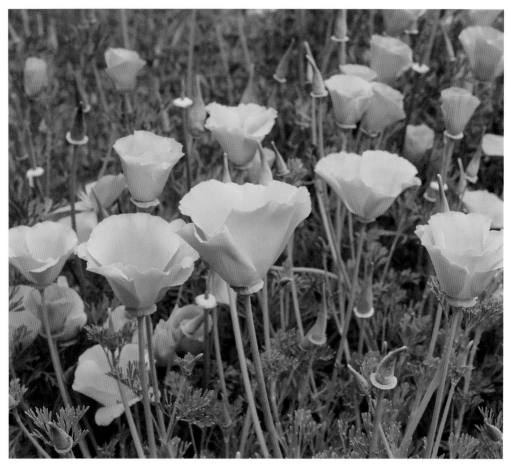

California poppy

Mid Summer

Open Meadows, Disturbed Soils, Sunny Areas, and the Edges of Sunny Areas

cow parsnip seed (until late summer)
goldenrod flowering tops (until mid autumn)
pearly everlasting leaf and flower (until early autumn)
red root leaf (until early autumn)
red root root bark (until late autumn)
sagebrush leaf (until early autumn)
sharptooth angelica seed (until early autumn)
sweetroot root (until mid autumn)
western peony root (until early autumn)

wild carrot seed (until late summer)
wormwood leaf and flower (until early autumn)

Wetlands, Riverbanks, Lakesides, Bogs

blue vervain leaf and flower (until early autumn)
field mint leaf (until early autumn)
Labrador tea leaves (until mid autumn)
northern bugleweed leaf (until early autumn)
yellow pond-lily root (until early autumn)

Late Summer

Open Meadows, Disturbed Soils, Sunny Areas, and the Edges of Sunny Areas

blue elder berry (until early autumn)
cow parsnip root (until mid autumn)
dandelion root (until early autumn)
Gray's lovage root (until mid autumn)
mullein leaf (until early spring)
sharptooth angelica root (until mid autumn)
Sitka valerian root (until mid autumn)
spreading dogbane root (until mid autumn)
waxy coneflower root (until mid autumn)
western juniper berry (until mid autumn)
yarrow root (until mid autumn)

Woodlands and Partially Shaded Places

cut-leaved goldthread whole plant (until mid autumn)
nettle seed (until early autumn)
red baneberry root (until mid autumn)
salal berry (until mid autumn)
thinleaf huckleberry berry (until early autumn)
western trillium leaf (until early autumn)
woodland strawberry root (until mid autumn)

Wetlands, Riverbanks, Lakesides, Bogs

California greenbrier root (until early autumn)
California mugwort leaf (until early autumn)
western aralia berry (until early autumn)
western aralia root (until mid autumn)
western skunk cabbage root (until mid autumn)

Seashore and Coastal Areas

California bayberry root bark (until late autumn)

AUTUMN

As late-season fruits mature, the job of procreation is mostly done. After a long season of expansion, the plants prepare to send the resources they've accumulated throughout the summer months downward into their roots, where vibrant energy for next season's growth is stored. During this time of renewal and giving back to the earth, the herbaceous plants begin to die back as the rains return to refresh and soften the soil. It's time for digging roots, gathering late-season berries, harvesting medicinal mushrooms, and preparing for the descent into the darkness of winter.

Early Autumn

Open Meadows, Disturbed Soils, Sunny Areas, and the Edges of Sunny Areas

alumroot root (until late autumn)
burdock root (until early spring)
burdock seed (until late autumn)
California bay seed (until mid autumn)
Fuller's teasel root (until early spring)
green ephedra stem (year-round)
mullein root (until early spring)
smooth sumac berry (until mid autumn)
wild carrot root (until early spring)
yellow dock root (until late autumn)

Woodlands and Partially Shaded Places

artist's conk fruiting body (until late autumn)
bald hip rose hips (until mid autumn)
devil's club root or stem bark (until late autumn)
false Solomon's seal root (until late autumn)
nettle root (until late autumn)
oneseed hawthorn berry (until mid autumn)
red-belted conk fruiting body (until late autumn)
wild ginger root (until late autumn)

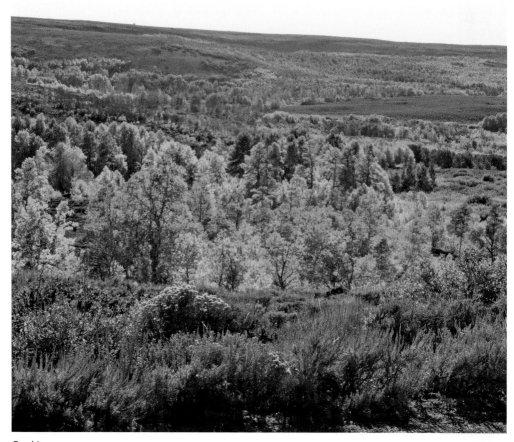

Quaking aspen

After the final harvests of the season, you can clean your tools, finish processing the herbs you've dried, attend to any macerating tinctures that need pressing, make yourself a warm cup of tea, and take a well-earned rest while you enjoy the bounty of your harvest. Prepare to enter a time of introspection and repose as the natural world gathers and firms its nascent energy for the renewal of life in spring. Even though the end of the harvest season may bring feelings of sadness, don't despair for the wildcrafting cycle will soon begin again.

WILD MEDICINAL PLANTS OF THE PACIFIC NORTHWEST

Pacific dogwood

alumroot

Heuchera glabra
alpine heuchera
PARTS USED root, leaf

*This resident of waterfall spray zones, stream banks, and other wet places is full
of tannins that dry out and tighten loose, boggy tissues.*

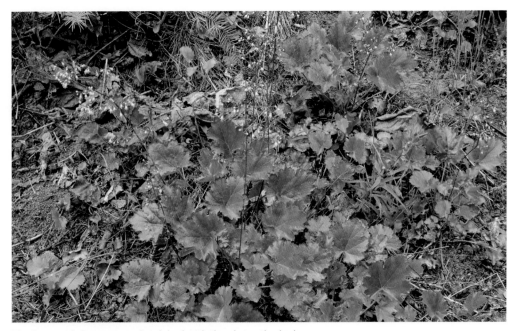

The leaves of alumroot are five-lobed with deeply toothed edges.

How to Identify

Wider than long, mostly basal, and palmately 5-lobed leaves attach to stout, scaly
rhizomes via long, hairless leaf stalks. Sticky
hairs may or may not cover the undersides
of the smooth-topped, deeply toothed leaves
that reveal cottony fibers along the veins
when torn cross-wise. Thin, wiry, reddish
stems with 1 or 2 bract-like leaves that are
much smaller than the basal leaves rise 6–24
inches above the foliage bearing sprays of
small, white, 5-petaled flowers on branching
stalks. Five orange-tipped stamens, the often
thread-like, male, pollen-bearing parts of a
flower, and the curled-back petals peek out
from the hairy calyx, the outer whorl of a
flower that is made up of the sepals, which
protect the flower while in the bud stage.
Egg-shaped capsules house elongated, brown
seeds lined with rows of spines. Dead leaves
from previous years often remain attached to
the plant.

Crevice alumroot (*Heuchera micrantha*)
has leaves that are longer than wide with
hairy undersides and can be used similarly as
medicine.

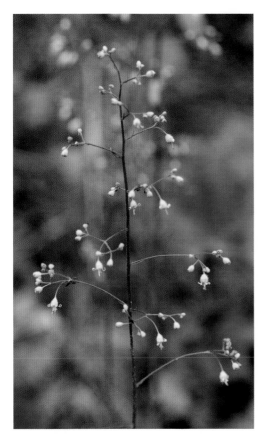
Wiry, reddish stems bear small white flowers with orange-tipped stamens.

Where, When, and How to Wildcraft

This plant inhabits wet and rocky places from the coast to beyond timberline throughout this region. It thrives in moist crevices, in rocky meadows, on stream banks, and near misty waterfalls.

Harvest the roots from early to late autumn after the leaves begin to die back. The leaves can be harvested any time before autumn for use in the field.

Medicinal Uses

Alumroot's astringent tannins tighten and dry tissues of the skin and internal mucous membranes that are damp from lack of tone. Gargle a decoction of the root or the tincture diluted in 1 fluid ounce of water to aid boggy sore throats. The same preparations, swished in the mouth, tighten inflamed gum tissue. Drink the tea to relieve diarrhea or to reduce gastrointestinal inflammation. For hemorrhoids, apply a wash of the tea to the anus. The powdered root or crushed leaves applied topically stop bleeding from cuts as well as nosebleeds.

Future Harvests

After digging the root, remove the leaves and cut off the crown along with the top 3–4 inches of the root. Replant the crown in the hole you've just dug, mulch it well with the discarded leaves, and give it some water.

HERBAL PREPARATIONS

Root Tea
Standard Decoction
Drink 2–3 fluid ounces up to 3 times per day.

Root Tincture
1 part fresh root
2 parts menstruum (75 percent alcohol, 15 percent distilled water, 10 percent glycerin)
or
1 part dried root
5 parts menstruum (50 percent alcohol, 40 percent distilled water, 10 percent glycerin)
Take 30–60 drops up to 3 times per day.

---

arrowleaf balsamroot

Balsamorhiza sagittata

PARTS USED root, leaf

Resin-filled roots soothe the throat and lungs, clear mucus, boost immunity, and lift the spirit. Arrow-shaped leaves speed the healing of wounds.

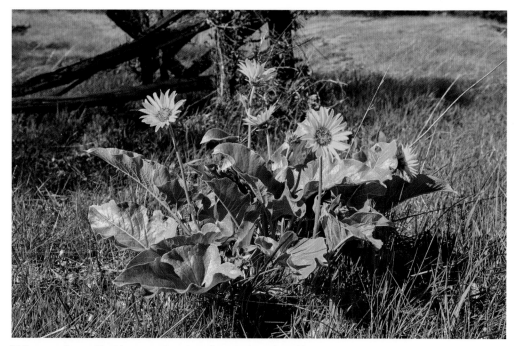

Yellow, sunflower-like blossoms rise above long, pointy-tipped leaves.

How to Identify

Large, multi-crowned, woody taproots filled with rich veins of golden resin and covered with corky, deeply furrowed bark twist deep into the earth. From the hairy crowns, long-stalked basal leaves, 8–24 inches long, with heart-shaped bases and spearhead-shaped blades, emerge smooth-edged and silvery. They are densely covered in fine wooly hairs and turn green with age. Many yellow ray and disk flowers on 1- to 1½-inch-wide sunflower-like heads that are cupped by whorls of white-haired, lance-shaped bracts bloom from mid spring to mid summer atop 8- to 36-inch tall, resinous, short-haired stems lined with few small, lance- to spoon-shaped leaves. Each flowering stalk usually bears a single head of flowers with occasional smaller heads present in the upper leaf axils, the points just above where the leaves emerge from the stem. Small, edible, ⅓-inch-long, sunflower-like seeds ripen in summer. The stem, leaves, and flower heads release a pleasant resinous aroma when rubbed.

Deltoid balsamroot (*Balsamorhiza deltoidea*), which is used similarly, has greener

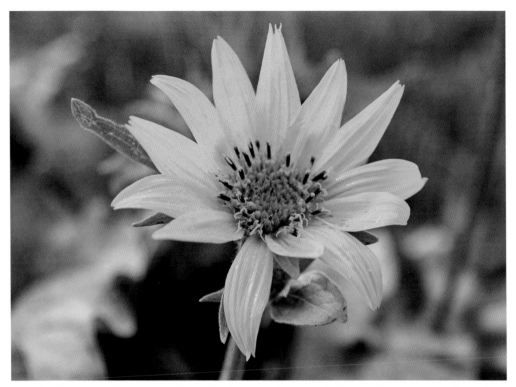

Arrowleaf balsamroot's composite flower heads are made up of petal-like ray flowers and small, tubular disk flowers.

and less hairy leaves. The leaves of the related mule's ears (*Wyethia* species), with which the balsamroots are sometimes confused, are hairless, lance-shaped, somewhat shiny, and lack a heart-shaped base. The root and leaf of mule's ears do not have medicinal properties similar to those of the balsamroots.

Where, When, and How to Wildcraft

This widespread plant grows in isolated patches or in large stands that carpet hillsides with vibrant yellow flower heads at low to middle elevations in open, sunny grasslands and on rocky slopes. Find it east of the Cascades from southern British Columbia to central Oregon and farther west into southern Oregon and California.

From late spring to mid summer while the plants are blooming, remove a few leaves from each plant and bundle them by the stalks to hang for drying. Dig the roots from mid spring to mid autumn; it's easier earlier in the year when the ground is still moist from the spring rains. Give yourself plenty of time for this harvest. Depending on the soil conditions and the size of the root, it can take several hours to remove one from the ground, and these large and woody roots can be difficult to process. It's possible with hand clippers, but it will strain the tool and your wrists. I use a hatchet.

Medicinal Uses

The root tincture in hot water promotes the flow of mucous secretions in the respiratory tract to soothe irritated tissues and clear mucus from the lungs. Use it as a less potent version of echinacea to stimulate the immune system and reduce recovery time from lung infections. Arrowleaf balsamroot stimulates white blood cell activity and, with its antimicrobial properties, makes the terrain less hospitable to infectious agents. A syrup of the roots soothes sore throats, and the leaf salve speeds the healing of wounds. A few drops of tincture lifts the spirits and relieves seasonal affective disorder and depression characterized by grief stored in the lungs. Think of it this way: the flower heads receive the golden nectar of the sun and send it to the roots, where it is concentrated as resin. In this same way, balsamroot brings joy and light to the dark places of our beings. Follow the direction of the upward-pointing, arrow-shaped leaves and allow yourself to be uplifted.

Future Harvests

Larger specimens of this slowly growing plant may attain ages of 40 to 80 years. Restrict your harvests to large, abundant patches and leave the roots of larger and obviously older individuals alone.

HERBAL PREPARATIONS

Root Tea
Standard decoction
Drink 6–8 fluid ounces 3 times per day.

Root Tincture
1 part dried root
5 parts menstruum (75 percent alcohol, 25 percent distilled water)
or
1 part fresh root
2 parts menstruum (100 percent alcohol)
Take 15–60 drops up to 4 times per day.

Leaf Oil and Salve
For leaf oil, follow directions for Dry Herb Infused Oil or Alternative Oil Method (page 64). For the salve, follow directions on page 65.

artist's conk

Ganoderma applanatum
PARTS USED fruiting body

Brown-spored conks inhibit tumor growth, stimulate the immune system, and calm the nerves.

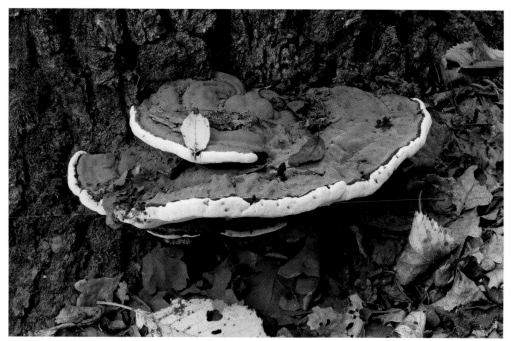

This fungus, which derives its name from the practice of etching drawings into the large, white, brown-staining underbelly, can grow to be quite large.

How to Identify

Light brown with wide, rounded, white lips at their front edges, fan-shaped or semicircular fruiting bodies with dense, woody, cinnamon brown, corky flesh emerge from dead trees as a network of white, thread-like mycelium, the vegetative part of a fungus, break down the decaying wood. As they age the outer lip narrows and the flat, wide cap darkens to a brown to grayish black color and develops concentric furrows that ripple across the hard, knobby, and dull upper-surface crust.

Whitish undersides made up of tiny, barely visible spore tube pores that generate as many as 4.5 trillion spores during the sporing season immediately and permanently stain brown when scratched. Each year a new $^{3}/_{16}$- to ½-inch spore tube layer forms separated from the previous by a thin, brown layer of tissue. Brown or reddish brown spores often dust the upper surface of these 2½- to 30-inch-wide, perennial, shelf-like conks that rarely have stems, smell somewhat meaty, and are rarely hoof-shaped. Determine the age of the fruiting body of these conks, which can live for up to 70 years, by counting the stratified spore tube layers.

With similar medicinal properties, varnished conk (*Ganoderma tsugae*), most often found growing on western hemlock trees, produces annual fruiting bodies with reddish brown to mahogany-colored, shiny, varnished tops that are pliable rather than hard.

Where, When, and How to Wildcraft

Growing mostly on hardwood trees throughout North America, this perennial polypore is most often found in the Pacific Northwest decomposing the wood of Douglas-fir trees. Find them alone or in small groups in the forest or in the city on stumps, dead standing and fallen trees, or occasionally on living but damaged or diseased trees.

Gather the conks when they are actively producing spores during the autumn rainy season. Apply downward pressure to dislodge them. Sometimes they cling tenaciously and need to be pried off. Cut them into 1-inch cubes as soon as possible. If you wait too long they become incredibly hard and you'll need a saw to chop them up.

Medicinal Uses

Containing similar immune-stimulating compounds as those of the famous reishi mushroom (*Ganoderma lucidum*), artist's conk benefits the immune, digestive, respiratory, and nervous systems. Drink the tea or make a soup stock from the fruiting bodies of this meaty, bitter, and sweet-tasting conk to lessen general inflammation, to reduce the size of and inhibit the growth of cancerous tumors, to stimulate white blood cell activity to boost immunity, or to protect the body from the harmful effects of radiation.

The tea or tincture aids digestion, settles an upset stomach, and dries up excessive mucus discharge from the lungs and sinuses. These preparations also calm the nervous system and inspire a deep, meditative state of consciousness that is timeless and free from thought, fear, and attachment. Tap into this mycelial awareness that for eons has witnessed the rise and fall of many forests and relax. The tea or tincture also antidotes the effect of ingesting too much caffeine.

Future Harvests

Two to four of these fairly common, perennial conks should be enough to supply a family with medicine for the year. Harvesting conservatively allows many spores to be produced and encourages the spread of these important, tree-decaying fungi throughout the forest.

HERBAL PREPARATIONS

Fruiting Body Tea
Long decoction

Add 1 tablespoon of coconut or olive oil per quart of water to increase the extraction of the inflammation-reducing and tumor-inhibiting constituents known as triterpenes. Simmer over very low heat for at least 2 hours. The tea makes a great addition to soup stocks.
Drink 4–6 fluid ounces twice daily

Fruiting Body Tincture
1 part dried fruiting body
10 parts menstruum (50 percent alcohol, 50 percent distilled water)

To get the full medicinal spectrum of this mushroom, add the tincture to the tea.
Take 30–60 drops up to 3 times per day.

baldhip rose

Rosa gymnocarpa
dwarf rose, wood rose
PARTS USED flower, hip

The pink flowers relieve sore throats, strengthen the uterus, and lift the spirit. Brilliant red hips, along with the flowers, reduce inflammatory conditions of the respiratory and digestive systems.

How to Identify

From a shallow, rhizomatous root system, spindly, grayish brown stems armed with thin, needle-like prickles sprawl or stand erect 1–5 feet tall. Alternately arranged compound leaves comprising 5–9, ½- to 1-inch-long leaflets unfurl round-tipped, double-toothed, and elliptic to egg-shaped. Glands on the leaves dot the stalks, undersides of midribs, and tips of teeth. Saucer-shaped, pale to deep pink, many-stamened, 5-petalled flowers borne singly or in clusters of 2 or 3 bloom at the ends of branches from late spring to mid summer.

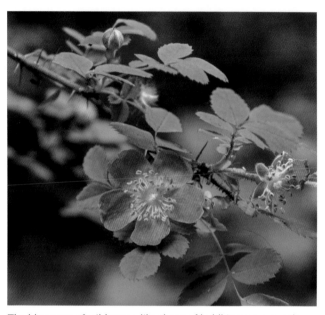

The blossoms of wild roses, like those of baldhip rose, open the heart and lift the spirit.

Triangular, green sepals taper into pointy, tail-like tips and fall off before the pear-shaped, brilliant red hips ripen. The hips encase smooth, ⅜-inch-long seeds tipped with long hairs and may remain on the plant through winter. Younger stems sometimes emerge prickle-free.

All of this region's wild native roses, including Nootka rose (*Rosa nutkana*), clustered wild rose (*R. pisocarpa*), and pearhip rose (*R. woodsii*), can be used medicinally in the same way as baldhip rose.

Where, When, and How to Wildcraft

More abundant at lower latitudes and elevations, this long-lived, deciduous, shade-tolerant shrub prefers somewhat drier sites in open-canopy forests, forest margins and clearings, thickets, and cutover areas. Its range extends from southern British Columbia to central California. Baldhip rose grows from sea level to upper middle elevations on both sides of the Cascades. Gather flowers and buds from mid spring to early summer and the hips after the first hard frost.

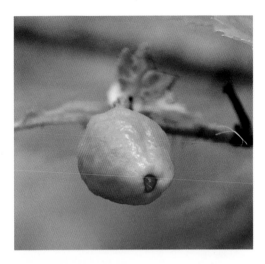

The name hip is derived from the botanical term *hypanthium*. After pollination this cup-shaped structure, formed by the fused bases of the calyx and corolla, enlarges and encases the seeds in a fleshy, berry-like structure.

Medicinal Uses

Both the aromatic flowers and the sour, flavonoid-rich hips are astringent and cooling. A tea of either reduces digestive and respiratory inflammation, clears the nasal passages, and stops the flow of watery mucus. Gargling an infusion of the flowers relieves sore throats, and swished in the mouth it speeds the healing of mouth sores and tightens bleeding gums. As a wash the flower tea soothes sore, tired, bloodshot eyes.

Drink baldhip rose flower tea to restore tone to the uterine muscles, to reduce pelvic congestion that may lead to painful periods or irregular bleeding, to clear vaginal discharges, or to relieve diarrhea.

The hips are high in vitamin C, and the flowers in any form calm the nerves, lift the spirit, and open the heart.

⚠ Caution

Before eating the hips, carefully remove the seed hairs, which can irritate the mouth and throat on the way in and the anus on the way out. Filter them out when making tea.

Future Harvests

When gathering flowers, leave plenty to produce a good crop of hips. When collecting hips, leave a large portion for the birds and other animals who depend on them for food during the cold, lean winter months. To propagate, collect hips in the early autumn and soak them in water to separate the seeds from the flesh. Clean the seeds and sow them immediately for best germination.

HERBAL PREPARATIONS

Flower or Hip Tea
Standard infusion
Drink as needed.

---

barestem biscuitroot

Lomatium nudicaule
Indian consumption plant
PARTS USED seed

Pungent seeds speed the healing of flus and other viral outbreaks.

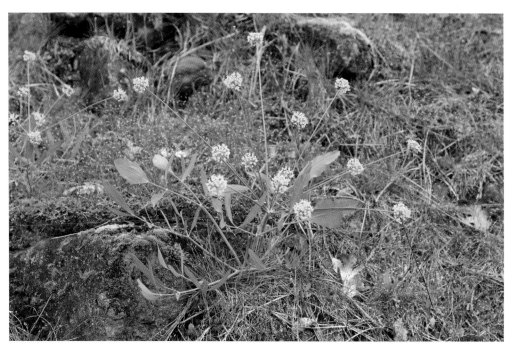

The small yellow flowers of barestem biscuitroot ripen into large, winged seeds.

How to Identify

Compound leaves, mostly basal and divided 1–3 times into 3–30 lance- to oval-shaped leaflets, arise from stout taproots. The leaflets are smooth edged or coarsely toothed near the tip and are arranged opposite each other on the leaf stem. From a swollen bulb at the top of the flower stem, stalks of unequal length hold widely spaced compound umbels of small, yellow or rarely purple flowers that bloom from mid spring to early summer. (An umbel is a grouping of flowers whose stalks, called rays, all originate from the same point. In a compound umbel, a secondary set of smaller umbels sits at the end of each ray rather than a single flower.) Oblong to elliptic, ½-inch-long seeds with wings that are shorter than the seed's width sometimes taper to a beak-like tip. The stems and leaves of this hairless, 10- to 28-inch-tall perennial are covered with a bluish waxy coating.

Where, When, and How to Wildcraft

Stands of barestem biscuitroot are found from southern British Columbia to central

California in dry, open spaces, sagebrush scrub lands, and on grassy, exposed mountain slopes at low to middle elevations. Strip ripe seeds from their stalks in summer when they are just turning from yellow to brown. If they are too young, the flavor will be overly sharp and pungent; too old, and they will have lost their aromatics. When just right, the chewed seeds emit a roundly pungent sensation that expands throughout the mouth and head.

Medicinal Uses

The seeds of barestem biscuitroot have an affinity for the upper respiratory tract, lungs, and stomach. Like the roots of desert parsley (*Lomatium dissectum*), they are strongly antiviral. Use the seed tincture or the tea to aid the body in recovering from flu and other viral infections. Although most research has focused on desert parsley, the seeds of barestem biscuitroot were and continue to be used extensively by native peoples for similar conditions.

Future Harvests

Take no more than a third of the seeds from each plant. If, as you harvest, you find mature brown seeds that are past their prime for use as medicine, sow some of them ½ inch deep in spots where they will get a little extra water to help their germination and initial growth.

HERBAL PREPARATIONS

Seed Tea
Standard decoction
Drink 3–4 fluid ounces up to 5 times per day.

Seed Tincture
1 part dried seed
5 parts menstruum (75 percent alcohol, 25 percent distilled water)
or
1 part fresh seed
2 parts menstruum (100 percent alcohol)
Take 15–20 drops up to 5 times per day.

black cottonwood

Populus trichocarpa
balsam poplar
PARTS USED bud, twig

Resinous buds expel mucus from the lungs, soothe sore muscles, and speed the healing of cuts, scrapes, and burns.

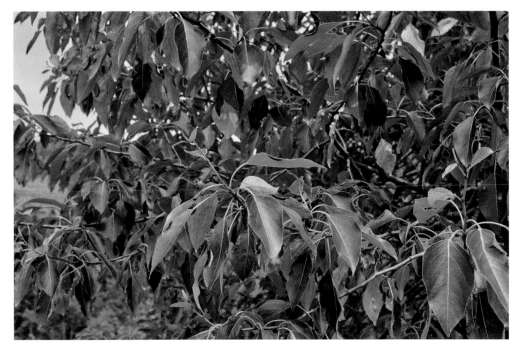

The sound of black cottonwood leaves fluttering in the wind brings joy to the heart.

How to Identify

From late winter to early spring, resinous buds swell and fill the air with their sweet fragrance. Hanging catkins (dense spikes of single-sexed flowers that lack petals), male and female on separate trees, emerge from early to late spring, followed by thick, dark green, heart-shaped leaves with pale undersides and pointed tips. Fine teeth and small hairs line the edges of the alternately arranged, deciduous leaves. After they ripen, hairy seeds burst out of 3-chambered capsules, filling the sky and covering the ground with the white fluff that gives the cottonwoods their name. Smooth bark thickens into deep furrows as the broad-trunked trees age, and brown twigs turn gray after their first year.

Where, When, and How to Wildcraft

Found throughout western North America from sea level to middle elevations, this rapidly growing tree (formerly *Populus balsamifera* subsp. *trichocarpa*) resides in wet forests

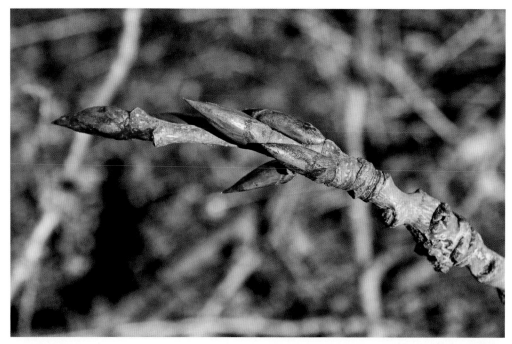

The first scent of the resinous, sweet-smelling buds heralds the arrival of spring and the beginning of the harvest season.

and along waterways from Alaska to California. At lower elevations west of the Cascades, black cottonwood often grows in large stands in the bottomlands of large streams and rivers. East of the Cascades its range is limited to protected valleys and canyons.

From mid winter to early spring, look for low-hanging branches or limbs that have fallen to the ground after a windstorm. Cut the bud-laden branch ends. Remove buds to make a fresh tincture, or place the bud-covered twigs in bags to dry for making oils or dry bud tinctures. Leaving the slow-to-dry buds on the twigs increases airflow to speed the drying process. Save the twigs for tea after you've removed the dried buds to make an oil or tincture.

Medicinal Uses

Warming and stimulating resins in the buds stimulate lung secretions to expel mucus, speed the healing of infections, and increase the circulation of blood to the exterior. Take the tincture in hot water to clear the lungs of hard stuck mucus that causes rattling unproductive coughs, to stimulate circulation to promote sweating and bring blood and warmth to the surface of the skin and extremities, and to help resolve nonviral lung infections.

Bitter salicylates in the buds and twigs reduce inflammation and relieve pain. Rub the oil on sore muscles and strains. The bud oil combines well with hairy arnica and/or Saint John's wort oil to reduce joint swelling and to ease the pain and inflammation of carpal tunnel syndrome. Drink a tea of the bitter twigs for added effect.

The bud salve or butter reduces swelling, prevents infection, and promotes rapid skin cell regeneration. I find the butter especially helpful for burns and chapped lips.

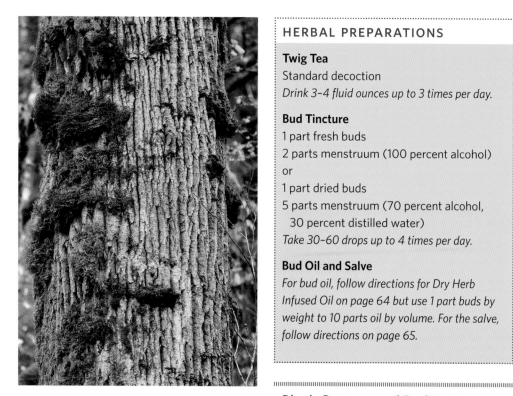
Growing upward of 100 feet, black cottonwood is this region's tallest native, deciduous tree.

On the emotional level, the deep anchoring and solidity of this tree is a signature for its ability to impart calmness. Black cottonwood teaches us to radiate a quiet dignity and to receive and transform chaotic energies. It has shown me that when I feel overwhelmed by life, there is often an internal process of change trying to take place. It asks me to stop resisting and go into the process so that the transformation can occur.

Future Harvests
Find large downed branches to harvest from, or take a few twigs from each tree. Stick branches in the ground where you harvest; they will root in and make new trees.

HERBAL PREPARATIONS

Twig Tea
Standard decoction
Drink 3–4 fluid ounces up to 3 times per day.

Bud Tincture
1 part fresh buds
2 parts menstruum (100 percent alcohol)
or
1 part dried buds
5 parts menstruum (70 percent alcohol, 30 percent distilled water)
Take 30–60 drops up to 4 times per day.

Bud Oil and Salve
For bud oil, follow directions for Dry Herb Infused Oil on page 64 but use 1 part buds by weight to 10 parts oil by volume. For the salve, follow directions on page 65.

Black Cottonwood Bud Butter

dried black cottonwood buds
clarified butter

1. Measure 1 part by volume of dried black cottonwood buds. Grind them with a coffee grinder or other device to the consistency of corn meal.
2. In a double boiler, heat 2 parts by volume of clarified butter (also known as ghee).
3. Add the ground buds and simmer for 4 hours on very low heat, stirring occasionally. Heating the mixture too high will ruin the medicine.
4. Into a clean, dry jar, pour the bud-infused butter through a cheesecloth-lined funnel to strain out the herb material.
5. Label accordingly, and store in a cool dry place.
Adapted from Michael Moore

bladderwrack

Fucus distichus
popweed, rockweed
PARTS USED thallus

*Easily identified by the gas-filled bladders at the tips of its blades, this iodine-
and mineral-rich seaweed is a specific remedy for underactive thyroid and goiter.
It also helps prevent thyroid cancer.*

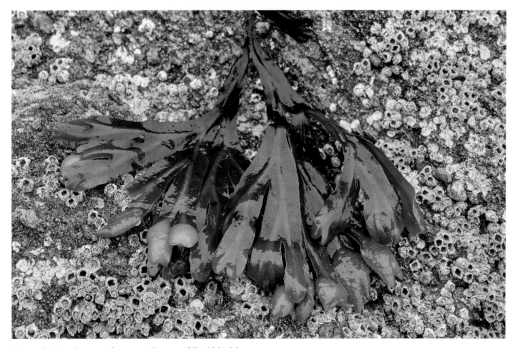

Reproductive bumps form on the gas-filled bladders.

How to Identify

Forming dense canopies that shelter other algae and invertebrates, this green to olive-brown seaweed attaches to rocks with a single, disc-shaped holdfast. Blades, ½ to 1 inch wide with raised midribs along the center, fork several times into Ys. Young blades may appear flat and lack bladders, but as they mature the tips turn yellowish green, swell up, and form small reproductive bumps. The mitten-shaped, gas-filled bladders allow the 4- to 20-inch-long thallus (the nonvascular, undifferentiated vegetative body of lichens and seaweeds) to float and stretch upward toward the sun.

Where, When, and How to Wildcraft

Often the dominant species of algae in the mid-intertidal zone, this hardy seaweed (formerly *Fucus gardneri*) inhabits exposed coastal waters and sheltered bays and estuaries. Because it tolerates a wide range of salinity, it can also be found at the mouths of streams that deposit freshwater into the sea. Find bladderwrack growing in dense bands on rocks and mussels all along the Pacific coast from the Bering Sea and Aleutian Islands in Alaska to Point Conception in central California. In sheltered areas bladderwrack can live for up to 5 years; those growing in exposed sites and battered by waves have an average life span of 2 to 3 years.

Harvest during a low tide from early to mid summer as the thalli mature and the bladders swell. Because bladderwrack grows in the mid-intertidal zone, from just below average sea level to the upper limit of the average lowest tides, they are underwater except during the twice-daily low tides. Consult a local tide table to plan an opportune harvest time. The most extreme low tides each month coincide with the new and full moons.

Collect from rocks rather than gathering specimens that have washed up on shore that have most likely deteriorated and lost their medicinal properties. Using a knife or scissors, trim 2–3 inches from the tips of the thalli. Wash away sand and other debris with ocean water and place the seaweed in a clean collecting bucket. Pour off water from the bucket before you leave the beach, and keep the seaweed covered and out of direct sunlight while transporting it home. Spread the seaweed out on screens to dry in the sun. If it's cloudy or raining, use a dehydrator on the lowest setting or set your screens indoors near a wood stove or other heat source. An electric fan will speed the process.

Medicinal Uses

Bladderwrack is high in a form of iodine that is easily converted into thyroid hormones. Ingest powdered bladderwrack daily for underactive thyroid gland (hypothyroidism)

or for goiter, an enlargement of the thyroid gland in response to inadequate supplies of iodine. Iodine 131 is released daily into the atmosphere by nuclear power plants and facilities all over the world. The human body readily absorbs this radioactive isotope and stores it in the thyroid gland, leading to increased risk of thyroid cancer. Daily intake of seaweeds including bladderwrack supplies the body with iodine 127, the natural form of iodine. If the thyroid has adequate supplies of iodine 127, it has no need to take up the radioactive form. Store dried seaweeds for 8–10 weeks prior to ingesting; based on iodine 131's rate of decay, this will ensure that the seaweeds are free of any accumulated radioisotopes.

Bladderwrack can also be taken to reduce prostate inflammation or to lower blood pressure. Apply a poultice or a hot compress to relieve joint pain.

Caution

If you are dealing with any type of thyroid condition, consult a physician or other qualified health practitioner before starting a treatment plan.

Future Harvests

Always leave at least 2 inches remaining at the base of the blade above the holdfast to ensure the regrowth of these perennial algae. Be mindful of your steps as you gather and avoid stepping on these seaweeds and other organisms.

HERBAL PREPARATIONS

Ground Thallus
Take 3–5 grams daily.

---

blue elder

Sambucus cerulea
blue elderberry
PARTS USED flower, berry, leaf

Fragrant flowers and tart berries speed the passage of colds and flus.

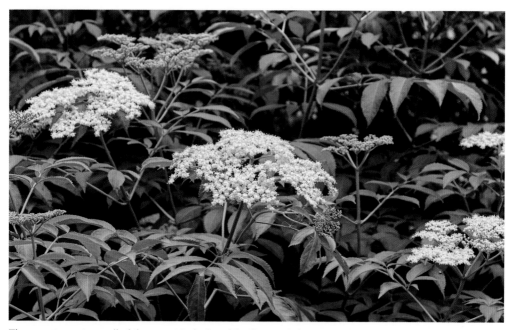

The sweet, musty smell of the sweat-inducing elder flowers is hypnotic.

How to Identify

Each year thick, purplish green stalks emerge from the base of this vigorously growing opposite-leaved perennial that grows as wide as it is tall, up to 13 feet. As the pith-filled stems age, they develop a reddish, warty bark that eventually becomes gray with linear ridges. Compound leaves are divided into 5–9 elliptic to ovate, serrated leaflets that emit a nutty smell when rubbed or crushed. Flat-topped clusters of white to cream-colored, musty-smelling flowers bloom from late spring to late summer and ripen into dark blue berries, whose whitish waxy coating gives them a lighter hue. Heavy clusters of mature berries weigh down the branches from late summer to early autumn.

Where, When, and How to Wildcraft

Find this shade-intolerant shrub on both sides of the Cascade Crest from southern British Columbia to California growing in dry well-drained soils along roads, in clear cuts, and in forest clearings.

Harvest the flowers from late spring to late summer before they are pollinated by taking the whole cluster. For a fresh plant tincture, clip the small stalks just below the tightest grouping of flowers. To dry the flowers for tea, put the whole and intact flower heads on screens, and remove and discard the larger stems after the material is dry. Gather clusters of berries when they are ripe and juicy. For tea, dry the berries in a dehydrator. For tincture, pick the fresh berries off the stalks individually. The leaves can be harvested throughout the growing season and are best used fresh to make oil.

Medicinal Uses

A tea of the flowers or the tincture in hot water promotes sweating and supports the body's natural response to fever. Blue elder is indicated for people with a bluish cast to the skin who may lack oxygen, as it opens the bronchioles and stimulates blood flow to the surface of the skin and extremities. It is also one of the safest and gentlest flu remedies, suitable for very young children and the elderly. A classic western herbal formula can be made by combining equal parts of blue elder flower, yarrow flower, and field mint leaves.

The berries are strongly antiviral and will significantly reduce the recovery time during a bout of flu. They can be consumed as a tincture, a decoction of the dried berries, or a syrup. An infused oil of the leaves relieves pain and inflammation from sprains, strains, and bruises. The salve is used to treat hemorrhoids.

Elder flower tincture develops a sweet, musty flavor that gets better as it ages. I see this as a signature for the way it helps us ripen into elders. It also resolves fear of death or transformation and helps with letting go and accepting change.

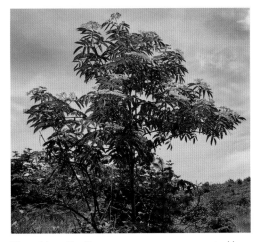

Blue elders like the open sunny spaces created by clear cuts.

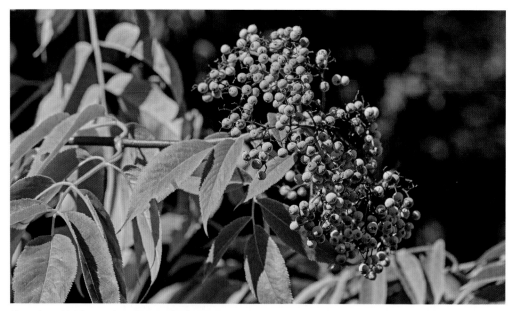
Note the whitish waxy coating on the berries.

 Caution

Due to the presence of hydrocyanic acid, the seeds may cause nausea and dizziness with vomiting and/or diarrhea. Some people can eat lots of berries without any adverse effect, whereas others eat just a few and begin to feel queasy. Test your own sensitivity by eating a few at a time to see what happens. When I eat the berries raw, I don't chew the seeds. Berries prepared as tea or tincture are perfectly safe to consume.

Future Harvests

When harvesting elder flowers or berries, I've come to an agreement with the birds, bears, and other creatures who receive nourishment from this tree. I take only what I can reach from the ground; ladders or other height boosters are not allowed. This leaves plenty of berries on each tree for all to ingest, enjoy, and participate in the dispersal of seed.

HERBAL PREPARATIONS

Flower Tea
Standard infusion
Drink 4–6 fluid ounces up to 5 times per day.

Berry Tea
Standard decoction
Drink 4–6 fluid ounces up to 5 times per day.

Flower Tincture
1 part fresh flowers
2 parts menstruum (75 percent alcohol, 25 percent distilled water)
Take 15–60 drops up to 5 times per day.

Berry Tincture
1 part fresh berries
2 parts menstruum (100 percent alcohol)
Take 15–60 drops up to 5 times per day.

Leaf Oil and Salve
For the leaf oil, follow the directions for Fresh Herb Infused Oil on page 63. For the salve, follow the directions on page 65.

blue vervain

Verbena hastata
swamp verbena
PARTS USED leaf and flower

Intensely bitter leaves and flowers help break fevers, stimulate digestion, relax tension, and soothe and nourish the nerves.

How to Identify

From short crowns slowly spreading rhizomes send up stiff, erect stems, often bristly, square, and branched above. Pairs of 1½- to 6-inch-long, short-stalked, roughly textured, lance-shaped leaves with acutely pointed tips, sharply serrated edges, and sometimes lobed bases ascend the green to reddish stems opposite each other. Many tiny, tubular, 5-lobed, purplish blue flowers bloom from bottom to top, just a few at a time, from mid summer to early autumn in densely packed, candelabra-like clusters of 1½- to 4-inch-long, erect, slender spikes with inconspicuous, awl-shaped bracts. Each pollinated flower produces 4 reddish brown nutlets.

Where, When, and How to Wildcraft

Widely distributed throughout North America and occupying a patchwork of counties in Washington, Oregon, and northern California, this moisture-loving, self-seeding biennial or short-lived perennial is found at lower

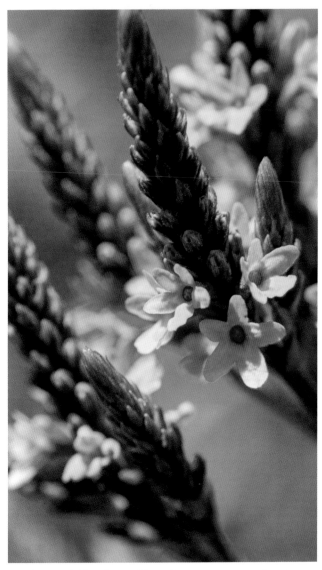

Small purplish blue flowers bloom from summer to early autumn.

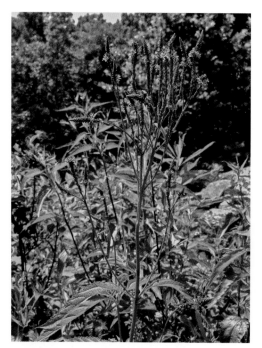

Rigid stalks hold candelabra-like clusters of summer-blooming flowers.

elevations in meadows, marshes, wetlands, ditches, disturbed areas, and along river and stream banks. It is common east of the Cascades in Washington and both east and west of the Cascades in Oregon but rare in southern British Columbia.

While in flower, clip stalks near the base. Use the leaves, flowers, and flexible upper parts of the stems for fresh tincture. Hang bundles to dry, and then strip the leaves and flowers; discard the rigid stems.

Medicinal Uses

Drink the tea hot or tincture in hot water to promote sweating at the first sign of fevers associated with colds and flus, to clear mucus from and reduce inflammation in the lungs and sinuses, or to initiate secretions in the uterus to treat delayed menses and suppressed postpartum discharge and bleeding. The cold infusion or tincture in small doses is a bitter tonic that increases appetite, stimulates digestion, and soothes and settles an irritated or nervous stomach. The tincture or tea drunk cold relaxes tension and nourishes the nerves to alleviate the effects of chronic stress, exhaustion, depression, and recovery from acute illness. It also fosters deep dreamless sleep and increases urine output to clear gravel from the bladder and kidneys. Used externally as a wash, the tea reduces swelling from sprains, strains, and contusions.

Caution

Because it stimulates uterine secretions, avoid ingesting this plant during pregnancy.

Future Harvests

Leave plenty of flowering stalks in each stand to ensure the production of seeds and the promise of future seedlings.

HERBAL PREPARATIONS

Leaf and Flower Tea
Hot or cold infusion
Drink 2–4 fluid ounces up to 3 times per day.

Leaf and Flower Tincture
1 part fresh leaf and flowers
2 parts menstruum (75 percent alcohol, 25 percent distilled water)
or
1 part dried leaf and flower
5 parts menstruum (50 percent alcohol, 50 percent distilled water)
Take 15–30 drops up to 3 times per day.

buckbean

Menyanthes trifoliata
bogbean, marsh trefoil
PARTS USED leaf

This bitter digestive tonic has a long history of use in Europe and North America for digestive stagnation, rheumatic joint pain, and headaches.

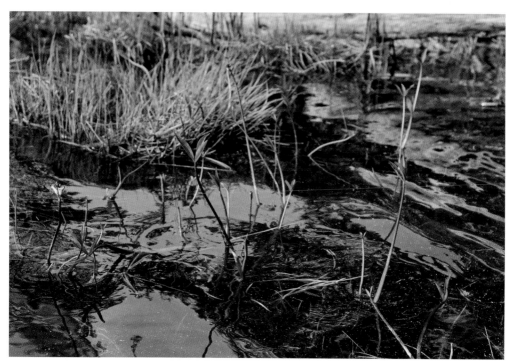

The three-parted leaves reach up out of the water on long stalks.

How to Identify

Remnants of the foliage from previous years persist on thick, colony-forming, underwater rhizomes. Hairless, green, 3-parted leaves rise above the water on 4- to 12-inch-long sheathing leaf stalks topped by elliptic to egg-shaped, short-stalked leaflets with smooth to coarsely toothed edges. Small clusters of short-tubed, rank-smelling flowers divided into 5 or 6 whitish, purplish to pinkish tinged, and frilly-topped petal lobes bloom from late spring to late summer at the ends of leafless flower stalks. Egg-shaped capsules house many shiny, brownish yellow seeds that float on the surface of the water.

Where, When, and How to Wildcraft

This perennial aquatic plant grows in ponds, lakes, and marshes throughout this region from low to middle elevations. The first time I found this plant it was growing in the middle of a lake, and the harvest required a boat.

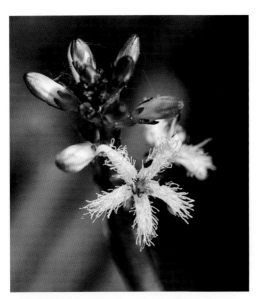

Frilly, rank-smelling flowers attract insects for pollination.

It's easier if you find a spot where it grows at the edge of the water. Gather the leaves along with their stalks from early to late summer.

Medicinal Uses

Take the bitter and somewhat spicy leaf tea or tincture 10–15 minutes before meals to stimulate appetite and relieve chronic indigestion with bloating and post-meal fatigue. Buckbean is particularly helpful for those with food allergies and sensitivities leading to sore, achy joints and/or headaches stemming from liver and digestive stagnation.

⚠ Caution

In large doses fresh plant preparations can be emetic. Do not use with acute intestinal inflammation.

Future Harvests

Leave the rhizomes alone to maintain the vigor of the colony, and harvest only one or two leaves from each plant.

HERBAL PREPARATIONS

Leaf Tea
Standard infusion
Drink 2-4 fluid ounces up to 3 times per day.

Leaf Tincture
1 part fresh leaf
2 parts menstruum (75 percent alcohol,
  25 percent distilled water)
or
1 part dried leaf (use recently dried herb
  that is less than 4 months old)
5 parts menstruum (50 percent alcohol,
  50 percent distilled water)
Take 10-15 drops up to 3 times per day.

---

burdock

Arctium lappa
greater burdock
PARTS USED leaf, root, seed

Nourishing roots support healthy gut flora and clean the blood to heal eruptive skin conditions. Bitter seeds cleanse the kidneys and bladder.

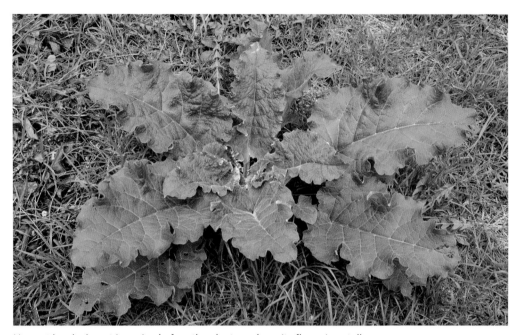

Harvest burdock root in spring before the plant sends up its flowering stalk.

How to Identify

Up to 20-inch-long, broadly oval to heart-shaped, undulating basal leaves, nearly smooth above and covered in white wooly hairs below, attach to long, fleshy, brown-skinned taproots via long fibrous leaf stalks. The whitish-fleshed roots taper as they extend up to 15 inches deep into the earth. In the second year of growth, 1½- to 10-foot-tall, juicy-fleshed stalks, hairy, furrowed, and with wide-spreading branches, shoot upward, lined with alternately arranged leaves that grow progressively smaller as they ascend the stem. Several whorls of overlapping, scale-like bracts with recurved or hooked tips encase globe-shaped composite flower heads lacking ray flowers that produce purple, tubular disk flowers that bloom from late summer to mid autumn. As the oblong, ribbed, dark brown, often black-spotted seeds crowned with short, bristly hairs ripen, the seed heads dry to become prickly burs, about ¾ inch wide, that detach easily from their stalks and stubbornly cling to the hair or clothing of those who brush up against them.

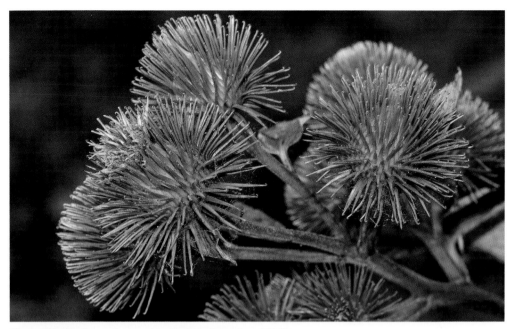

The hooked barbs on the burs inspired the invention of Velcro.

Where, When, and How to Wildcraft

Growing on disturbed ground, in forest openings and pastures, and along roadsides at lower elevations throughout North America (except the central United States), this introduced Eurasian biennial is mainly found near urban centers in Washington and Oregon and rarely found in southern British Columbia.

Gather leaves before the flowering stalks emerge. Dig the roots of this biennial as they enter their second season of growth: between early autumn and early spring. After the flowering stalks emerge, the leaves and roots dry out and lose their medicinal value. Collect seeds in autumn after the heads turn brown. The burs will stick together and wad up into a big ball. Place fully dried burs in a sturdy bag and beat the wadded mass with a stick to break up the seed heads. Winnow by pouring the seeds from one bucket to another in front of a fan to blow away the chaff and separate the seeds.

Medicinal Uses

Nourishing, sweet, and slightly bitter, burdock root, a classic alterative or blood purifier, helps the body process and eliminate waste products by strengthening the kidneys, liver, and lymphatic system. It is especially useful for long-term skin conditions such as eczema, psoriasis, and acne or for abscesses and boils because when the other modes of elimination are compromised, the body sends metabolic waste products to the skin for elimination. Take the root tea or tincture daily for several weeks or months to restore proper functioning to the organs responsible for ridding the body of toxins. As the burdock root and seed preparations restore balance to the body's eliminatory functions, skin conditions may initially worsen before they resolve.

Containing the prebiotic inulin, burdock root feeds the gut flora to boost immunity and restore the integrity of the intestinal ecology after courses of antibiotics or

What Is an Alterative?

Many herbs with varying actions are considered alterative. They have an overall balancing effect on the system as a whole. Alteratives have traditionally been considered blood purifiers because they were thought to eliminate toxins from the body, but a more precise definition is that they improve the functioning of the liver, kidneys, skin, bowels, and/or lymphatic system to help the body better excrete metabolic waste products and improve the body's ability to absorb nutrients.

Some Alteratives Found in the Pacific Northwest

- burdock
- California greenbrier
- chickweed
- cleavers
- dandelion
- nettles
- Oregon grape
- red alder
- red clover
- red root
- yellow dock

---

chemotherapy. Eat it raw or cooked, drink the tea, or take the tincture for this effect and to increase digestive function, relieve constipation, or moderate blood sugar levels.

Like the roots, the very bitter and somewhat tingly seeds aid the organs of elimination and strongly promote urination. Take the tincture to help cleanse the kidneys and bladder of gravelly deposits, to relieve edema, or to resolve pain and irritation caused by urinary tract obstruction.

Steam the bruised leaves and apply as a poultice to draw out infection, speed the healing of wounds, or clear fungal infections.

⚠ **Caution**

Preparations of the seed should not be consumed during the first and second trimesters of pregnancy.

Future Harvests

The clinging burs do an excellent job of distributing seeds far and wide. If you'd like to help, collect seeds in autumn, and sow them the following spring or summer.

HERBAL PREPARATIONS

Root Tea
Standard decoction
Drink 4–6 fluid ounces up to 3 times per day.

Root Tincture
1 part fresh root
2 parts menstruum (75 percent alcohol, 25 percent distilled water)
or
1 part dried root
5 parts menstruum (50 percent alcohol, 50 percent distilled water)
Take 30–60 drops up to 3 times per day.

Seed Tincture
1 part dried seed
4 parts menstruum (75 percent alcohol, 25 percent distilled water)
Take 5–20 drops up to 3 times per day.

California bay

Umbellularia californica
California laurel, Oregon myrtle
PARTS USED leaf, seed

Pungent, spicy leaves relieve sinus infections, headaches, and sore joints.

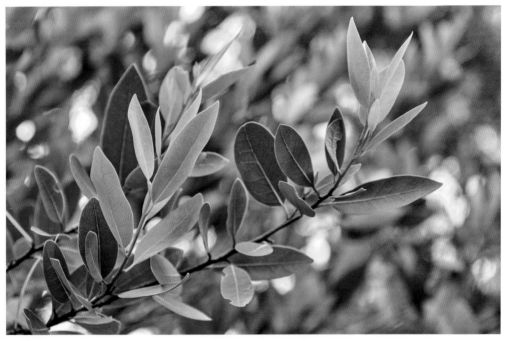

Crush the leaves between your fingers to release their sharp and clarifying aromatics.

How to Identify

Reddish brown or green bark covers the trunks of evergreen shrubs or trees. Thick, yellow-green to dark green, alternately arranged, highly aromatic, smooth-edged, lance-shaped, and short-stalked leaves remain on the tree for several seasons before turning brown and falling to the ground. Yellow-green flowers, clustered in groups of 6–10, produce 1-seeded, ¾- to 1-inch-wide, green, avocado-shaped fruits that ripen from mid to late autumn and turn dark purple as they dry. With favorable conditions these single- to multi-trunked, round-crowned trees can grow to 100 feet.

Where, When, and How to Wildcraft

Found in the southernmost coastal areas of the Pacific Northwest, California bay tolerates some shade and grows on forested slopes, ridges, and bluffs and in small canyons and chaparral shrub lands. Along canyon creeks, it attains its greatest heights, whereas in exposed, rocky soils it has a shrubby habit.

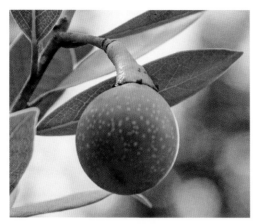
The roasted seeds have a stimulating, caffeine-like effect.

Pluck the leaves singly or snip branch ends from mid spring to early autumn. Gather the edible seeds from early to mid autumn as the husks soften or after the fruits have fallen from the tree.

Medicinal Uses

Sniff the crushed leaves or tincture, take the tincture in hot water, or inhale a steam of the leaves to treat sinus infections, clear nasal passages, or relieve headaches. Apply a rubbing alcohol liniment or compress of the tea or tincture to aid rheumatic conditions or to reduce nerve and joint pain.

For its antifungal effect, apply the oil externally to athlete's foot, ringworm, and jock itch. The smoke of the dried leaves will clear infections as well as negative energies from homes and other spaces.

Those looking for local stimulants or a substitute for caffeine can seek out the stimulating seeds. Roasting them drives off the too-intense volatile oils and prepares them for consumption.

⚠ Caution

While processing the leaves for medicine, be careful to avoid touching your eyes or mucous membranes; after processing, wash your hands well. Too much of any of the herbal preparations inhaled or taken internally can cause irritation or headaches. Start with small doses and increase slowly until the desired effect is achieved.

Future Harvests

Even though California bay is abundant with leaves, harvest from different trees to minimize your impact.

HERBAL PREPARATIONS

Leaf Tea
Standard infusion
For external use or as a steam.

Leaf Tincture
1 part fresh leaf
2 parts menstruum (100 percent alcohol)
Take 5–10 drops up to 5 times per day.

Leaf Oil
Follow directions for Dry Herb Infused Oil or Alternative Oil Method (page 64).

How to Roast California Bay Seeds

The pungent oils in the seeds make them too strong to consume raw. Roast them to cook off the pungent and irritating oils.

1. Remove the fleshy husks and discard.
2. On a baking sheet, roast seeds in the shell at 450°F for 20–25 minutes. Stir often.
3. They're ready when they turn a creamy brown. It takes a bit of experimentation: if under-roasted they will be too spicy, but when over-roasted they get bitter.
4. Remove the shells before consuming.

California bayberry

Morella californica
Pacific bayberry, Pacific wax myrtle
PARTS USED root bark

Spicy, astringent root bark provides medicine to clear clogged nasal passages,
relieve sore throats, and invigorate and tighten gum tissue.

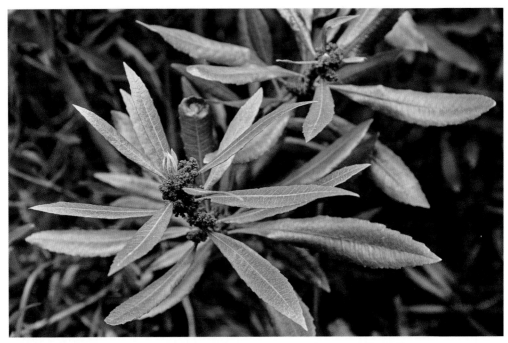

Catkins of reddish brown female flowers ripen into purplish waxy berries traditionally
used to make candles.

How to Identify

Smooth, light gray to brownish bark envelops
the reddish brown wood of the several arching trunks and their branches. Small hairs
cover new-growth twigs, and black glands dot
the dark green, coarsely serrated, aromatic,
lance-shaped leaves. Alternately arranged,
glossy, and hairless, these somewhat sticky
leaves grow 2–4 inches long. Mostly uni-
sexual, ½- to 1-inch-long catkins, male and
female on the same shrub or tree, bear small

flowers that bloom in spring. Pollinated
female flowers form purplish berries covered
in white wax that ripen in early autumn.
Occasionally this 7- to 30-foot-tall, multi-
branched, coastal evergreen shrub will take
on the habit of a small tree.

Where, When, and How to Wildcraft

Find this woody perennial (formerly *Myrica
californica*) along the coast in canyons,
on slopes, and in sandy-soiled forests at

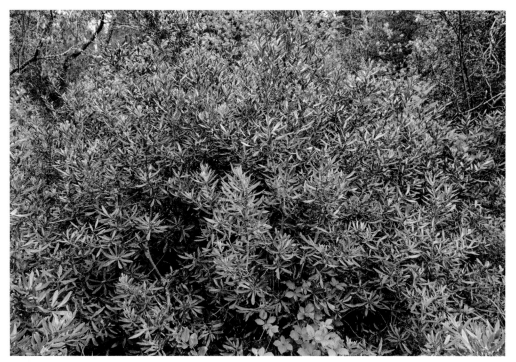

Harvesting California bayberry is a great excuse for a visit to the coast in autumn.

elevations below 500 feet. California bayberry's range extends from Gray's Harbor, Washington, to the Santa Monica Mountains of southern California, with some isolated stands on the west coast of Vancouver Island in British Columbia.

Harvest the root bark from late summer to late autumn. This is easier said than done, as the roots can be quite large. Bring a good shovel and a sharp saw for the job, and give yourself plenty of time—not just for digging but also for stripping the bark, which can be thick, especially around the crown, and difficult to remove.

Before you start digging, remove a few of the branching trunks so you can get to the base of the shrub, and carefully excavate around the root crown with a small shovel or digging knife to determine which direction the lateral roots spread. Use a large shovel to dig up the soil and follow the lateral roots to

their ends. Saw them off where they connect to the crown to ease their removal, and if you plan to take the whole root, dig some more until you are able to extract the whole root ball. After you finish, replace the soil and cover the area with the trimmed branches.

Medicinal Uses

California bayberry root bark is spicy, astringent, and resinous. It's so spicy that taking more than a few drops of the tincture undiluted will burn your tongue. The aromatic resins stimulate blood and lymph flow to damp, stagnant tissues. This stimulating effect coupled with the astringency of bayberry's tannins is especially useful for boggy sore throats and spongy, inflamed, and/or bleeding gums.

For a sore throat, gargle the diluted tincture (5–10 drops in ½ fluid ounce of water); for inflamed gums swish it around in the mouth for 1 minute. Take the tincture or powdered herb in hot water to relieve sinus congestion, to clear mucus from the lungs, or to restore tone to lax, over-secreting tissues in the stomach or intestines.

Caution

The spicy dust that billows out of the grinder may sting your eyes, burn your nasal passages, and bring about fits of coughing and choking. Avoid this by wearing a mask and grinding in a well-ventilated area. Bayberry is reported to be emetic at larger doses.

Future Harvests

For most, a few lateral roots ought to provide enough medicine for the year. Dig up one side of a shrub and remove one or two of the large side roots. Trim off an equal-sized portion of the corresponding aerial parts to avoid stressing the plant.

HERBAL PREPARATIONS

Root Bark Tea
Drink ¼ teaspoon of the ground root bark in 4 fluid ounces of hot water up to 3 times per day.

Root Bark Tincture
1 part fresh root bark
2 parts menstruum (100 percent alcohol)
or
1 part dried root bark
5 parts menstruum (70 percent alcohol, 30 percent distilled water)
Take 5–10 drops up to 5 times per day.

California greenbrier

Smilax californica
California sarsaparilla, California smilax
PARTS USED root

Somewhat sweet-tasting, saponaceous roots nourish the adrenals, help maintain hormonal balance, and support the liver's hormone processing function.

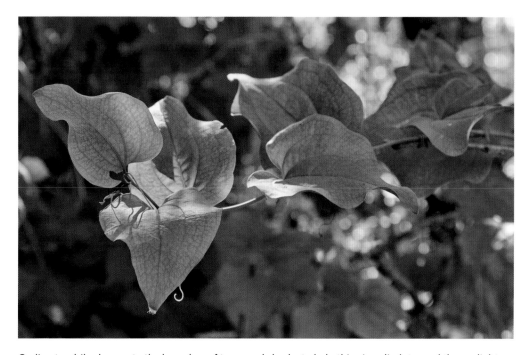

Curling tendrils clasp onto the branches of trees and shrubs to help this vine climb toward the sunlight.

How to Identify

Dense, woody-barked, and ridged rhizomes, segmented and with somewhat fleshy nodular growths, run through sandy soil to form thickets of prickly green stems that extend 6–16 feet from a short woody base to climb into neighboring trees or shrubs or to trail along the ground. Alternately arranged, oval to heart-shaped, evergreen leaves, dull green and hairless, unfurl pointy-tipped, 2–4 inches long, and strongly parallel-veined. Dangling in many-flowered clusters from the leaf axils, male and female flowers bloom on separate plants from late spring to early summer. The greenish flowers are made up of 6 reflexed tepals (the name given to the outer parts of a flower when the sepals and petals are indistinguishable). Each tepal is much longer than it is wide. Female flowers produce fleshy, black, round to ovoid, 3-seeded berries. The vining stems attach themselves via tendrils,

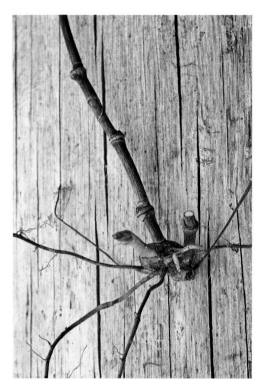

California greenbrier roots are male reproductive tonics. Note the doctrine of signature correspondence related to this root's form.

relieve impotence, reduce prostate swelling, or to increase fertility by supporting the thickening of the uterine lining after ovulation. Before and during menstruation these preparations reduce pain and swelling in the breasts and moderate mood swings, and they regulate the production of sexual hormones to ease periods of hormonal transition such as puberty or menopause.

The tea or tincture of the root promotes urination and helps the liver break down unprocessed hormonal waste products that can lead to chronic eruptive skin conditions or inflammation, pain, and stiffness of the muscles and joints.

Future Harvests

Take only a small portion of root from each plant for medicine. Divide roots while harvesting, and transplant pieces with at least two nodes in the area where you are harvesting to expand the colony or to another location with wet sandy soil to establish a new one.

are armed with up to ½-inch-long flexible prickles, and lack a central pith.

Where, When, and How to Wildcraft

Residing in seeps or along the banks of slow-moving streams and rivers from southwestern Oregon to northwestern California, this perennial vine can be found growing in open to partially shaded coniferous forests at low to middle elevations. Dig the roots from late summer to early autumn.

Medicinal Uses

California greenbrier root nourishes the adrenals and reproductive system. Take the tea or tincture to revive interest in sex,

---

HERBAL PREPARATIONS

Root Tea
Cold infusion or standard decoction
Drink 2–4 fluid ounces up to 3 times per day.

Root Tincture
1 part fresh root
2 parts menstruum (75 percent alcohol, 25 percent distilled water)
or
1 part dried root
5 parts menstruum (50 percent alcohol, 50 percent distilled water)
Take 30–60 drops up to 3 times per day.

California mugwort

Artemisia douglasiana
Douglas mugwort, Douglas' sagewort
PARTS USED leaf, flower

Aromatic and bitter leaves increase the digestibility of fats, reduce inflammation in the digestive system, and stimulate dreaming. Flowers make a potent antifungal oil.

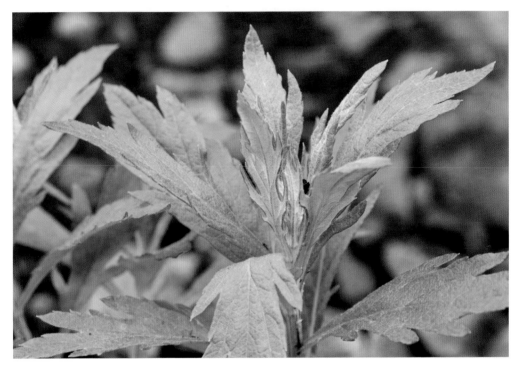

California mugwort's wooly-haired leaves stimulate dreaming.

How to Identify

In spring, ridged stems emerge from perennial, colony-forming rhizomes and extend upward 1½ to 5 feet tall. Green to grayish green, very aromatic, elliptic to lance-shaped leaves, 2¾ to 6 inches long, alternate up the stalks with white-wooly undersides. Sometimes smooth-edged, the leaves may develop lobes and coarse teeth that give them a shape somewhat like the flames you might see painted on the side of a hot rod. Drooping clusters of composite, disk-like flower heads with tubular, pale yellow flowers bloom from late summer to early autumn on leafy stalks atop the stem or in the leaf axils below. The outer 6–10 flowers bear female parts only; the inner 10–25 are hermaphroditic. Pollinated flowers produce dry naked seeds lacking a crown of feathery hairs. Pay close attention when identifying mugworts;

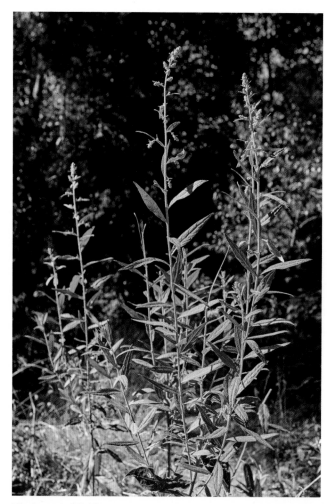

The leaves of California mugwort can be smooth edged (like this one), toothed, or lobed.

Artemisia is a very large genus and sometimes difficult to discern at the species level, and not all *Artemisia* species have similar medicinal properties.

Where, When, and How to Wildcraft

Growing along stream banks and in river flood plains throughout the western United States, California mugwort is found mainly east of the Cascades in Washington, on the western side of the Cascade Crest in Oregon, and south into California. It is listed as extirpated in British Columbia, where it is no longer found in the wild.

While the plant is in flower, harvest whole stalks (four or five per clump). Snip at the base and discard brown or damaged leaves. Bundle and hang to dry out of direct sunlight. After the herb is fully dried, remove the leaves and flowers separately. Reserve the flowers for oil and use the leaves for tea or tincture.

Medicinal Uses

For those with difficulty digesting fats and oils, as indicated by excessive cravings for fatty foods, dry skin, floating stools, and/or post-meal headaches, the cold infusion or tincture of the aromatic and bitter leaves increases the body's ability to properly break down and assimilate fats and prevents the fat molecules from being dumped into the bloodstream where they may cause the aforementioned health issues. The cold infusion before bed or the tincture before meals helps reduce inflammation throughout the digestive system. Take either preparation for stomach ulcers, to mitigate the effect of inflammatory bowel disease, and for stomach inflammation with nausea, bloating, indigestion, a burning sensation in the stomach, and/or loss of appetite.

The leaf tea drunk hot encourages sweating to break a fever and acts as a warming menstrual stimulant to relieve cold uterine cramping.

Associated with the moon, the leaves hung above the bed, placed under the pillow, or ingested as tea, tincture, or smoke promote vivid dreams and help uncover, access, and transform areas of psychic unconsciousness. The flower oil rubbed on the middle of the forehead works the same and also possesses antifungal properties.

Apply the flower oil or a wash of the leaves topically to red itchy areas affected by ringworm, athlete's foot, jock itch, and other fungal infections of the skin. Smoke the leaves alone or mixed with other herbs for their mentally stimulating effect. The wadded leaves rubbed between the palms fluff up to make an excellent slow burning smudge to clear negative energies from a space. Burned on or near the skin as moxa, the fluffed leaves dissolve energetic blockages in the meridians.

 Caution

Preparations of California mugwort stimulate the uterus, so don't use them during pregnancy.

Future Harvests

Divide the spreading rhizomes to create new colonies by digging up a portion of the root system, removing the aboveground portions, and breaking the roots into smaller chunks before replanting. Be sure that each chunk you plant has at least one new-growth bud.

HERBAL PREPARATIONS

Leaf Tea
Cold or hot infusion
Drink 2–3 fluid ounces up to 3 times per day.

Leaf Tincture
1 part dried leaf
5 parts menstruum (50 percent alcohol, 50 percent distilled water)
Take 20–45 drops up to 3 times per day.

Flower Oil
Follow directions for Dry Herb Infused Oil or Alternative Oil Method (page 64).

California poppy

Eschscholzia californica

PARTS USED whole plant

All parts of this alkaloid-rich plant calm and sedate the nervous system to relieve anxiety, insomnia, and pain.

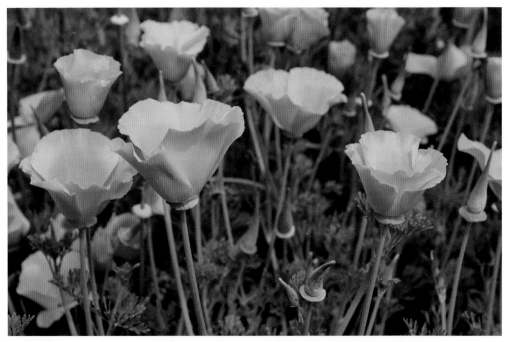

The first European scientific expeditions arriving on the Pacific coast witnessed the native peoples using California poppy and learned about its medicinal properties from them.

How to Identify

From opaque, orange taproots, many times divided, bluish green basal leaves splay out, terminating in narrow linear segments. Sitting atop 6- to 16-inch-long stalks rising directly from the root crown, single, pale yellow to orange flowers unfurl from slightly curved, conical, and pointy buds. A pair of sepals forms a wizard-hat-shaped enclosure that is shed as 4 egg-shaped petals emerge, luminous-sheened and wedge-shaped at the base. Rimmed receptacles (the thickened parts of a stem upon which the flower parts grow) extend outward and cup the bases of the saucer-shaped, many-stamened flowers. Brown to black, round to ellipsoid seeds ripen in 1¼- to 3½-inch-long, narrow, and strongly ridged capsules. Alternately arranged stem leaves, similar in shape to the basal leaves, become smaller as they ascend the stalk. These annual or perennial plants are hairless, sometimes waxy-coated, and all parts exude a clear sap when crushed or cut. The flowers bloom from late spring to early autumn.

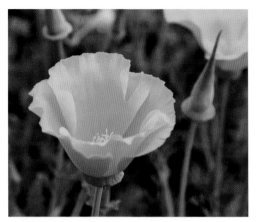

Alkaloid-rich California poppy is much gentler in action than its cousin, the opium poppy, and it does not depress the central nervous system in the same way.

Where, When, and How to Wildcraft

California poppy prefers open sunny locations and sites with dry, rocky soil: roadsides, grasslands, and waste places. Find it at lower elevations on both sides of the Cascade Mountains from southern British Columbia to California. Harvest the whole plant when in flower and, preferably, when immature seed pods are present.

Medicinal Uses

Even though California poppy contains opiate-like alkaloids, it is gentle acting and suitable for use with children and the elderly. Take or administer the whole-plant tincture to calm overstimulated, irritable, and inconsolable children of all ages, to soothe frazzled nerves, or to relieve anxiety. Take the tincture before bed if you wake in the morning feeling unrested, as it will smooth out nervous system static and deepen your sleep. Keep a bottle of tincture by the bed in case you wake in the middle of the night or too early in the morning with your mind spinning.

The whole-plant tincture or a more potent root-only preparation relaxes muscle spasms, both skeletal and smooth, and relieves the pain of headaches, toothaches, and menstrual cramps. Mix the tincture with honey or use a glycerin tincture (known as a glycerite) if your child dislikes the taste of this bitter, strongly flavored medicine.

⚠ Caution

Do not use during pregnancy or with pharmaceutical medications. California poppy alkaloids in your urine may trigger a false positive result for opiate-screening drug tests.

Future Harvests

California poppies readily self-seed. Harvest just a few plants from each abundant stand to ensure that ample seed is deposited for the yearly successional cycle to continue. Leaving many plants also maintains the genetic diversity of a stand and allows them to thrive for many generations.

HERBAL PREPARATIONS

Whole Plant Tea
Standard infusion
Drink 2–4 fluid ounces 4 times per day.

Root or Whole Plant Tincture
1 part fresh root or whole plant
2 parts menstruum (75 percent alcohol,
  25 percent distilled water)
Take 20–60 drops up to 4 times per day.

Glycerin Tincture
1 part fresh root or whole plant
2 parts menstruum (100 percent glycerin)
*Take 40–120 drops up to 4 times per day,
10–30 drops for children*

Cascade Oregon grape

Berberis nervosa
Cascade barberry, dwarf or dull Oregon grape
PARTS USED root

This spiny-leaved plant spreads through the forest via rhizomes that speed the healing of intestinal infections, improve liver and digestive function, and clear itchy skin conditions.

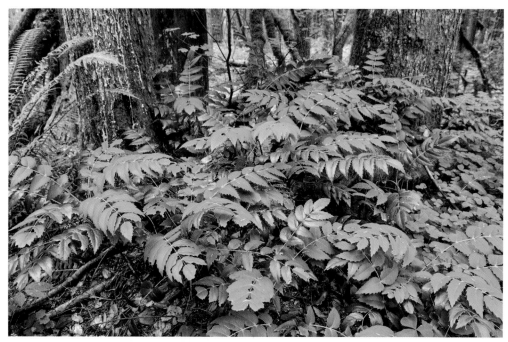

Cascade Oregon grape often forms dense stands in the forest understory.

How to Identify

Stems, whose tops are lined with persistent, pointy-tipped bud scales, ascend to a height of 4–24 inches from woody rhizomes that spread laterally just under the surface of the soil. Tufts of alternately arranged, pinnately compound leaves made up of 9–19 thick, dark green, oval to lance-shaped, holly-like leaflets with spiny, coarsely saw-tooth edges top the woody stems. Leaflets are dull-surfaced above and below and borne on long, wiry stalks. Bracted, yellow-flowered clusters up to 8 inches long sit above the leaves. Three greenish yellow outer bracts, 6 bright yellow sepals, and 6 bright yellow, 2-lobed petals alternate in 5 whorls of 3 to make up flowers that bloom from early spring to early summer and ripen into purplish blue, blush-covered, sour-tasting berries containing large black seeds. The inner bark of the rhizomes is deep orange-yellow, the wood is yellowish, and the evergreen leaves turn orange to reddish in autumn.

The Pacific Northwest is home to two other species of Oregon grape, both of which have the same medicinal properties as Cascade Oregon grape. Shining Oregon grape, *Berberis aquifolium*, has 5–9 shiny-topped leaflets, grows up to 4 feet tall, and prefers open areas. Trailing Oregon grape, *B. repens*, maxes out at 8 inches and has 5–7 dull-surfaced, egg-shaped leaflets.

Where, When, and How to Wildcraft

This shade-tolerant plant (formerly *Mahonia nervosa*) often forms dense stands in mixed evergreen forests west of the Cascades from southern British Columbia to central California. It prefers open to semi-open forests from sea level to middle elevations.

Collect rhizomes from mid spring to mid autumn. From a good-sized stand, find a non-flowering plant that calls out to you. Grasp its stem and give a gentle tug. If the rhizome moves easily, continue pulling and follow it until the rhizome breaks or until you reach a junction point where you can cut the rhizome free. Remove the leaves and replant the crown. Cut the rhizomes into ½- to 1-inch-long pieces to dry for tea or for making a dry root tincture. For a fresh root tincture, cut them into ¼-inch-long pieces before adding to the menstruum. Process the rhizomes as soon as possible, as they become increasingly hard and difficult to cut as they dry.

Medicinal Uses

Bitter, earthy, and slightly sweet, Cascade Oregon grape root, which gets its yellow color from the alkaloid berberine, speeds the healing of intestinal infections and acts mainly on the liver, skin, and digestion. Although berberine is known to be a potent antibiotic alkaloid, it is best to think of Cascade Oregon grape's antimicrobial action this way: it alters the internal mucosa and speeds

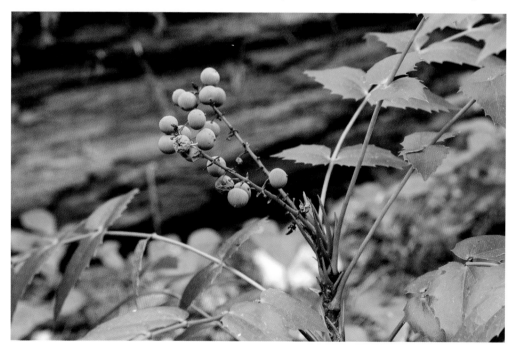

Oregon grape gets its name from these edible, blush-covered berries.

the removal of waste products in the blood to make the terrain less hospitable to infectious agents.

Take Oregon grape root tea or tincture for giardia, staph, or salmonella infections. These preparations also stimulate liver metabolism, cleanse the blood, and clear damp heat. Take them if you have food sensitives or allergies, are prone to constipation, wake up feeling groggy and listless in the morning, have bad breath with a coated tongue, and/or have chronic itchy skin conditions.

Skin conditions are often related to liver congestion or impaired hepatic function; if the liver cannot adequately filter toxins and other impurities from the blood, the unprocessed waste products are eliminated through the skin. Cascade Oregon grape root remedies dry itchy skin conditions like psoriasis as well as red, inflamed skin eruptions like acne and eczema and fungal outbreaks such as athlete's foot, ringworm, and jock itch that result from systemic damp heat. In addition to taking preparations of Oregon grape, eliminate sweets, stimulants, and alcohol from the diet, as consuming them worsens conditions of damp heat.

When taken before meals, the tincture acts as a bitter tonic that stimulates the digestive juices. This improves the body's ability to break down food, especially fats and oils, and maximizes the assimilation of nutrients.

Future Harvests

Harvest from large, healthy stands and replant the crowns. Cut off all of the leaves before replanting and make sure to include a portion of the rhizome with small rootlets attached.

HERBAL PREPARATIONS

Root Tea
Standard decoction
Drink 6–8 fluid ounces 3 times per day.

Root Tincture
1 part fresh root
2 parts menstruum (75 percent alcohol, 25 percent distilled water)
or
1 part dried root
5 parts menstruum (50 percent alcohol, 50 percent distilled water)
As a bitter tonic, take 15–20 drops 10–15 minutes before meals; as a liver stimulant, take 15–45 drops 3 times per day.

cascara sagrada

Frangula purshiana
cascara buckthorn, chittum bark
PARTS USED aged bark

Bitter bark strengthens the colon, relieves constipation, and improves digestion.

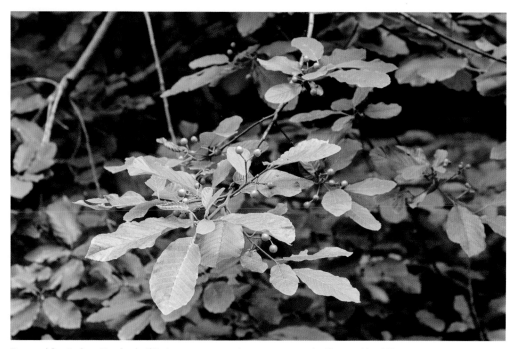

Revered for its laxative bark, this tree was named cascara sagrada ("sacred bark") by Spanish missionaries.

How to Identify

Mottled grayish white bark covers a thin layer of yellowish brown inner bark. Nascent leaves, brownish and fuzzy, lacking scales to protect them through winter expand in spring to form green, 3- to 5-inch-long, oblong leaves. Ten to 12 prominent veins radiate out directly opposite each other from along the midrib of the alternately arranged leaves. Greenish white, star-shaped, 5-petalled flowers produce purplish black, 3-seeded berries.

Where, When, and How to Wildcraft

This shade-tolerant tree (formerly *Rhamnus purshiana*) grows up to 35 feet tall in the understory or along the edges of wet forests at low to middle elevations west of the Cascades from southern British Columbia to northern California. It can also be found further inland in wetter places as far east as Idaho and Montana.

Remove thumb-sized or larger branches in spring when the sap is running. The bark will peel more easily if you strip it soon after

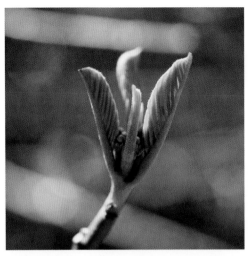

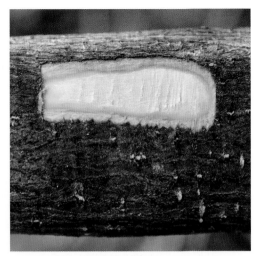

Easy to identify in winter, cascara sagrada is the only Northwest tree with naked buds.

The yellowish brown inner bark tastes quite bitter.

harvesting. Wear gloves if you are handling large quantities of bark, as the constituents responsible for its laxative effect can be absorbed through the skin. Dry the stripped bark in bags or on screens; once it is fully dry, place it in a burlap sack or paper bag and let it sit for at least 1 year before making medicine. Fresh or recently dried bark is too potent and can cause intense intestinal upset.

Medicinal Uses

Bitter constituents in the bark known as anthroquinone glycosides strengthen the bowels and increase peristalsis in the colon to relieve acute or chronic constipation. Take the aged bark tincture before going to bed. It usually takes about 8 hours to move the bowels. You can take larger doses, up to 60 drops, but smaller doses will tonify and support the normal action of the colon, whereas larger doses will force an action in the body that, especially for the aged and ill, may weaken the bowels. Combine cascara sagrada with carminative herbs like sweetroot or angelica root or seed to ease the stimulating effect of the bark.

Take small doses of the bark tincture 10–15 minutes before meals to stimulate digestion or mix it into formulas to support the body's eliminative function.

Some people with chronic constipation have trouble letting go of emotional issues and can be tightly wound up. Cascara can also help bring about a cathartic release for people who find themselves stuck in this way.

Caution

Age the bark for at least 1 year before making medicine. Ingesting the fresh bark will lead to intestinal griping. I've tried it. It's not fun unless you enjoy having your guts wrung out with intense cramping, gurgling gas, and diarrhea followed by the lower intestinal equivalent of dry heaves.

This plant should not be used during pregnancy. Some women report the onset of out-of-cycle menstruation when ingesting very small quantities of the fresh bark. A tolerance can be built up with frequent and continued use.

Cascara Sagrada: A Sad Story with a Happy Ending

Before World War II cascara sagrada, which only grows in this region, was the main laxative plant in the United States. Large quantities of the highly sought after bark were harvested each year from Pacific Northwest forests. The standard practice was to remove all of the bark from a standing tree. This unsustainable approach made it easier to harvest large quantities of bark but led to the death of the trees. The once-plentiful trees became increasingly scarce. A more sustainable approach, based on an understanding of the growth habit of trees, would have been to cut the trees down before stripping the bark so that they could resprout from the base.

In the end it was the pharmaceutical revolution that spared this precious tree. The arrival of new synthetic laxatives lowered the demand for botanical medicines like cascara sagrada. Today cascara sagrada trees are popping up everywhere, thanks to the birds who consume the berries and spread their seeds far and wide.

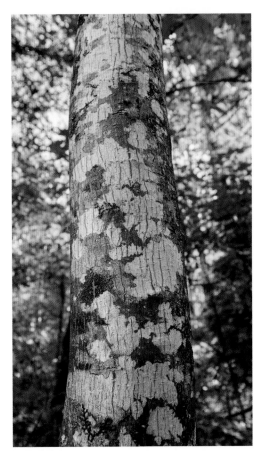

Cascara sagrada bark is the Pacific Northwest's strongest and most reliable laxative.

Future Harvests

Most people will only need a handful of decent sized branches to make a year's supply of medicine for friends and family. As you walk through the forest, look for cascara sagrada trees with broken but still-living branches to harvest. Otherwise, harvest crossing branches, which often lose bark as the branches rub against each other, and branches growing into the center, which eventually die for lack of light. Consider the artful pruning of such branches a mutually beneficial harvest that improves the health of the tree.

HERBAL PREPARATIONS

Aged Bark Tincture
1 part dried aged bark
5 parts menstruum (50 percent alcohol, 50 percent distilled water)
Take 10–20 drops before bed as a laxative or 1–5 drops up to 3 times per day as a bitter tonic.

chickweed

Stellaria media
PARTS USED herb

This small, ground-hugging plant cools and soothes hot inflamed tissues, dissolves cysts and fatty deposits, and increases the body's ability to receive nourishment.

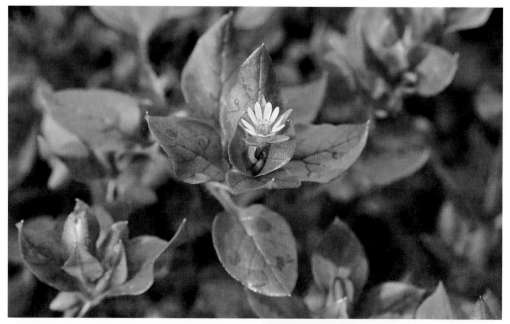

Often overlooked, this humble, star-flowered annual is fragile yet tenacious.

How to Identify

Held loosely in the soil by a slender taproot, succulent, fragile, 3- to 15-inch-long stems trail lightly across the ground to form dense mats. A line of hairs alternates from one side of the stem to the other between the nodes of oppositely arranged, evenly spaced leaves. Oval-shaped, smooth-edged, and flat, the leaves are sometimes hairy at the base, and each of the 5 white petals is deeply cleft to the base. Together the petals are cupped by a 5-sepalled, star-shaped calyx.

Where, When, and How to Wildcraft

Originally from Europe, this sometimes overwintering, small, prostrate annual can be found throughout this region and all over North America in woodlands, gardens, meadows, and disturbed areas. Chickweed prefers cool weather, moist and shady places, and rich soil.

Harvest the aerial parts—leaf, stem, and flower—year-round before the plants set seed. Chickweed grows under the cover of snow, but in the heat of summer you'll have to search for it in wet, shady spots.

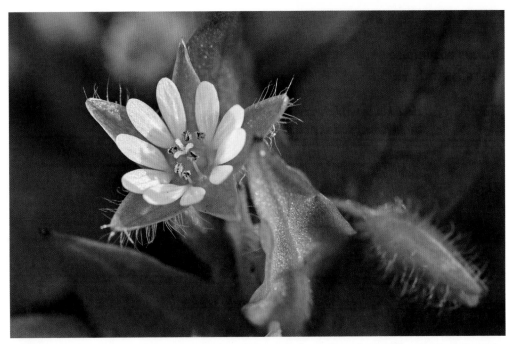

At first glance there appear to be ten petals, but chickweed's flower is made up of five deeply cleft petals.

Medicinal Uses

Chickweed herb is cooling and moistening. Ingest it as a food, take the tea or tincture, apply the infused oil, or make a poultice to relieve skin inflammations and rashes or to soothe dry, red, itchy skin conditions such as eczema. A poultice of the fresh plant draws out infections, and a wash of the fresh herb tea speeds the healing of pink eye. The saponins in chickweed dissolve cysts and fatty deposits and increase cellular membrane permeability, allowing the body to receive nourishment and rid itself of wastes more easily.

Future Harvests

Sow seeds in rich, moist soil in the shade.

HERBAL PREPARATIONS

Herb Tea
Standard infusion of the fresh or very recently dried herb (no older than 2-3 months)
Drink 4-6 fluid ounces up to 5 times per day.

Herb Tincture
1 part fresh herb
2 parts menstruum (50 percent alcohol, 50 percent distilled water)
Macerate no more than a week to retain the taste of the fresh plant. The tincture lasts longer with a higher percentage of alcohol, but the flavor of this delicate plant is lost. Take 30-60 drops up to 5 times per day.

Herb Oil
Follow directions for Fresh Herb Infused Oil on page 63.

chokecherry

Prunus virginiana
PARTS USED bark

Chokecherry, a close kin to wild cherry, is a cooling sedative that relieves spasmodic coughs, stimulates appetite, and reduces gastric irritability.

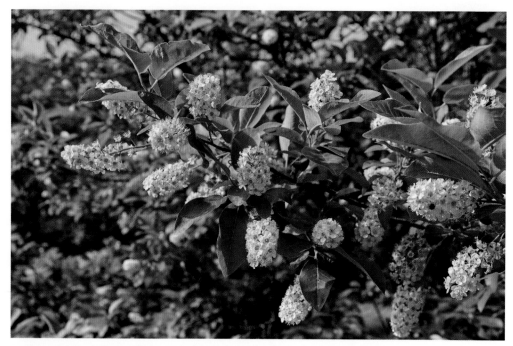
Bottlebrush-like clusters of flowers produce tart, edible fruits.

How to Identify
Many slender, reddish to grayish brown, smooth-barked stems, branching at the base or upright and spreading, rise up from a network of sucker-forming rhizomes. Finely serrated leaves, 1–4 inches long and oval to egg-shaped with a usually sharp-pointed tip, unfold bright green and smooth above and paler and smooth to slightly hairy below. The leaf stalks have 1 or 2 glands near the top. Long, multi-flowered terminal clusters bloom like bottlebrushes from late spring to mid summer. The 5-petalled, creamy white flowers ripen into fleshy, red, purple, or black 1-seeded fruits. These edible, ½-inch-long, stone-filled cherries are tart and astringent. The young twigs of this thicket-forming, deciduous shrub are usually hairy, and the outer bark does not easily peel as in other *Prunus* species. Chokecherry sometimes grows as a small tree and ranges in height from 3 to 20 feet tall.

Where, When, and How to Wildcraft
This shade-intolerant shrub prefers the wetter areas of dry landscapes. Find it growing along

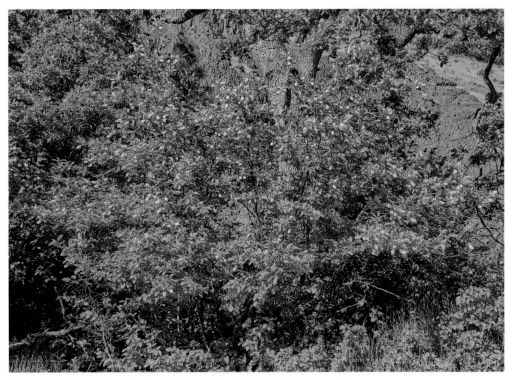

Chokecherry forms shrubby thickets throughout the Pacific Northwest.

stream banks and in forest clearings, canyons, and wooded ravines and gullies at low to middle elevations throughout this region.

Cut thumb-sized or larger stems and branches in spring after the leaves have emerged, and strip the bark promptly for drying. Good, quality medicine will be strongly almond-scented.

Medicinal Uses

The tincture, cold infusion, or syrup of chokecherry bark is a cooling sedative for the cardiac and respiratory systems. It is best indicated for persistent and spasmodic irritating coughs with rapid pulse and breathing or for fevers with large, daily spikes in temperature known as hectic fevers. Take the tea or tincture to stimulate the appetite or reduce gastric irritability.

Future Harvests

Take only a few branches or stems from each shrub to minimize your impact.

HERBAL PREPARATIONS

Bark Tea
Cold infusion (decocting will drive the hydrocyanic acid, which gives the medicine its cooling and sedative qualities, from the bark)
Drink 2–4 fluid ounces up to 3 times per day.

Bark Tincture
1 part dried bark
5 parts menstruum (50 percent alcohol, 50 percent distilled water)
Take 30–60 drops up to 5 times per day.

cleavers

Galium aparine
goose grass, stickywilly
PARTS USED herb

*Cleavers herb cools and clears the lymphatic system and reduces pain and
inflammation in the urinary tract.*

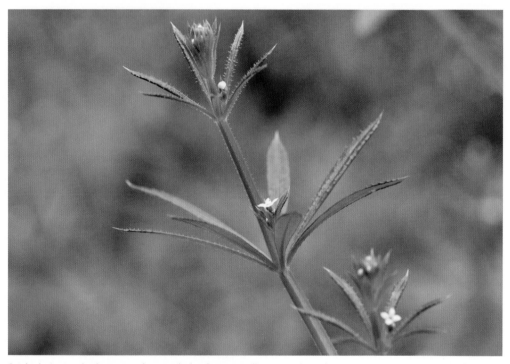

Sticky hairs on the leaves and stems help cleavers adhere to other plants to support its upward growth.

How to Identify

From a shallow, branching taproot, weak
and sprawling square stems climb upward
using hooked hairs to attach themselves to
other plants. Linear leaves, ½ to 3 inches
long, with sharp points at their rounded ends
are arranged in whorls of 6–8. Branchlets
attached to the leaf joints hold 3–5 whitish
to greenish flowers. Each ripens into a pair of
small seeds covered in sticky, hooked hairs.
When cleavers has nothing to climb on, it
forms a short, ground-hugging mat. The
stems and seeds cling to clothing and animal
fur to aid in dispersal.

Where, When, and How to Wildcraft

Find this sprawling annual in gardens, disturbed lands, and forest clearings. It grows
in moist, shady places from low to middle
elevations throughout this region.

Harvest while in flower by gently disen-
tangling it from the plant or plants that it

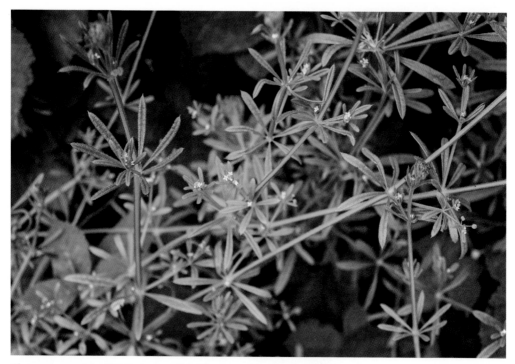
Cleavers sprawls until it finds something to support its climbing habit.

is trellised upon. If drying for tea, loosely wad the herb and dry it in a bag or lay it on a screen.

Medicinal Uses

Cleavers herb tea or tincture reduces heat in the lymphatic system and clears obstructions in swollen glands. It is especially indicated when there is heat with rashes, eczema, or psoriasis.

The tea or tincture has a diuretic effect that promotes urination and helps clear deposits from the bladder and kidneys. These same preparations soothe soreness and inflammation in the bladder and urethra, relieve infections of the urinary tract, and are particularly useful in clearing obstructions that lead to painful urination.

Roast the caffeine-containing seeds for use as a coffee substitute.

Future Harvests

Cleavers is self-sufficient in sowing its seed. You'd be hard pressed to get rid of it even if you tried, but leave some to set seed to ensure that there will be a continuous and abundant supply of medicine.

HERBAL PREPARATIONS

Herb Tea
Standard infusion
Drink 4–6 fluid ounces up to 5 times per day.

Herb Tincture
1 part fresh herb
2 parts menstruum (75 percent alcohol, 25 percent distilled water)
Press after 1 week to retain the fresh plant's taste.
Take 30–60 drops up to 5 times per day.

coastal hedgenettle

Stachys chamissonis var. *cooleyae*
Cooley's hedgenettle, great hedgenettle, woundwort
PARTS USED herb, root

Fuzzy leaves relieve headaches, lessen inflammation, and stop bleeding.

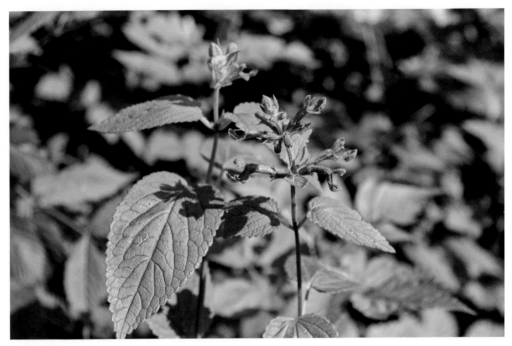

Vibrant flowers, sweet with nectar, are a favorite of hummingbirds.

How to Identify

Square, mostly unbranched, bristly-edged stems stand erect 25–60 inches from creeping rhizomes. Aromatic, long-stalked, oppositely arranged leaves, 2½ to 6 inches long, triangular to egg-shaped, coarsely blunt-toothed, and hairy above and below, grow somewhat smaller and shorter-stalked as they ascend the stem. From early to late summer, deep red to magenta, tubular, 2-lipped flowers, 1–2 inches long and hairy, bloom in bracted whorls from the upper leaf axils. The flower's hood-like upper lip wraps around the 4 stamens, and the often white-spotted lower lip spreads 3-lobed. Clusters of 4 nutlets mature in persistent 5-lobed calyces tipped with spiny teeth. The smell of the leaves, pleasant to some, is distasteful to others.

Where, When, and How to Wildcraft

Growing mainly west of the Cascade Crest in Oregon and Washington, this perennial mint (formerly *Stachys cooleyae*) makes its home in wet, sunny locations at low to middle elevations from Alaska to California. Find coastal hedgenettle in meadowy areas, below seeps, along streams and roadsides, and in forest margins and clearings.

Gather the aboveground portions while in flower. Process fresh for tincture or hang in bundles to dry for tea.

Medicinal Uses

Take the tea or tincture to relieve headaches or to reduce urinary tract and joint inflammation. Gargle the tea or diluted tincture for sore throats. Externally a compress or poultice of the leaves stanches bleeding, speeds the healing of wounds, reduces pain and swelling from sprains, and soothes headache pain. Out in the field use the pounded roots for the same.

Future Harvests

Sow seeds or divide the roots in spring to create new colonies of this beautiful, hummingbird-attracting plant.

HERBAL PREPARATIONS

Herb Tea
Standard infusion
Drink 4–6 fluid ounces up to 5 times per day.

Herb Tincture
1 part fresh herb
2 parts menstruum (75 percent alcohol,
    25 percent distilled water)
or
1 part dried herb
5 parts menstruum (50 percent alcohol,
    50 percent distilled water)
Take 30–90 drops up to 4 times per day.

comfrey

Symphytum officinale
knitbone
PARTS USED leaf, root

Soothing, moistening leaves and roots speed the healing of broken bones, seal wounds, and reduce swelling and bruising.

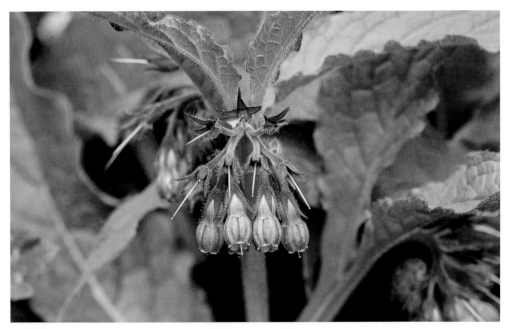

The thread-like styles persist after the petals fall.

How to Identify

Thick and branching, dark-skinned and white-fleshed taproots spread to form dense colonies of bristly haired plants. Deeply veined, oblong to oval-shaped, smooth-edged basal leaves grow 6–12 inches long. Alternately arranged stem leaves become gradually smaller and stalkless as they climb, taper to long-pointed tips, and from their bases form ridges that run down the stems. Bractless flowering clusters uncoil at the branch tips bearing several to many yellowish white to dull blue to purplish, bell-shaped, drooping flowers that bloom from late spring to mid summer. Five hairy lobes with backward-bending tips crown each fused tube of petals. The tubular corolla falls after pollination, leaving a protruding, thread-like style (the female reproductive stalk that extends from the ovary). Four shiny, brownish black nutlets mature attached to the base of the 5-lobed calyx.

The closely related prickly comfrey (*Symphytum asperum*), which lacks ridges on the stem, has the same medicinal properties as *S. officinale*.

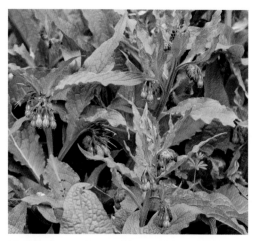
Vigorously growing comfrey spreads quickly in gardens and disturbed areas.

Where, When, and How to Wildcraft

Introduced from Europe, this garden escapee is found throughout much of North America in disturbed areas, pastures, and gardens. Although comfrey is uncommon in southern British Columbia, you will find it at low to middle elevations west of the Cascades in Washington and northwestern Oregon. Harvest the roots and leaves throughout the growing season.

Medicinal Uses

Filled with sticky mucilage, comfrey root and leaf contain allantoin, a compound that stimulates cell growth and helps repair damaged tissues. Use a poultice of the leaf or root to speed the healing of abraded skin, broken bones, injured tendons and ligaments, or to repair damaged cartilage. A poultice also soothes the pain and reduces inflammation and bruising from blunt force traumas.

A poultice or salve seals gaping wounds as it literally knits the skin back together, but be aware that comfrey heals wounds from top to bottom. If the wound isn't cleaned well, it may become infected. Before applying comfrey be sure to cleanse and disinfect the wound site or consider using yarrow or Saint John's wort, which heals wounds from the bottom up.

⚠ Caution

Because comfrey root and leaf work so quickly, fractured bones must be set immediately, or they may heal poorly. Comfrey may also cause tissue overgrowth if used excessively, resulting in lumps or calluses at the site of the break.

Although people have been using comfrey internally for centuries without noticing any adverse effects, recent evidence shows that ingesting comfrey root or leaf preparations may have serious consequences. Comfrey roots and leaves contain pyrrolizidine alkaloids that are known to cause a severe and life-threatening disorder known as hepatic veno-occlusive disease, the lethal effects of which are not noticeable unless an autopsy is performed. Based on our current understanding of the dangers, comfrey should not be used internally at all.

Future Harvests

Once comfrey has been established, it will never go away. Even the tiniest bit of root will sprout and form a new plant.

HERBAL PREPARATIONS

Root or Leaf Oil and Salve
For root or leaf oil, follow directions for Dry Herb Infused Oil on page 64. For the salve, follow directions on page 65.

---

common mallow

Malva neglecta
cheeseweed
PARTS USED root, leaf, fruit

*Soothing and cooling, all parts of this plant reduce inflammation,
soothe irritated tissues, and benefit sore throats.*

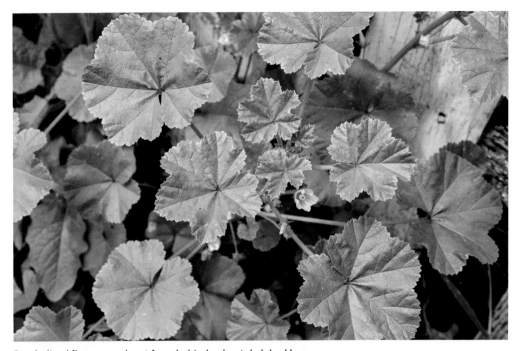

Purple-lined flowers peek out from behind palmately lobed leaves.

How to Identify

From taproots branching stems spread
to form ground-covering mats. Scalloped
edges and 5 or more shallow lobes line the
periphery of 2- to 3-inch-diameter, round
to kidney-shaped, alternately arranged, and
long-stalked leaves. During the summer
months stalks along the stems produce 1–3
white to pinkish purple flowers. Each of the
5 petals is slightly notched and often has
pale purple lines running along its length.
Many stamens fuse around the pistil. The
distinctive round and flattened fruits look
like miniature cheese wheels held in green,
5-sepalled wrappers.

Where, When, and How to Wildcraft

This spreading annual, originally from
Europe, grows in gardens, in disturbed soils,
along roadsides, and from cracks in the sidewalk throughout this region and across most
of North America. Harvest the whole plant
or individual parts from late spring to early
autumn.

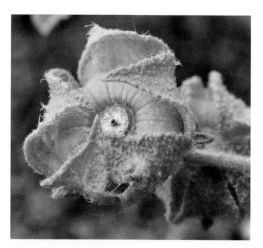

This relative of marshmallow is easily recognized by its cheese-wheel-shaped fruits.

Medicinal Uses

All parts of the plant contain a soothing mucilage, a thick, gelatinous substance produced by plants that aids in water storage. Steep the chopped fresh plant or dried herb overnight in cold water to extract its soothing and moistening properties. Use externally for bug bites, burns, stings, and other skin inflammations and internally for upset stomach, urinary tract irritation, constipation, and lung inflammation. Its slight astringency makes common mallow particularly useful for sore throats.

Ingesting the plant as a food will also impart its medicinal benefit. The young leaves and flowers of this common edible make a great addition to salads. Older leaves, roots, and the cheese-wheel fruits can be added to soups and stews.

Future Harvests

Sow seeds in disturbed ground to ensure a yearly harvest.

HERBAL PREPARATIONS

Root, Leaf, or Fruit Tea
Cold infusion
Drink 4–6 fluid ounces up to 5 times per day.

cow parsnip

Heracleum maximum

common cowparsnip

PARTS USED seed, root

Oily aromatic roots reduce digestive upset, clear mucus from the lungs, and may reverse the effects of nerve damage. Pungent seeds do much of the same and bring numbing relief to painful toothaches.

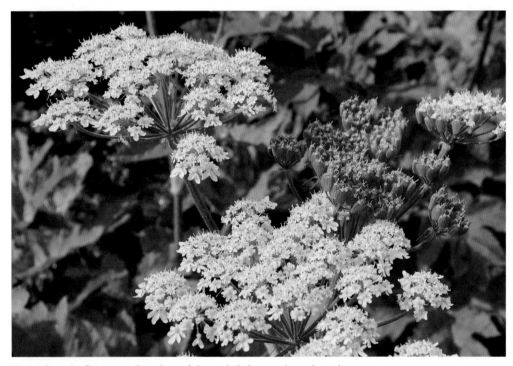

Notice how the flowers at the edges of the umbels have enlarged petals.

How to Identify

Irregularly toothed and growing up to 12 inches long with thinly hairy undersides, large leaves with hairy, 4- to 16-inch, widely sheathing stalks divide into 3 distinct, egg-shaped to roundish leaflets that in turn may become 3-lobed. Broad, flat-topped flowering heads sit atop 3- to 10-foot-tall erect, hollow, strongly ridged, and usually branching stalks that arise from clusters of fibrous roots or from fleshy taproots. Blooming from late spring to early summer, each compound flower head, growing up to 10 inches wide, comprises many white, male or hermaphroditic flowers that are grouped into 15–30 umbels borne on stalks, known as rays, that grow up to 4 inches long. Five to 10 narrow, deciduous bracts extend from beneath each terminal umbel, and flowers along the outer rim of the flower head have enlarged and irregularly shaped outward-facing petals. Flattened and winged seeds, egg- to heart-shaped, hairless to slightly hairy, and ¼ to ½ inch long, narrow toward the base with reddish brown stripes descending from the top as they mature during the summer months. The entire plant is highly aromatic and covered with long hairs, and 1–4 secondary umbels may sprout from side shoots on the flowering stalk.

Do not confuse cow parsnip with its introduced relative giant hogweed, *Heracleum mantegazzianum*. Oils in this plant can elicit a very strong reaction that causes intense blistering and scarring of the skin. It is a much larger plant than cow parsnip, from 5 to 15 feet tall, and has 50–150 umbel rays and seeds that are blunt and rounded toward the base.

Where, When, and How to Wildcraft

Widely distributed throughout North America, this single-stemmed native perennial (formerly *Heracleum lanatum*) prefers moist areas at low to high elevations on both sides of the Cascades. It grows in grasslands, meadows, open woodlands, disturbed areas, and riparian zones across the Pacific Northwest.

Collect cow parsnip seeds from mid to late summer as the seed bodies begin to turn from green to brown and the reddish brown markings darken. Immature green seeds are overly sharp and pungent, and brown dried out seeds will have lost their aromatics. When harvested at their peak, the flavor of the chewed seeds is roundly pungent and feels expansive and opening. To kill insect eggs or larvae that will eat up your harvest when they mature, place well-contained seeds in the freezer for 2 weeks. Harvest the roots from late summer to mid autumn after the leaves begin to die back.

Medicinal Uses

The seeds and preparations of the dried root reduce spasms in the digestive tract; relieve gas, bloating, and nausea; and expel mucus from the lungs. The seed tincture, applied either directly or on a piece of gauze or cotton, numbs and relieves the pain of a toothache. Because of its nerve irritating and stimulating properties, the fresh root tea in a bath or the fresh root tincture applied topically was

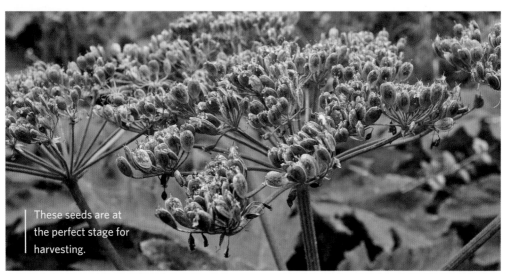

These seeds are at the perfect stage for harvesting.

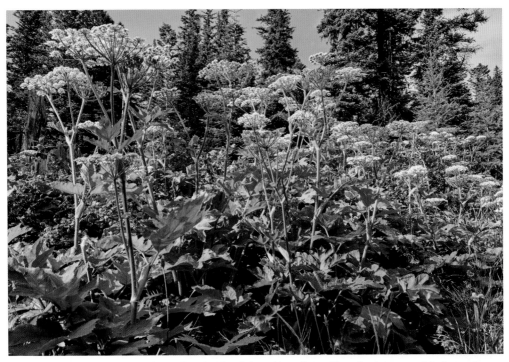

Cow parsnip was named *Heracleum* after the Greek hero Heracles or Hercules because of its large size and great vigor.

traditionally used to reverse recent cases of paralysis. Cow parsnip was similarly used for Bell's palsy, trigeminal neuralgia, or other twitching, pain, or paralysis caused by damage to the facial nerves. Starting at the spine, repeatedly apply the tincture along the entire pathway of the affected nerve.

Caution

Do not use preparations of the seed or root internally while pregnant. The fresh root, which contains an oil that irritates the mucosa, should only be used externally. Oils in the plant that contact the skin may cause a photosensitive reaction leading to a rash or blistering.

Future Harvests

Replant root crowns, and sow mature seeds as you harvest.

HERBAL PREPARATIONS

Seed or Dried Root Tea
Standard decoction
Drink 4–6 fluid ounces 3 times per day.

Root Tincture
1 part dried root
5 parts menstruum (65 percent alcohol, 35 percent distilled water)
Take 15–30 drops up to 4 times per day.
or
1 part fresh root
2 parts menstruum (100 percent alcohol)
For topical use only

Seed Tincture
1 part fresh seed
2 parts menstruum (100 percent alcohol)
Take 15–30 drops up to 4 times per day.

curl-leaf mountain mahogany

Cercocarpus ledifolius

PARTS USED leaf, twig

Leaves and twigs make a useful first aid wash when out in the field, gargle for sore throats, and remedy for diarrhea and constipation.

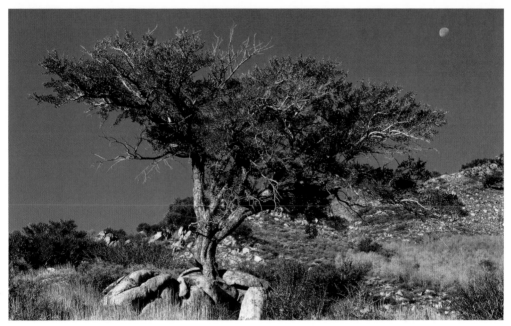

A large old curl-leaf mountain mahogany in its preferred habitat of dry, rocky slopes.

How to Identify

An extensive and shallow root system housing nitrogen-fixing bacteria in nodules feeds the growth of this many-branched and often multi-trunked tree or shrub. Slightly hairy, reddish barked new growth twigs become hairless as they age and form a canopy of gray tangled branches growing at odd angles. Narrowly elliptic, resinous leaves arranged alternately in clusters at the stem tips curl strongly at the edges to become linear in outline. Dark green with paler undersides, the ⅜- to 1⅛-inch-long evergreen leaves persist for 2–3 years and develop a thick outer covering and sunken pores to reduce water loss. From mid spring to early summer, many-stamened, petal-less, wind-pollinated flowers with tubular, 5-lobed, wooly calyces form singly or in groups of as many as 5 in the leaf axils of second-year branches. Wind-dispersed, sharp-tipped seeds fly on 1- to 3-inch-long, corkscrew-shaped, feathery tails. Stunted trees growing in extreme conditions may top out at 3 feet tall; larger individuals may take up to 100 years to reach their maximum height of 35 feet. Thick, furrowed bark on older specimens allows them to survive light fires.

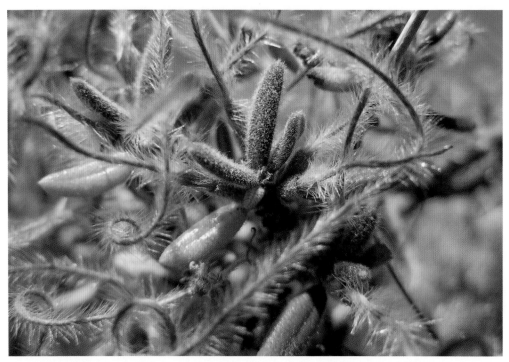

The curled leaf edges and feathery corkscrewing seed tails make this tree easy to identify.

Birchleaf mountain mahogany (*Cercocarpus montanus* var. *glaber*), with fuzzy birchlike leaves, has similar medicinal properties.

Where, When, and How to Wildcraft

Long lived, slow growing, and drought tolerant, this highly variable and most widely distributed species of mountain mahogany inhabits dry, rocky, nutrient-poor slopes at middle to high elevations. From its northern limit in the southeastern corner of Washington, its range in this region extends southward and moves increasingly westward through Oregon into California and beyond. Gather branches and leaves throughout the growing season.

Medicinal Uses

Apply a tea of the astringent leaves and/or twigs to cuts, wounds, and burns to reduce inflammation, speed healing, and prevent infection. Swish the tea in the mouth to tone lax, sore, and bleeding gums; gargle it to alleviate a sore boggy throat; and take it internally to reduce stomach inflammation or to allay the effects of diarrhea. It also promotes bowel movements to relieve constipation.

Future Harvests

Trim branches in a way that encourages bushier growth by cutting just above an outward-facing bud.

HERBAL PREPARATIONS

Leaf Tea
Standard infusion
Drink 3–4 fluid ounces up to 3 times per day.

Twig Tea
Standard decoction
Drink 3–4 fluid ounces up to 3 times per day.

cut-leaved goldthread

Coptis laciniata
canker root, Oregon goldthread
PARTS USED whole plant

Denizen of the deep forest, this unassuming, golden-rooted plant is a bitter tonic that provides medicine to stimulate digestion, reduce stomach inflammation, and heal mouth sores and herpes lesions.

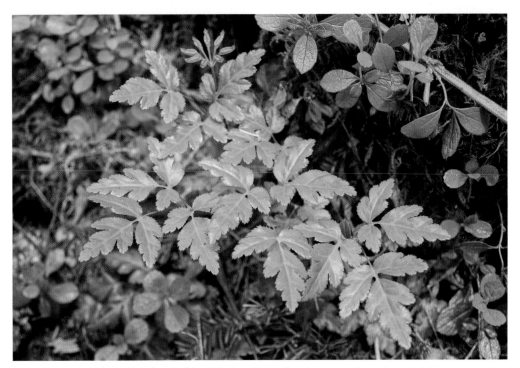

The leaves are easily confused with those of other plants, but the canoe-shaped seed pods are unmistakable.

How to Identify

Thin, brown-barked, and deeply golden yellow rhizomes creep underground. Leathery, long- and wiry-stalked, evergreen basal leaves, dark green and shiny, divide into 3 sharply toothed 3- to 5-lobed and deeply cleft ¾- to 1½-inch-long leaflets. Attaching directly to the rhizome, 3- to 10-inch-long, leafless flowering stalks, shorter than the leaves, bear 1 or 2 flowers with 5–7 small, lance-shaped and slenderly clawed, whitish petals that quickly detach after the flowers open from mid spring to early summer. Five to 8 linear sepals, petal-like and greenish, many thread-like stamens, and 5–10 pistils make up the rest of the flower. Radiating out in circular fashion on short stalks, small, dry, canoe-shaped fruits taper to curled tips with seams running across their tops. The seams split after the fruits mature, and splashing rain disperses the seeds.

Coptis aspleniifolia, spleenwort-leaved goldthread, has fern-like leaves with 5 leaflets and flowering stalks that are taller than the leaves. It grows from northwestern Washington north into Alaska. Although this plant has similar medicinal properties, it is listed as a sensitive species by the U.S. Forest Service and should not be harvested.

Where, When, and How to Wildcraft

This uncommon plant thrives in old-growth and wet, shady coniferous forests west of the Cascade Crest from southwestern Washington to California. Find it growing below seeps, near waterways and wetlands, or on north-facing slopes in areas of high precipitation at low to middle elevations below 3000 feet. Collect the whole plant—roots, rhizomes, and leaves—from late summer to mid autumn.

Medicinal Uses

To make best use of this small, precious plant, it is best prepared as a tincture. The berberine-rich roots and leaves of goldthread are bitter and cooling to the digestive tract. Take the tincture as a bitter tonic to increase the appetite and stimulate the digestive juices. Use it to relieve indigestion and to reduce chronic stomach inflammation. Gargle the diluted tincture (30 drops in 1 fluid ounce of water) to speed the healing of ulcerations of the mouth or to treat thrush. Apply it directly to herpes lesions or cold sores.

Future Harvests

This somewhat rare and difficult to find plant deserves great respect. Its shallow roots are sensitive to soil disturbance, so be mindful of your steps. Restrict your harvests to large healthy stands, and take only a few plants from each area. Consider using this region's more commonly found and widespread berberine-containing plant, Oregon grape (*Berberis* species), in its place.

HERBAL PREPARATIONS

Whole Plant Tincture
1 part fresh whole plant
2 parts menstruum (75 percent alcohol, 25 percent distilled water)
or
1 part dried whole plant
5 parts menstruum (50 percent alcohol, 50 percent distilled water)
As a bitter tonic, take 15–20 drops 10–15 minutes before meals; as a stomach remedy, take 15–45 drops 3 times per day.

---

dandelion

Taraxacum officinale
PARTS USED root, leaf

Don't throw that dandelion weed into the compost pile. Receive it with gratitude. It is full of vitamins and minerals, improves digestion, and is a potent remedy for liver and kidney ailments.

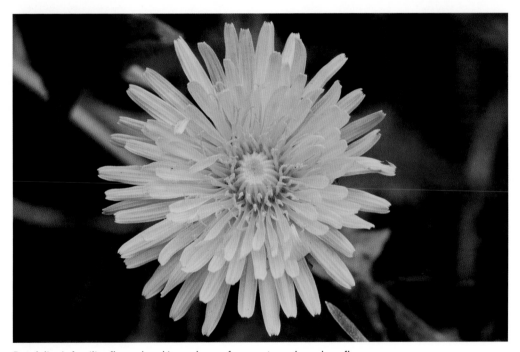

Dandelion's familiar flower head is made up of many strap-shaped ray flowers.

How to Identify

Below a rosette of toothed, basal leaves, a whitish taproot dives into the ground up to 6 inches deep. Arising from the center of the leaves at ground level, a hollow, naked stem, up to 24 inches tall, holds a single flower head containing between 100 and 300 yellow, strap-shaped ray flowers. Many oval to lance-shaped, backward-bent bracts cup the composite head from below. Small, dry seeds connected to a parachute of slender white bristles form a white, globe-shaped seed head. Stems, leaves, and roots exude a milky sap when cut or broken.

Where, When, and How to Wildcraft

This introduced, European perennial tolerates a wide variety of site and soil conditions. Find it just about everywhere from sea level to high elevations. You've probably seen it around in vacant lots, disturbed areas, cracks in the sidewalk, lawns, gardens, forests, and floodplains.

Harvest the leaves in spring when the plant is flowering and the roots in spring or

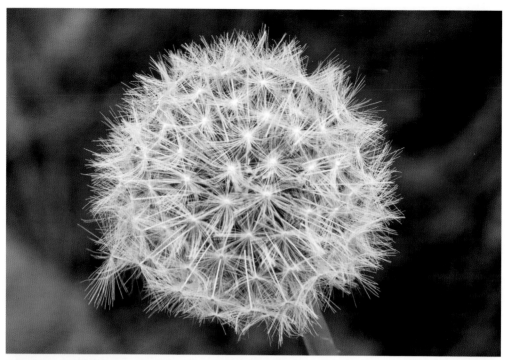

Dandelion seeds can travel many hundreds of feet in the wind.

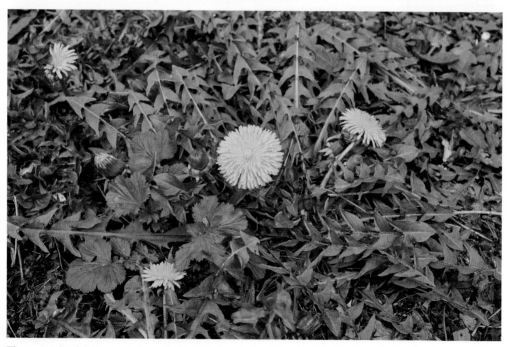

The name dandelion comes from the French *dent de lion* ("tooth of the lion") and refers to the teeth on the leaves.

in late summer and early autumn. Spring-dug roots are sweeter and less medicinally active for cleansing the liver and stimulating digestion, but they are more nourishing and rich in inulin.

Medicinal Uses

Dandelion root, eaten raw or cooked or taken as a tea or tincture, is a digestive bitter that stimulates the secretion of bile and increases the supply of hydrochloric acid in the stomach. The roots are a good source of iron and contain inulin, which balances blood sugar levels, increases absorption of minerals, and supports the immune system. Preparations of the root clean the liver to reduce hepatic congestion and inflammation, prevent gallstones, and relieve inflamed bile ducts. Take the root tea or tincture for hepatitis, cirrhosis, to clean toxins from the blood and liver due to exposure to chemical pollutants or to clear heat from the liver that may give rise to acne, abscesses, and boils.

The strongly diuretic leaves help relieve swelling in the legs, ankles, and feet, a condition known as edema, by expelling excess fluids via the urine. Unlike pharmaceutical diuretics, which deplete the body's potassium reserves, mineral-rich dandelion leaves replenish the potassium lost through urination. To help flush out deposits in the kidneys, drink 1 quart of leaf tea first thing in the morning.

Mix the bitter leaves into salads, add them to soups, or eat them alone to stimulate digestion and receive a healthy dose of vitamins and minerals. Along with many other essential nutrients, they contain especially large amounts of vitamin A, vitamin C, potassium, and calcium. Apply the sap several times per day for 7–10 days to dissolve warts.

 Caution

Ingesting large quantities of the root may cause diarrhea.

Future Harvests

Dandelions hardly need our assistance, but if you are unable to contain yourself, blow the seeds into the wind and make a wish.

HERBAL PREPARATIONS

Root Tea
Standard decoction
Drink 4–6 fluid ounces up to 3 times per day.

Leaf Tea
Standard infusion
Drink 4–6 fluid ounces up to 5 times per day.

Root or Leaf Tincture
1 part fresh root or leaf
2 parts menstruum (75 percent alcohol, 25 percent distilled water)
Take 30–60 drops up to 5 times per day.

---

desert parsley

Lomatium dissectum
fernleaf biscuitroot, lomatium
PARTS USED root

The strongly antiviral properties of this long-lived, slow-growing perennial are best reserved for serious cases of pneumonia or influenza.

How to Identify

Thick, hollow, and lightly ribbed stems thrust upward from a stout taproot with shiny, reddish brown to gray outer skin. In older individuals, this skin peels off in horizontal strips like cherry bark; when cut, a sticky white sap oozes from the soft, fibrous, and cream-colored flesh. The fern-like, mostly basal leaves are 6–14 inches wide and divided into 3 finely dissected leaflets whose ultimate segments are thin and narrow. Leaves growing on the stem connect via sheathed attachments. Small clusters of purple or yellow flowers bloom from mid spring to mid summer and radiate out in compound umbels of 10–30 rays. The large, flat, and oval seeds, ½ to ⅔ inches wide, are lined with barely visible oil tubes, and the width of their wings is less than the width of the seed body. The foliage of this 1- to 6-foot-tall, long-lived perennial begins to die back and turn brown in mid summer, and the pungent roots taste like a strong, bitter, and somewhat citrusy-scented disinfectant.

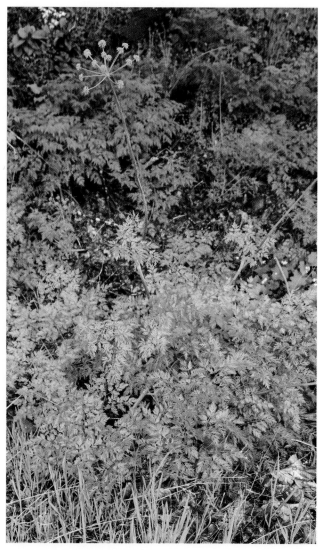

Finely dissected leaves and tall arching stems distinguish desert parsley from others in its genus.

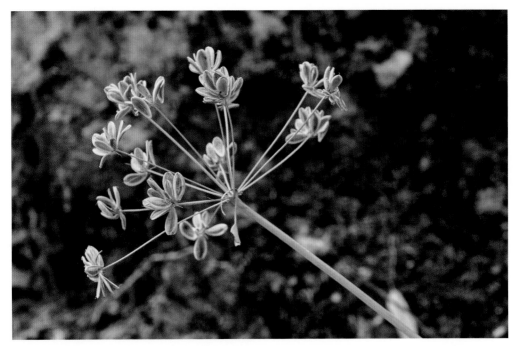

Loma means "fringe" or "border" in Greek. The lighter colored winged edges of these mature desert parsley seeds are characteristic of the genus *Lomatium*.

Where, When, and How to Wildcraft

This slow-growing plant inhabits wooded, brushy, or rocky slopes at low to high elevations from southern California to British Columbia and eastward to the Rocky Mountains. Very conservatively dig the roots from late spring to early autumn.

Medicinal Uses

The roots of desert parsley, often simply called lomatium by herbalists, are strongly antiviral and immune stimulating. Because the oils in the roots are not soluble in water, this medicine is best prepared as a tincture. The tincture aids the body in recovering from colds, flus, pneumonia, and other viral infections. It has an affinity for the upper respiratory tract, lungs, and stomach and has been used by some to reduce the need for antiretroviral HIV medications. This plant is very slow growing and its habitat is being lost to human development, so it should only be used for serious cases. For everyday diseases like simple colds and flus, use one of the many other herbs like elderberry, elderflower, Saint John's wort, or yarrow that can be sustainably harvested in larger quantities.

There are some seventy species of *Lomatium* growing in the western United States. Many are still being used as food and medicine by the native people of this region. More research into the medicinal properties of this rich genus of plants is in order.

⚠ Caution

Don't exceed the recommended dose. Some people develop a rash after taking desert parsley. Some have speculated that this reaction results from a strong bacterial or viral die-off, while others believe it occurs in individuals whose liver may have trouble processing the strong aromatic oils. The rash usually disappears within 2 weeks and does not appear to be caused by an allergic reaction. Whatever the cause, it is best to take desert parsley in conjunction with herbs that support liver metabolism like Oregon grape root or dandelion root.

Future Harvests

Due to its slow rate of growth, loss of habitat, and increasing popularity as a medicine, desert parsley is on the verge of becoming endangered in the wild. Even after 10 years of growth, a plant may only form two leaves and a pencil-sized root. Larger individuals may reach ages of 100 years or more and weigh as much as 20 pounds. These older plants should never be harvested. Before considering a harvest please consult a local herbarium or native plant society to find out if desert parsley is threatened in the area. Gather very, very conservatively, and respect this precious resource by reserving its use for very serious cases of viral infection.

After you've harvested roots, replant the root crown and sow seeds. The seeds germinate best when planted at a depth of ½ inch.

HERBAL PREPARATIONS

Root Tea
Standard decoction left to sit covered for
 1 hour after removing from heat
Drink 3–4 fluid ounces up to 3 times per day.

Root Tincture
1 part dried root
5 parts menstruum (70 percent alcohol,
 30 percent distilled water)
or
1 part fresh root
2 parts menstruum (100 percent alcohol)
Take 15–30 drops up to 3 times per day.

devil's club

Oplopanax horridus
PARTS USED root bark, stem bark

Preparations of the spicy root and stem bark warm the lungs and clear mucus, moderate blood sugar levels, support the adrenals, and provide energetic protection.

How to Identify

Sprawling stalks, 3–10 feet long, armed with ⅛- to ⅜-inch-long spines, grow tall, fall over, root into the soil, and sprout new stems to form large, rhizomatous, and outward spreading colonies. Large, maple-like leaves with 7–9 irregularly toothed lobes and long, spiny stalks extend 4–14 inches wide. An erect spike-like stalk of small, whitish green, very fragrant flowers emerges from a protective nest of spiny leaves from mid spring to early summer, and red, saponaceous, 2- to 3-seeded berries ripen later in summer. Long spines line the leaf veins, and white pith fills the center of the stalks.

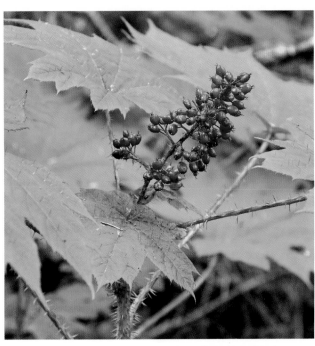

Devil's club teaches about energetic boundaries. It helps those who are affected by and may feel overwhelmed by external energies and is particularly beneficial for people practicing the healing arts.

Where, When, and How to Wildcraft

Devil's club grows in boggy places, along streams and creeks, on wet hillsides, or in places that are wet at least during the rainy months. Its range extends from the southern edge of the Willamette Valley west of the Cascades in Oregon, eastward into northern Washington, and northward into Alaska. Isolated stands can also be found in northern Idaho, northwestern Montana, and on several northern Lake Superior islands in Michigan.

The root bark and stem bark can be harvested in spring, preferably before the leaves emerge, or in autumn. Take care, as getting poked by the tough spines may lead to a nasty infection. The toughest spines are the green ones protecting the new spring growth.

The common-sense method for harvesting from stands that spread outward is to dig roots from the outer edges. This certainly works, but I was guided by the plant to seek out the center of the stand where the largest plants with the thickest roots grow. As they age, the bark on these older and thicker roots begins to rot. I often find roots as thick as my wrist that show initial signs of decay or with a portion of the root bark gone to rot. If you find one like this, scrape off the soft, rotting sludge and use the part that remains to make really good, strong medicine. In addition to the root bark, include the true roots whole.

Medicinal Uses

Quite useful during this region's cold, damp rainy season, spicy and pungent devil's club root or stem bark, drunk hot as a tea or the tincture taken in hot water, dispels cold and dampness from the lungs, loosens stuck mucus, and speeds the healing of respiratory infections.

Take the tea or tincture to help moderate blood sugar levels and—along with changes in diet and lifestyle—to reverse the effects of Type II diabetes. Apply the salve or oil externally to speed the healing of skin infections such as staph.

Bitter, sweet, and saponaceous, the adaptogenic tea or tincture of the root or stem bark also supports the adrenals by moderating the body's reaction to stress. Devil's club is well known as a spiritually protective plant and aids those with adrenal burnout who have suffered major traumas in their lives. Those who have been sexually, verbally, or physically abused often live in a state of constant vigilance, and being on guard all of the time is draining. Take the tea or tincture to nourish the adrenals and relax the hypervigilant nervous system.

Devil's club teaches us to trust our ability to perceive when a response to true danger

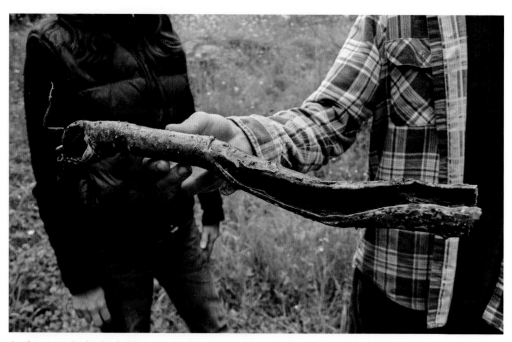

As they age, the bark of older roots in the center of the stand begins to rot. Using these roots for medicine is a wise and sustainable way to wildcraft.

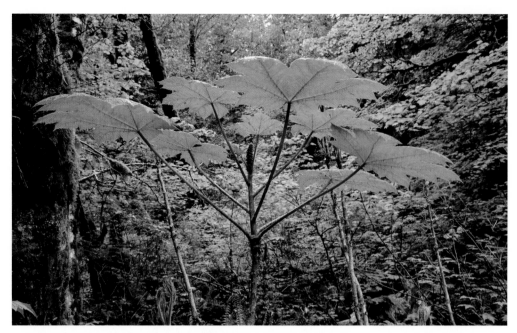

This tall imposing member of the ginseng family is a protector of the forest and is one of the most important shamanic plants of the Northwest native peoples.

is necessary, helps us see that our greatest gifts come from the places of our deepest wounding, and provides a protected healing sanctuary for those new sprouts to emerge.

⚠ Caution

The berries are reported to be toxic.

Future Harvests

Find two well-established root nodes. Test the strength of their rootedness by pulling on the stalk before you dig. If they are well-rooted and will support the weight of the stalks, you can safely cut out the chunk of root between them. Also, if you are left with stalks that you won't use for medicine, bury them horizontally a few inches under the ground. They will root in and send up stalks from the former leaf nodes.

HERBAL PREPARATIONS

Root Bark or Stem Bark Tea
Standard decoction
Drink 2–4 fluid ounces up to 3 times per day.

Root Bark or Stem Bark Tincture
1 part fresh root bark or stem bark
2 parts menstruum (75 percent alcohol,
   25 percent distilled water)
or
1 part dried root bark or stem bark
5 parts menstruum (50 percent alcohol,
   50 percent distilled water)
Take 15–30 drops up to 3 times per day.

Root Bark or Stem Bark Oil and Salve
For root bark or stem bark oil, follow directions for Dry Herb Infused Oil or Alternative Oil Method (page 64). For the salve, follow directions on page 65.

Douglas-fir

Pseudotsuga menziesii
Oregon pine
PARTS USED bark, needle, pitch

Astringent and resinous bark relieves diarrhea and heals wounds.
Wound-healing pitch prevents infections and clears congested lungs.

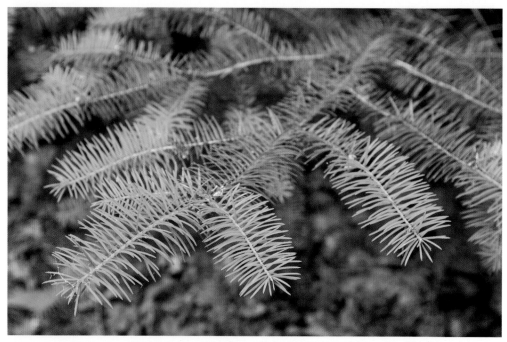

The young branch tips of Douglas-fir are an easily gathered source of vitamin C.

How to Identify

Thick, heavily furrowed, dark brown bark, up to 1 foot thick, reveals a corky textured pattern of light and dark brown bands when cut in cross section. In spring, sour-tasting and pliant, light green new-growth needles emerge from sharp-pointed buds encased in dark brown, overlapping scales. As they age, the flat needles, growing up to ½ to 1 inch long, turn from yellowish green to bluish green with 2 white stripes running the length of their undersides. They are pointy-tipped and spread around the twig. Yellow to reddish, pollen-bearing male cones attach stalkless to the undersides of branches. Oval, somewhat pointed, seed-bearing female cones, yellowish to purplish green when young, hang down 1½ to 4 inches long, bear 3-lobed bracts, and turn reddish brown before falling to the ground. The center lobe is longer than the outer ones. Resin blisters dot the smooth-barked younger trees that have pyramidal crowns and more or less whorled branches. Mature trees with drooping

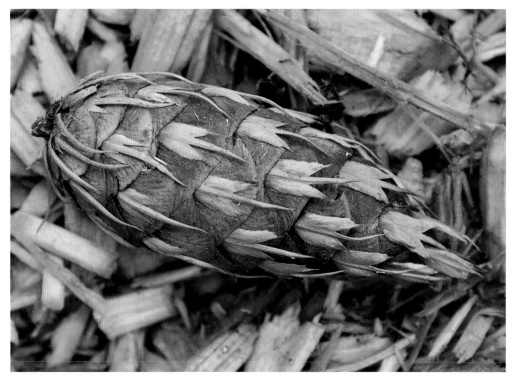

The cones are easily identified by their bracts with three-lobed tips, which are described as "mouse tails" in local folklore.

branches and rounded or flattened crowns may reach heights of 200 feet or more.

Where, When, and How to Wildcraft

Douglas-fir (the name hyphenated because it is not a true fir) dominates forests from southwestern British Columbia to California. Find it growing in dry to moist, mixed-conifer forests from sea level to middle elevations.

From mid to late spring, gather the fresh, light green growing tips. This is also a good time to harvest branch bark. Remove thick, lower branches, and strip the bark promptly to dry in bags or on screens.

Throughout the year be on the lookout for pitch. The trees exude this resin, which varies in consistency from the thickness of honey when fresh to almost as solid as a rock when dried out, to protect and seal

their wounds. Pry chunks off with a knife or scrape the ooze into a jar. Don't take pitch directly from an active wound or you will hinder the tree's natural mechanism of healing and protection. Instead take pitch that has flowed down below the damaged part of the trunk.

Medicinal Uses

Drink the bark tea to stop intestinal tract bleeding and to relieve diarrhea. Use an external wash of the tea to heal cuts, abrasions, or burns. Apply the pitch directly to wounds to speed healing and prevent infection. Rub the pitch-infused oil on sore muscles. Use the salve for healing wounds or as chest rub for colds, flus, and chest and sinus congestion. The spring tips, eaten fresh or brewed as a tea, are high in vitamin C.

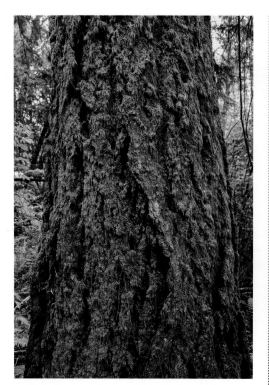

As Douglas-fir bark ages, it becomes deeply fissured.

HERBAL PREPARATIONS

Needle Tea
Standard infusion of the young tips
Drink 4–6 fluid ounces up to 3 times per day.

Bark Tea
Standard decoction
Drink 2–4 fluid ounces up to 3 times per day.

Bark Tincture
1 part fresh bark
2 parts menstruum (75 percent alcohol,
    25 percent distilled water)
or
1 part dried bark
5 parts menstruum (50 percent alcohol,
    50 percent distilled water)
Take 15–30 drops up to 3 times per day.

Pitch Oil or Salve
For pitch oil, follow directions for Dry Herb Infused Oil (page 64) but use 1 part pitch by weight to 10 parts oil by volume. For the salve, follow directions on page 65.

Future Harvests

Fire suppression throughout the western United States has resulted in a broadening of Douglas-fir's historical range; in many places it outcompetes less shade tolerant native trees, such as ponderosa pine. A respectful bark harvest will have little impact on its populations.

false Solomon's seal

Maianthemum racemosum subsp. *amplexicaule*
dragon root, feathery false lily of the valley, plumed Solomon's seal
PARTS USED root

Sweet, bitter, and saponaceous roots moisten connective tissue,
regulate hormones, and soothe sore throats.

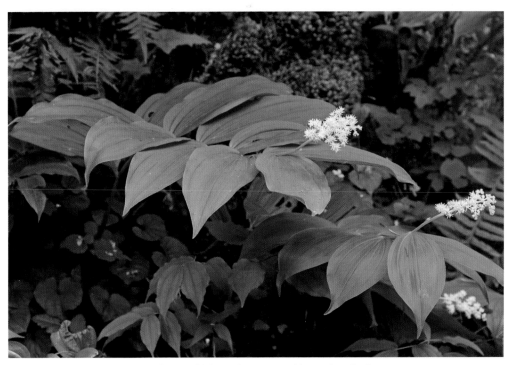

Gracefully arching and fragrant-flowered false Solomon's seal beautifies the forest in spring.

How to Identify

From white-fleshed, brownish skinned, knuckled, and sometimes branching rhizomes, 1- to 3-foot-long unbranched stalks arch out, lined with 5 to 12 alternately arranged, 3- to 8-inch-long leaves with parallel veins and smooth edges. Hairless above and with short stiff hairs below, the oblong-elliptic to egg-shaped stalkless leaves often taper at the base to clasp the stem. In mid spring, branched, many-flowered, pyramidal clusters of highly fragrant, creamy-white flowers with 6 distinct tepals (indistinguishable petals and sepals) bloom at the ends of the stalks. Globe-shaped, 1- to 2-seeded berries start out green with golden brown mottling and become bright red as they mature.

The roots of star-flowered false Solomon's seal (*Maianthemum stellatum*), a related but smaller species with 10 or fewer flowers, darker colored berries, and much smaller roots, may be used similarly.

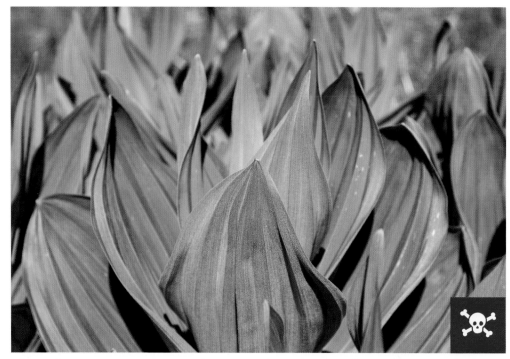

When its leaves emerge in early spring, the poisonous look-alike false hellebore (*Veratrum* species) may be mistaken for false Solomon's seal.

As they emerge in early spring, the leaves of false Solomon's seal may be confused with those of the highly toxic plant false hellebore (*Veratrum* species). The leaves of false hellebore are distinctly creased lengthwise, and their rhizomes are stout and lack the knuckles found on the rhizomes of false Solomon's seal. As the season progresses these plants are easily distinguished: false hellebore stands erect, 3–6 feet tall, with leaves that overlap as they ascend a thick stem.

Where, When, and How to Wildcraft

Growing from sea level to middle elevations, false Solomon's seal (formerly *Smilacina racemosa*) inhabits moist, forested areas with nutrient-rich soils from Alaska to California. Dig the rhizomes in autumn after the tops begin to die back.

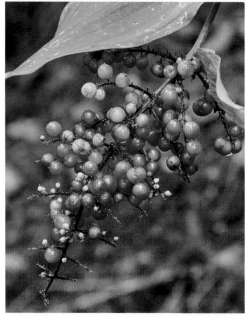

Bright red berries of false Solomon's seal ripen in autumn.

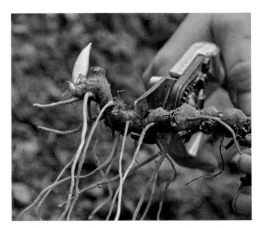

After harvesting false Solomon's seal roots, be sure to replant the end with the white pointy bud.

Medicinal Uses

This lovely plant nourishes the waters of the body. Constant stress, overwork, or the normal process of aging can deplete the body of moisture and leave the joints and connective tissue dry. Without proper lubrication the tendons and ligaments lose their elasticity and shorten. A tea or tincture of the roots of false Solomon's seal moistens the connective tissue of the joints and restores flexibility, leaving the joints less susceptible to injury, and allows bones that have been pulled out of place by tightened ligaments or tendons to pop back into place.

Perhaps due to its steroidal saponin content, the root tincture also helps regulate the menstrual cycle and moderate hormonal swings. Saponins, made up of both fat-soluble and water-soluble constituents that make them foam up like soap, are compounds that closely resemble and act as natural precursors to hormones in the human body.

The moistening properties of the root combined with its astringency and saponin content make this remedy useful for sore throats. Take it as a syrup or gargle the tea or diluted tincture. An external wash or poultice reduces inflammation from insect bites and stings and promotes skin cell regeneration to speed the healing of wounds and burns.

Future Harvests

Harvest a few plants from each healthy, abundant stand. After digging the roots, remove the aboveground parts and replant a 3-inch-long chunk of the bud-containing front portion of the rhizome. Sow seeds soon after the berries ripen in autumn.

HERBAL PREPARATIONS

Root Tea
Standard decoction
Drink 6–8 fluid ounces up to 4 times per day.

Root Tincture
1 part fresh root
2 parts menstruum (50 percent alcohol, 50 percent distilled water)
Take 15–60 drops up to 4 times per day.

---

feverfew

Tanacetum parthenium
PARTS USED leaf and flower

*Cooling and bitter leaves and flowers break fevers, prevent migraines,
and relax the uterus to relieve pain and cramping.*

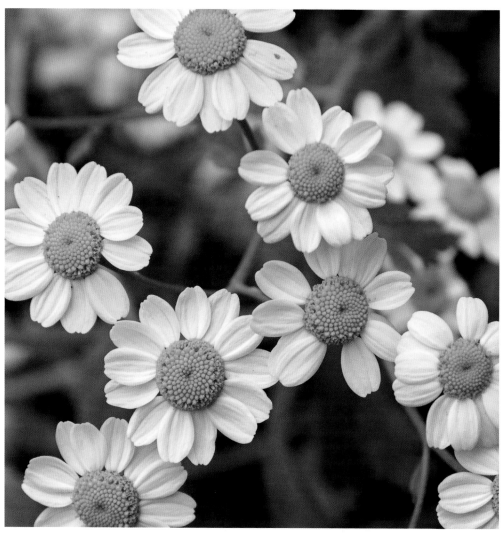

White ray flowers encircle a central button comprising many yellow disk flowers.

How to Identify

From a taproot with 1 to several branches, finely haired stems stand erect, 12–32 inches tall, carrying yellow-green aromatic leaves divided once or twice into broad segments. Fine, white-wooly hairs cover the alternately arranged and somewhat round- to pointy-tipped leaves. White, petal-like ray flowers and many small, yellow disk flowers make up daisy-like composite flower heads that gather in flat- to round-topped clusters at the tops of the branches. Two to 3 whorls of slightly hairy, ridged, lance-shaped bracts with translucent edges adorn the green receptacle, a swollen upper portion of the stem that provides a foundation for the flowers to grow. Blunt-tipped seeds, dry and cylindrical with 8–10 veins running their length, may ripen with tiny crowns of bristly hair.

Where, When, and How to Wildcraft

This hardy European perennial (formerly *Chrysanthemum parthenium*) is a garden escapee that has made a home in much of the eastern and western portions of North America. In the Pacific Northwest, it inhabits disturbed sites and gardens from British Columbia to California at low to middle elevations.

When the plant is in full bloom, cut the stems at the base and hang them in bundles or lay them on screens to dry. Strip the leaves and flowers, and store them in airtight bags or jars in a cool, dry place. Discard the stems.

Medicinal Uses

Cooling and bitter feverfew leaf and flower together relieve pain and inflammation and, as the name suggests, remedy fevers. Drink a hot tea to break fevers with aches and pains from colds and flus. While they may or may not provide relief during acute migraine episodes, taking the tea or tincture daily helps prevent them. The tea or tincture also helps relieve tension headaches.

The leaf and flower tea or tincture relaxes the uterus to relieve painful menstruation and cramping and brings on delayed bleeding. A cold infusion calms an upset stomach.

Caution

Because it causes uterine contractions, do not use during pregnancy.

Future Harvests

If your garden or nearby wasteland lacks feverfew, the easily sprouted seeds are readily available commercially.

HERBAL PREPARATIONS

Leaf and Flower Tea
Standard or cold infusion
Drink 2–4 fluid ounces up to 3 times per day.

Leaf and Flower Tincture
1 part fresh leaf and flower
2 parts menstruum (75 percent alcohol,
 25 percent distilled water)
or
1 part dried leaf and flower
5 parts menstruum (50 percent alcohol,
 50 percent distilled water)
Take 30–60 drops up to 4 times per day.

---

field mint

Mentha arvensis
brook mint, wild mint
PARTS USED leaf

Stimulating leaves soothe digestive upset, relax intestinal cramping, and promote sweating to speed the healing of colds and flus.

How to Identify

Rhizomes spread and send up square-stemmed, single or branched stalks that stand 8–32 inches tall. Lining the slightly hairy stems opposite each other, pointy-tipped, smooth to hairy leaves with coarse- to sharp-toothed edges and rounded bases unfurl 1–3 inches long and vary from lance-shaped to nearly round. The minty-scented, short-stalked, and prominently veined leaves gradually become stalkless as they ascend the stem. Tubular, 4-lobed flowers bloom white to pink to violet in compact whorls in the upper leaf axils from mid summer to early autumn. Clusters of 4, egg-shaped nutlets mature in persistent, slightly hairy, 5-lobed calyces.

Where, When, and How to Wildcraft

Common throughout much of the upper half of the northern hemisphere, this water-loving perennial thrives in marshes, meadows, and along the edges of ponds, lakes, and streams. Find it at low to middle elevations just about anywhere in the Pacific Northwest from Alaska to California. While the plants are flowering, clip stalks at the base just above a leaf node, discard damaged leaves, and hang to dry in a shaded area with ample airflow.

Medicinal Uses

Field mint is slightly less potent than peppermint but can be used in similar ways. Drink the stimulating and pleasant-tasting tea to relieve indigestion, gas pain, colic, heartburn, nausea, and stomach and upper intestinal cramping. At the first sign of a cold or flu, drink the tea alone or with equal parts of yarrow flower and blue elder flower to promote sweating to help cleanse and clear the body of infection.

⚠ Caution

This plant, with constituents similar to those of the uterine-stimulating pennyroyal, is contraindicated during pregnancy.

Future Harvests

Divide roots in spring or autumn. Plant in a suitable wet habitat where the spreading rhizomes have plenty of room to roam.

HERBAL PREPARATIONS

Leaf Tea
Standard infusion
Drink as needed or desired.

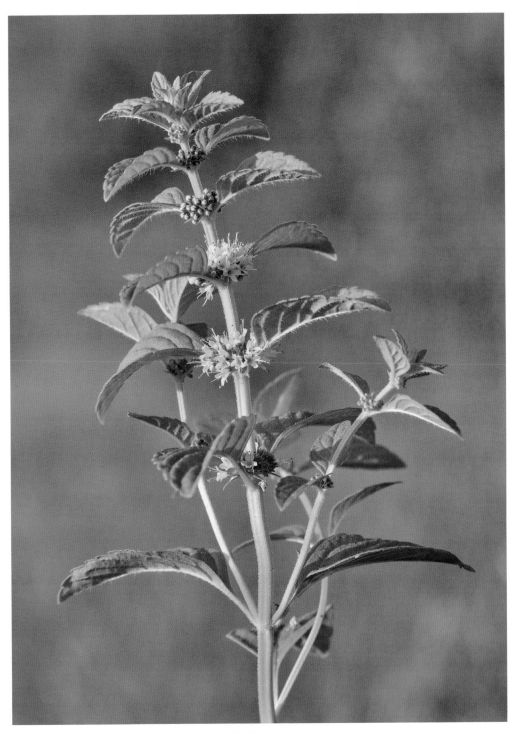

Field mint is the only *Mentha* species native to North America.

Chamerion angustifolium
great willow-herb
PARTS USED leaf

Astringent leaves soothe intestinal inflammation and tighten the colon to prevent dehydration during episodes of diarrhea.

How to Identify
Straight, unbranched, sometimes reddish stems, 3–7 feet tall, arise from a colony-forming root system bearing alternate, 4- to 8-inch, lance-shaped leaves with distinctly veined and pale undersides. Long-stalked flowers, blooming from early summer to early autumn with 4 sepals and 4 deep pink to magenta petals, are borne in terminal clusters of 15 or more. Longer than each of the 8 pollen-producing stamens, a 4-lobed pollen-receiving protuberance known as a stigma tops the female reproductive organ in the center of each flower. Long and narrow, green- to red-colored capsules split open to release fluffy, white-haired seeds.

Where, When, and How to Wildcraft
This weedy native (formerly *Epilobium angustifolium*) grows from Alaska to California, inhabiting clear cuts, roadsides, burn sites, and other disturbed areas from the lowlands to the mountains. Gather leaves when

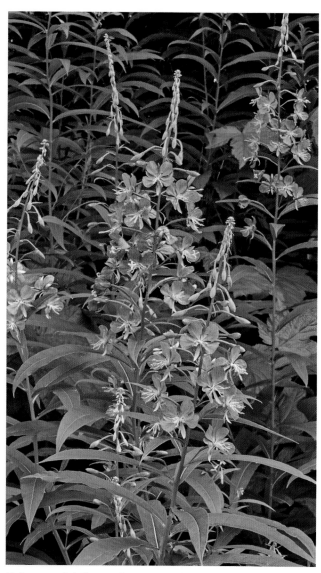

Pink to purplish flower plumes top tall, graceful stalks.

the plant is in flower. Cut the stalk at the base and discard brown or wilted leaves. Use the flexible upper part of the stem and flowers along with the leaves. Dry them together on a screen for teas or process them fresh for tincture.

Medicinal Uses

Fireweed contains tannins that tighten and dry out tissues. Imagine the feeling on your tongue when you drink a cup of strong black tea. The same thing happens when you ingest a high-tannin plant like fireweed: the tissues shrink, pucker up, and dry out. Fireweed also contains compounds that soothe irritated tissues and reduce inflammation in the intestines. It is this combination that makes fireweed so useful during bouts of diarrhea.

Diarrhea has many causes, but the most common cause is a viral infection of the gut. Rather than suppress the expulsion of the infection by plugging things up, it's best to wait a few days and let the body do its thing. If the diarrhea continues, take the tea or tincture to minimize the loss of fluids. The soothing mucilage in fireweed also soothes intestinal tissues that are irritated and inflamed by the infection. Always drink lots of fluid during an episode of acute diarrhea to prevent dehydration.

An external wash or poultice of the leaves speeds the healing and soothes burns, rashes, cuts, and skin inflammation.

Future Harvests

As they ripen from late summer to early autumn, break apart mature seed pods and scatter the seeds into the wind.

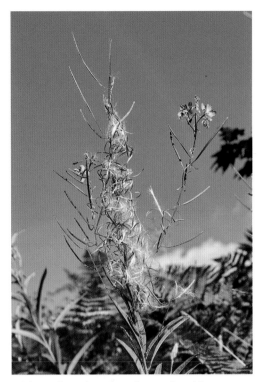

With its plumed seeds and spreading rhizomes, fireweed is well-adapted to rapidly colonizing disturbed areas, especially those scarred by fire or logging.

HERBAL PREPARATIONS

Leaf Tea
Standard infusion
Drink 4–6 fluid ounces up to 5 times per day.

Leaf Tincture
1 part fresh leaf
2 parts menstruum (75 percent alcohol, 25 percent distilled water)
Take 30–60 drops up to 5 times per day.

Fremont's silktassel

Garrya fremontii
bearbrush
PARTS USED leaf

Bitter leaves with an apple-skin-like aftertaste relax smooth muscles to reduce the pain of intense menstrual cramping or to ease gall bladder spasms.

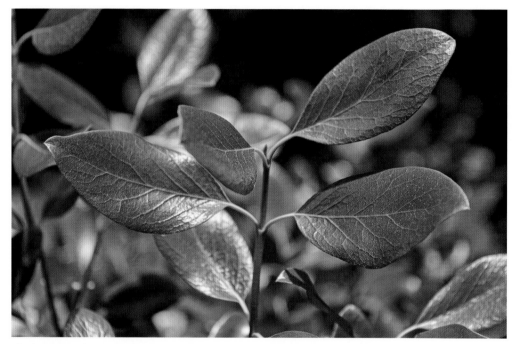

Thick, oppositely arranged leaves provide a potent medicine that relieves spasms.

How to Identify

Pairs of tough, leathery evergreen leaves, smooth and shiny above and sometimes slightly hairy below, rotate 90 degrees opposite each other along the smooth-barked stems of this 3- to 10-foot-tall dryland shrub. The leaves are generally flat without wavy margins, elliptic to egg-shaped, dark green above, and yellowish green below. At the ends of branches or from the upper leaf axils, catkin-like clusters (male and female on separate plants) hang pendulous and bear small flowers lacking petals that bloom in groups of 3 from mid winter to late spring in oppositely arranged, cup-like bracts. Flowers on the female plants, cupped by densely silky-haired bracts, form green, fleshy, berry-like fruits that ripen dark purple with age.

Don't confuse this spreading, opposite-leaved shrub with the similar-looking but alternate-leaved manzanitas (*Arctostaphylos* species) and canyon live oaks (*Quercus chrysolepis*), with which Fremont's silktassel shares its scrubland habitat.

Other Medicinal Silktassels

A few other medicinally active silktassels can be found in the Pacific Northwest. Wavyleaf silktassel (*Garrya elliptica*), with long hanging catkins and a graceful growing habit, grows along the coast from southern Oregon into California. It is a favored ornamental plant. Boxleaf silktassel (*G. buxifolia*) is a compact bush that inhabits the southern portions of this region. Its leaves, smaller than those of the other species, have densely haired undersides.

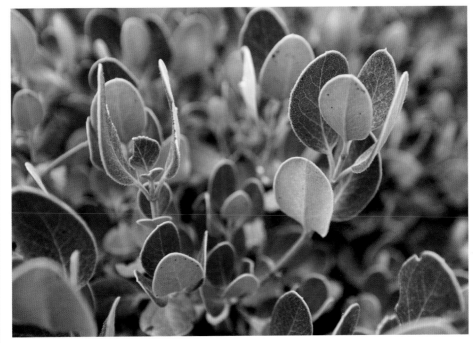

Boxleaf silktassel has small leaves with wooly undersides.

Where, When, and How to Wildcraft

From California northward through Oregon on the western side of the Cascade Crest, Fremont's silktassel occupies chaparral and mixed coniferous forests in dry, lowland foothills and middle-elevation mountains. Its range narrows in the northern half of Oregon until it reaches its northernmost limit in Skamania and Klickitat Counties on the Washington side of the Columbia River Gorge.

Clip the branch ends from early spring to late summer. Process the leaves fresh, or dry them on the stems on screens or in bags. Discard the stems after you've stripped the dried leaves. Some people recommend using the trunk or root bark for medicine, but the leaves are sufficiently strong.

Medicinal Uses

The leaves of Fremont's silktassel, so bitter they make you shiver, relax smooth muscles and relieve spasms. The leaf tincture is a specific and reliable remedy for intense menstrual cramping.

Take the tincture also to relieve intestinal cramping and gas pains or to reduce pain and

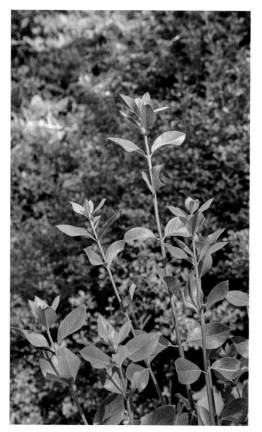

Fremont's silktassel has an upright growth habit.

Because it is so relaxing, a small dose of the tincture before lying down to rest will make even the shortest break seem like a long, deeply rejuvenating nap.

⚠ Caution

Some people are sensitive to this plant. Start by taking 5–10 drops and increase the dosage until you reach the desired effect. Do not exceed the recommended dosage. Ingesting large quantities may lead to strained breathing or cause your skin to break out in a cold sweat.

Silktassel is neither for use during pregnancy nor appropriate for children, and it should not be mixed with over-the-counter or prescription drugs.

Future Harvests

Gather leaves from several different plants to minimize your impact.

spasms in the gallbladder when stones are present.

Some people eat plenty of good, nourishing food and drink plenty of water but find themselves nutrient or moisture deficient. If the lack of nourishment or moisture results from tension that constricts the gut, take 5–10 drops of the leaf tincture before meals to relax the digestive organs. Often this inability to receive nourishment or moisture stems from traumas stored deep in the body. Work with silktassel to release this stored tension to receive nourishment of all kinds on deeper and more refined levels.

HERBAL PREPARATIONS

Leaf Tincture
1 part dried leaf
5 parts menstruum (50 percent alcohol, 50 percent distilled water)
or
1 part fresh leaf
2 parts menstruum (75 percent alcohol, 25 percent distilled water)
The tincture is much easier to stomach than the intensely bitter tea, and it's easier to regulate the dosage of this potent medicine. Take 5–30 drops up to 5 times per day.

Fuller's teasel

Dipsacus fullonum

PARTS USED root

Spiky, spiny Fuller's teasel provides roots to remedy Lyme disease, reduce joint pain, and strengthen bones, joints, and tendons.

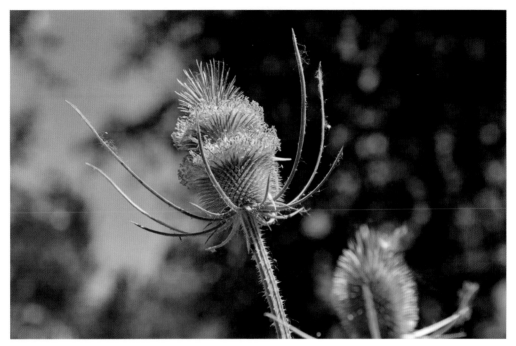

With its long spiny bracts and egg-shaped flower head, there is no mistaking Fuller's teasel.

How to Identify

Reaching a depth of 2 feet or more, a stout taproot produces a rosette of prickly basal leaves. In the plant's second year of growth, a hollow, prickle-lined stem with erect branches rises up 2–6½ feet tall to produce an egg-shaped head of flowers. Oppositely arranged, lance-shaped leaves up to 12 inches long with toothed or wavy edges and spiny midribs clasp the stem and fuse together to form water-collecting cups. A whorl of long, spine-tipped, linear bracts juts out from underneath stiff, 1½- to 4-inch-tall flower heads. Pinkish purple flowers, each blooming for a day, form a narrow ring around the center of the flower head. The central ring of flowers separates into 2 belts: one spreads toward the top, the other toward the bottom. As the seeds mature, the flower head dries brown and spiny. If conditions are unfavorable for growth, the plants will delay flowering and live longer than the normal, 2-year biennial cycle. The basal leaves die early in the flowering season, and after flowering the entire plant dies.

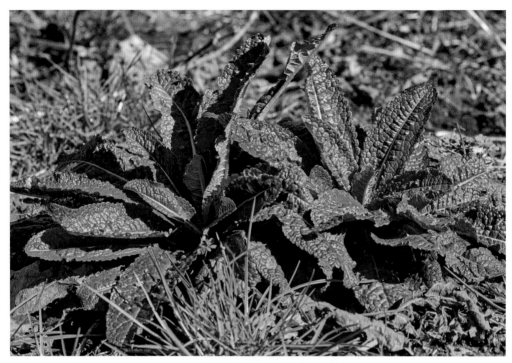

Harvest roots before the plant sends up its flowering stalk.

Where, When, and How to Wildcraft

This introduced Eurasian and North African biennial grows at low to middle elevations throughout much of North America in waste areas, pastures, meadows, and along roadsides. In this region, find it on both sides of the Cascades from British Columbia to California.

Dig the roots as they enter their second season of growth between early autumn and early spring. Look for lush, dense rosettes of large, ground-hugging leaves. The newly sprouted first-year plants, which are not ready for harvesting, will have much smaller leaves. After the flowering stalks begin

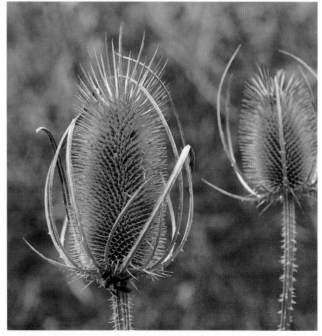

For much of the year, the long-lasting dried seed heads lead you to stands of teasel.

to emerge, the roots become woody and can-not be used for medicine.

Medicinal Uses

Until it was popularized as a remedy for Lyme disease by Matthew Wood, teasel was seldom used in western herbalism. In tradi-tional Chinese medicine, the similar species *Dipsacus asper* and *D. japonicus* have been used for centuries to tonify the liver and kidney systems to strengthen bones, joints, and tendons. Fuller's teasel may be used sim-ilarly. Take the tea or tincture for knee and lower back pain, stiff joints, and weakness in the legs.

Take the tea or tincture for at least 1 month to make the body inhospitable for the Lyme spirochete and to reduce Lyme-related joint pain. Sensitive people may get results from a dosage of 5 drops 3 times per day; others may need 10 drops or more. Start with the lower dosages and work your way up.

Future Harvests

Although Fuller's teasel is a weedy plant that doesn't need help maintaining its popu-lations, be sure to leave enough plants to produce seed for the seasons to come.

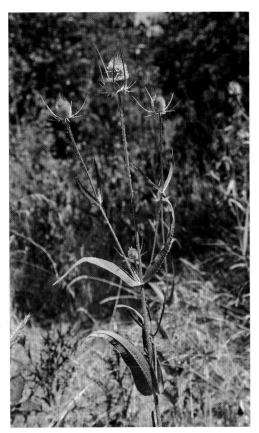

Spiny, stem-clasping leaves make water-holding cups. The captured water, up to 5 inches deep, deters the movement of insects along the stalk.

HERBAL PREPARATIONS

Root Tea
Standard decoction
Drink 4–6 fluid ounces up to 3 times per day.

Root Tincture
1 part fresh root
2 parts menstruum (75 percent alcohol, 25 percent distilled water)
Take 5–60 drops up to 3 times per day.

Monotropa uniflora
convulsion plant, corpse plant, fairy smoke, Indian pipe
PARTS USED flowering stalk

Ghostly white plants yield a dark purple tincture that increases pain tolerance, reduces the debilitating effects of acute anxiety attacks, and relieves spasms and seizures.

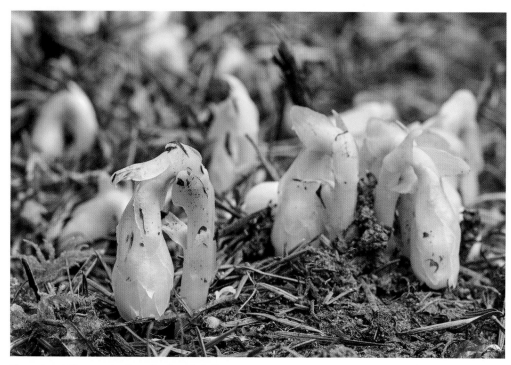

Flowering stalks emerge from the forest duff.

How to Identify
Receiving nutrients from mycorrhizal associations with trees, a fleshy root mass pushes several stalks upward through the forest humus. These black-flecked stalks lined with linear, sometimes wavy-edged, scale-like leaves emerge from early to late summer and terminate with downward-nodding, solitary, ghostly white flowers. Hairs line the inner surface of each flat-tipped, overlapping petal, and upper stem bracts enfold the narrowly bell-shaped, 5-petaled flowers. As the seed capsules mature, they turn upward to the sky. Slits open lengthwise along the dried, ¼-inch-long capsules to release the very tiny, wind-borne seeds. Entirely translucent white and waxy textured, this 2- to 11-inch-tall perennial plant exudes a clear, gelatinous fluid when cut, blackens with age or injury, and persists in dried form with all parts

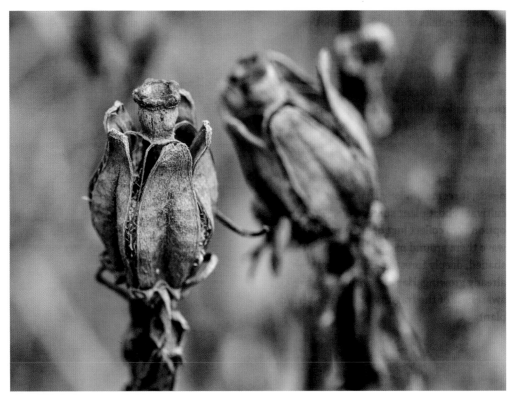

Seed pods split open to release tiny seeds.

perpendicular to the earth after dispensing its seed.

Where, When, and How to Wildcraft

This shade-tolerant, perennial mycohetero-troph—a non-photosynthetic plant that receives its nutrients from a photosynthesizing plant via a fungal relationship—occurs sporadically in deep, closed-canopy coniferous forests at low to middle elevations from southeastern Alaska south to California and beyond. It is more common at lower latitudes and west of the Cascades in Washington and Oregon.

Before they begin to set seed, gather no more than one-third of the flowering stalks from each clump by lightly grasping the stalks, one at a time, and pulling upward until they break free of the root mass. Process the plants fresh as tincture.

Medicinal Uses

Ghost pipe was used by early American botanical doctors for its antispasmodic properties, its calming effect on the nervous system, to encourage sweating to break a fever, and as a substitute for opium to relieve pain. They also used the juice of the fresh plant, by itself or combined with rosewater, to soothe chronically inflamed eyes. Modern herbalists use this acrid, slightly sweet, and sticky-astringent plant in much the same way.

Take the fresh tincture to increase pain tolerance, both physical and emotional, and to relieve muscle spasms, convulsive jerky movements, and seizures including those brought on by fevers. It helps ground and calm those who are mentally overstimulated, reduces the debilitating effects of acute anxiety attacks, and allows those experiencing or reliving traumas to do so in an emotionally detached way.

As an eyewash, ghost pipe relieves pink eye or conjunctivitis, an inflammation of the mucous membranes that cover the whites of the eyeball and the insides of the eyelids. It is especially indicated for crusty, pus-filled eyes.

Future Harvests

Because the plant has such specific site needs, it seems unlikely that you'd be able to cultivate ghost plant successfully. The best option is to collect just opened seed pods and wave them around mature conifers in the shaded, deeply forested areas where they are already growing. Harvest with great care and awareness of the fragility of this mysterious plant.

HERBAL PREPARATIONS

Flowering Stalk Tincture
1 part fresh flowering stalk
2 parts menstruum (75 percent alcohol, 25 percent distilled water)
Take 5–30 drops up to 5 times per day.

goldenrod

Solidago canadensis
Canada goldenrod
PARTS USED flowering top

Aromatic and bitter leaves and flowers support the urinary tract,
relieve seasonal allergies, and stimulate digestion.

How to Identify

Fibrous-rooted rhizomes creep to form large stands. Finely haired and branching near the top, solitary stems stand 1–7 feet tall and are alternately lined with sharply toothed, lance-shaped leaves. Three prominent veins mark the 2- to 5-inch-long, smooth to finely hairy leaves. Blooming between mid summer and mid autumn in clusters of many, sticky-bracted, yellow composite flower heads at the ends of the stems, 10–17 short ray flowers surround a center of few disk flowers. Sparsely haired, wind-dispersed seeds ripen crowned with many white, hair-like bristles. The basal leaves and lower stem leaves fall before the plants flower, and the leaves in the middle of the stem are longer than those above or below.

Where, When, and How to Wildcraft

Widespread throughout North America, this long-lived perennial can form sometimes dominant stands at all elevations

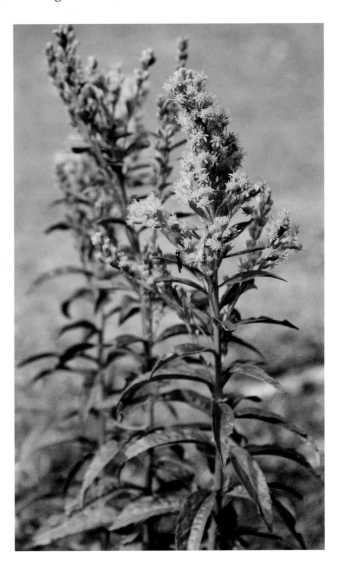

Sprays of yellow flowers are a signature for goldenrod's affinity for the urinary tract.

in this region from Alaska to California in meadows, grasslands, ditches, fields, roadsides, and forest openings. Clip the top third of plants that are flowering, discard the stems, and process the leaves and flowers fresh or dry on screens or in bags.

Medicinal Uses

The flowering top tea or tincture increases urine output, strengthens the bladder, and speeds the healing of urinary tract infections. Take it to resolve water swelling in the lower extremities or to rid the body of waste products that lead to skin eruptions such as psoriasis, eczema, or acne. Containing a host of allergy-relieving and inflammation-reducing flavonoids, these same preparations alleviate seasonal allergies.

The tea or tincture also stimulates the digestive juices and warms the stomach to relieve gas and stagnation in the gut. An external wash aids the healing of wounds and helps resolve pink eye.

Future Harvests

Goldenrod is an important late-season source of nectar and pollen for bees and other insects. Harvest conservatively from large stands and propagate plants to increase the size of or establish new colonies. In spring, sow seeds or transplant sections of rhizome.

HERBAL PREPARATIONS

Flowering Top Tea
Standard infusion
Drink 4–6 fluid ounces up to 3 times per day.

Flowering Top Tincture
1 part fresh flowering top
2 parts menstruum (75 percent alcohol,
  25 percent distilled water)
or
1 part dried flowering top
5 parts menstruum (50 percent alcohol,
  50 percent distilled water)
Take 30–60 drops up to 3 times per day.

Gray's lovage

Ligusticum grayi
Gray's licorice-root, kishwoof, oshala
PARTS USED root

Pungent and oily roots relieve sore throats, speed recovery from viral infections, and open and clear the lungs.

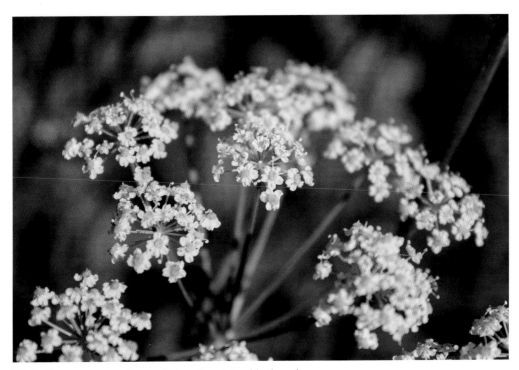

White flowers on secondary umbels mature into ribbed seeds.

How to Identify

Long, fibrous, and highly aromatic taproots, brown skinned and hairy topped, anchor 8- to 36-inch-tall hairless perennials to the earth. The mostly basal, 4- to 10-inch-long, parsley-like compound leaves are 3-times divided into ½- to 1½-inch leaflets with sharp narrow tips. Small white flowers are borne in compound umbels. The terminal umbel is made up of 7–14 unequal stalks or rays. Concave, ¼-inch-long seeds are lined with slightly winged ribs. There are no bracts beneath the flowers and few or no leaves on the stem.

Make positive identification before harvesting this plant or any other in the parsley (Apiaceae) family. Look for the hairy root crown, distinctive smell, and consult a botanical key to positively identify via the seeds to distinguish from potentially deadly carrot family look-a-likes such as poison hemlock (*Conium maculatum*). See "Toxic Plants" (page

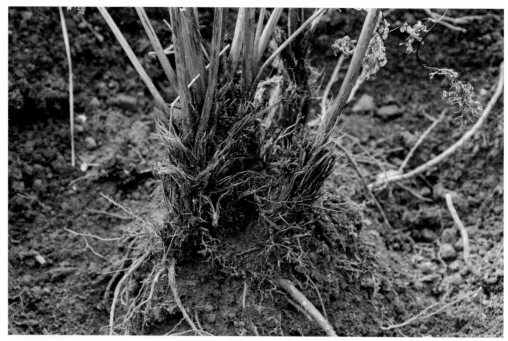

Tough fibers at the bases of the leaf stalks persist to form a hairy crown.

32) for tips on identifying poison hemlock and other poisonous umbels.

Where, When, and How to Wildcraft

This cousin to the Rocky Mountain plant oshá (*Ligusticum porteri*) is present throughout much of the western United States. Find it on open or wooded slopes and in dry meadows at middle to high elevations in scattered counties in central and eastern Washington, across a wide swath of Oregon on both sides of the Cascades, and in northern California.

Conservatively dig the roots from late summer to mid autumn after the seeds mature and the tops begin to die back. Sometimes you will find several roots intertwined. If so replant one or two of the intertwined roots and take the rest.

Medicinal Uses

Because the resins are not soluble in water, this plant is best prepared as a tincture or syrup. The pungent, bitter, and numbing roots, chewed or taken as tincture, open the bronchioles, clear the lungs of mucus, and help the body recover from colds, flus, and other viral infections affecting the lungs and stomach. The syrup, tincture, or chewed root numbs, soothes, and stimulates healing for sore throats made raw and dry from too much coughing or singing. Chew the root to protect yourself from airborne illnesses.

Although the root also relieves gas and stimulates digestion, choose different but equally effective remedies, like field mint, angelica seed and root, or sweetroot, which grow more abundantly and in less environmentally sensitive areas.

Gray's lovage embodies wildness. It resists cultivation and refuses to grow in gardens. To help themselves wake up from their winter hibernation, bears dig, eat, and rub these roots all over their bodies. Take small doses of the tincture and develop a relationship with this plant to awaken the wild, instinctive self and to learn how to cultivate a proper relationship with anger.

⚠ Caution

Gray's lovage can stimulate the uterus and initiate menstrual bleeding. Use with caution during pregnancy.

Future Harvests

In 1999 in response to fears of over-harvesting, the U.S. Forest Service issued a 3-year moratorium on digging oshá root. Although Gray's lovage is not a part of the commercial herbal trade and therefore not subject to the same harvesting pressures as its cousin, it is a similarly slow-growing plant that inhabits a specific ecological niche. Harvest with extreme care and use other, less environmentally sensitive plants whenever possible.

While harvesting, sow seeds in the wild using terraced garden techniques. After digging a root, use some rocks to create a small barrier on the downhill side of your hole. Level the dirt behind the barrier, shallowly plant seeds, and mulch with leaves and stems. This terrace not only captures and retains moisture to help the seeds germinate, but it marks the spots where you've planted seeds. Check in on them in subsequent years to follow their progress.

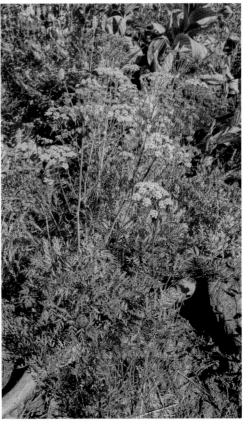

With its parsley-like leaves and white-flowered umbels, Gray's lovage shares features common to other parsley family plants, some of which are quite toxic.

HERBAL PREPARATIONS

Root Tea
Standard decoction
Drink 4–6 fluid ounces up to 3 times per day.

Root Tincture
1 part dried root
5 parts menstruum (70 percent alcohol, 30 percent distilled water)
or
1 part fresh root
2 parts menstruum (100 percent alcohol)
Take 30–60 drops up to 3 times per day.

Ephedra viridis
joint fir, Mormon tea
PARTS USED stem

Resinous and astringent stems open the bronchioles and clear mucus to aid asthmatic conditions and soothe seasonal allergies.

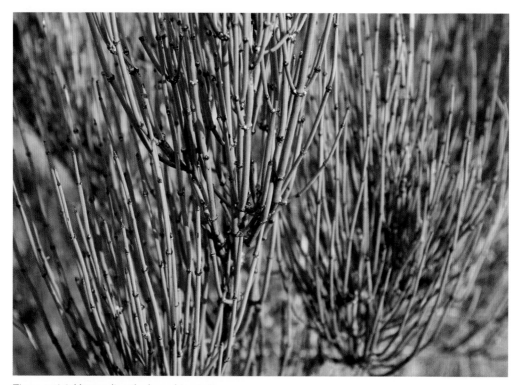

Tiny, vestigial leaves line the branching twigs.

How to Identify

Green to yellowish green young stems, jointed and grooved, emerge from grayish or reddish brown woody branches in broom-like bundles and become yellow with age. Filled with a reddish brown pith, the photosynthesizing stems of this seemingly leafless, scraggly looking shrub produce tiny, vestigial, scale-like leaves, 2 per node, that attach opposite each other along the stem. For 2 weeks between mid spring and early summer, small female cones receive pollen carried on the wind from clusters of yellow pollen sacs on the male cones. Male and female cones form on separate plants. Two-seeded beaked nutlets ripen from early summer to early autumn. A fibrous root system spreads from deeply descending taproots to stabilize the soil and prevent erosion.

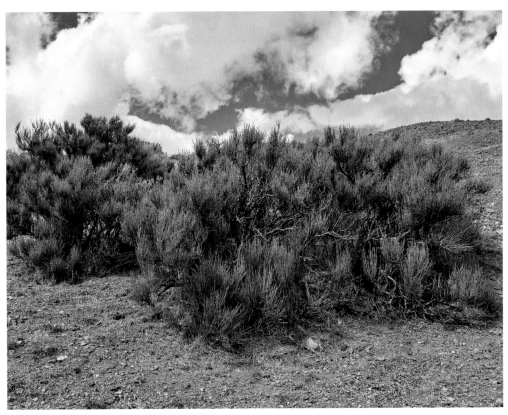

Green ephedra occupies harsh, high desert landscapes.

This 1½- to 5-foot-tall woody perennial grows up to 10 feet wide.

Where, When, and How to Wildcraft

Mostly a plant of middle to high elevations in the Great Basin sagebrush scrublands, green ephedra's range barely extends into the high desert of deep southeastern Oregon. Harvest throughout the year by snipping off bunches of twigs at the ends of branches.

Medicinal Uses

Unlike other *Ephedra* species from around the world, green ephedra contains no ephedrine or pseudo-ephedrine, but it is still warming, stimulating, and astringent. Resins in the stems help to open the bronchioles and clear mucus from the lungs. Use the tea or tincture for damp, asthmatic conditions or as part of a protocol for seasonal allergies of similar character.

Green ephedra, a diuretic, also has an astringent and slightly anti-inflammatory effect on the urinary tract. Drink at least 1 quart of tea daily along with 1 pint of unsweetened cranberry juice to speed the healing of urinary tract infections. Green ephedra tea is one of this region's most pleasant beverage teas.

This initiatory plant, strongly connected with fire and the sun, burns away anything that impedes the embodiment of one's mission in life.

⚠ Caution

Some people may find green ephedra overly stimulating. If so, cut back on the dosage or try something else.

Future Harvests

This is slow-growing plant inhabits harsh environments. Take only a few branch ends from each bush, and limit your cuts to the newer green growth to ensure stem regeneration. Do not cut the woody branches.

HERBAL PREPARATIONS

Stem Tea

Standard decoction; each batch of herb can be decocted 3 or 4 times.

Drink 4–6 fluid ounces up to 3 times per day for lung issues or 1 quart throughout the day for urinary tract infections.

Stem Tincture

1 part dried stems

5 parts menstruum (50 percent alcohol, 40 percent distilled water, 10 percent glycerin)

The fibrous stems (which are too tough to process fresh) grind into a mass of fluff that completely fills the jar. The plant material will absorb the liquid and form a gooey wad. Check frequently during the first couple of days of maceration. If the herb material is exposed, add a bit more menstruum to cover it.

Take 30–60 drops up to 3 times per day.

gumweed

Grindelia hirsutula
PARTS USED bud

Immature flower heads exude a bitter resin that alleviates asthma and spasmodic coughs, speeds the healing of urinary tract infections, and relieves poison oak rashes.

How to Identify

Red to yellowish green, few- to several-branched stems stand 8–32 inches tall alternately lined with somewhat resinous, smooth-edged to slightly toothed leaves. Lance-shaped and yellowish to reddish green, the leaves may be resinous and hairless or covered with densely matted woolly hairs. Composite flower heads in a resinous, green, bell-shaped cup lined with 4–7 whorls of strongly reflexed and pointy-tipped bracts bloom from late spring to early autumn. Initially the flowers, whose tops are covered with a thick white resin, appear to lack ray flowers. As the resin dissipates, the yellow ray flowers emerge, and soon after the disk flowers begin to bloom. Dry seeds tipped with 2–4 narrow, bristle-like appendages mature to a light to reddish brown color. The upper leaves become stalkless and somewhat oblong but not much smaller than the lower leaves, and the basal leaves may or may not persist during flowering.

Recently several distinct species, some hairy and some not, of the highly variable genus *Grindelia* have been grouped under the name *G. hirsutula*. Though this may seem confusing, rest assured that any species of gumweed you encounter in this region will make good medicine.

Where, When, and How to Wildcraft

Growing from the coast to middle elevations in the mountains, this short-lived perennial is found from the extreme southern portion of southwestern British Columbia to California. Gumweed inhabits coastal bluffs; dry hillsides with sandy, clay, or serpentine soils; and roadsides or other disturbed areas east of the Cascades in Washington and on both sides of the Cascade Crest in Oregon. Pluck the sticky buds one by one before the yellow

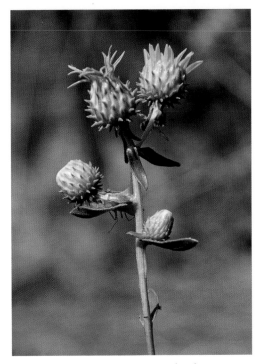

At this point in the upper flowers' development, as the ray flowers are emerging, the amount of resin is beginning to lessen. Harvest at this stage or earlier for the best medicine.

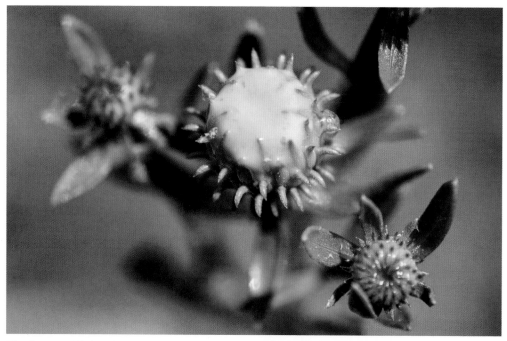

This flower is filled to the brim with white, medicinally active resin.

ray flowers emerge and when the indented tops are filled with white resin.

Medicinal Uses

The bitter, resinous buds clear mucus from the lungs, relax and open the bronchial passages, and relieve spasmodic coughs. Take the tincture in hot water for seasonal allergies, damp asthmatic conditions with chest pain and labored breathing, chronic or acute bronchitis, or harsh dry coughs such as whooping cough.

Add the tincture with its kidney-stimulating oils to water and drink throughout the day to increase urine output, speed the healing of urinary tract infections, and clear mucus from the bladder.

Apply the diluted tincture (1 part tincture to 6 parts water) directly or via compress to soothe poison oak rashes or to stimulate circulation, reduce inflammation, prevent infection, and promote skin cell growth to aid the healing of wounds and ulcers.

Future Harvests

On individual plants there are often flowers in various stages of development. Picking only the perfectly resinous buds will leave many flowers to set seed and allow future generations of gumweed to flourish.

Gather and dry ripe seeds in autumn. In spring sow seeds just below the surface of well-drained soil (directly or in pots) for later transplanting.

HERBAL PREPARATIONS

Bud Tincture
1 part fresh buds
2 parts menstruum (100 percent alcohol)
or
1 part dried buds
5 parts menstruum (70 percent alcohol, 30 percent distilled water)
Take 15–45 drops up to 5 times per day.

hairy arnica

Arnica mollis

PARTS USED flower

Aromatic resinous flower heads speed the healing of sprains, strains, and bruises.

How to Identify

Spreading by rhizome, single stems stand erect, 8–24 inches tall, and bear 2–4 pairs of lance-shaped to elliptic, oppositely arranged leaves with smooth or shallowly and irregularly toothed edges. Smaller than the stem leaves, the generally elliptic basal leaves usually fall before the plant flowers. From early to late summer, a single daisy-like, composite flower head cupped by sticky and hairy bracts blooms with 12–20, ½- to 1-inch-long yellow ray flowers that are toothed at the tips. Small yellow disk flowers fill the center of the flower head and ripen into small wind-borne seeds crowned with feathery, yellowish brown hairs. Two smaller flower heads usually emerge later on shorter stalks below the central flower head. The entire plant is covered with sticky resinous hairs, and after pollination the flower heads quickly turn into balls of white fluff.

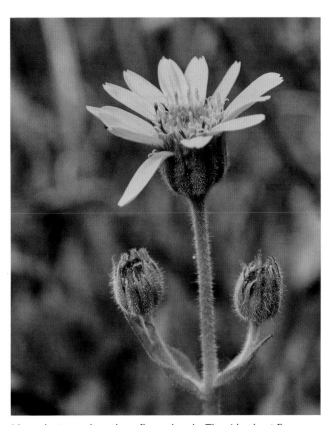

Most plants produce three flower heads. The side-shoot flower heads bloom later than the central one.

Several other species of *Arnica* can be found in this region. The two most common are heartleaf arnica (*Arnica cordifolia*), which has (as you might guess) heart-shaped leaves, and broadleaf arnica (*A. latifolia*), which is shorter than hairy arnica and has lance-shaped leaves. Neither of these forest-dwelling species have sticky hairs, but their flowers make good medicine.

Where, When, and How to Wildcraft

Inhabiting wet, subalpine to alpine meadows and growing along streams in open-canopied forests at middle to high elevations in the mountains, this herbaceous perennial can be found on both sides of the Cascades from British Columbia to California.

The bloom time of hairy arnica varies depending on location, elevation, and climactic factors. Each year the timing is different and seems increasingly erratic as weather patterns shift. The ideal time to harvest ranges from the late budding stage to the time just before the disk flowers are about to open. The window is small, as the plants develop rapidly from bud to flower to fluffy white seed head. The flowers will make good medicine after they've been pollinated but lose their potency rapidly as the seeds develop. Visit your stands early to see how the plants are progressing. Pluck the flowers from the stems by hand. Process fresh for oil or tincture.

Medicinal Uses

The stimulating flowers of hairy arnica are the most aromatic of this region's native species and make an excellent topical remedy for bruises, achy joints, and sore muscles. Apply the flower oil or liniment to any sprain, strain, or bruise to speed the removal of waste products from the site of the injury. If applied soon after a blunt force trauma occurs, a bruise may not even form. These same preparations also relieve joint inflammation and carpal tunnel syndrome.

Small doses of the tincture open the circulation to relieve restless leg syndrome, open the heart to bring joy and release tightness in the chest, and especially after major physical traumas like a car or bike accident, increase the effectiveness of external applications.

 Caution

This is a low-dose botanical. Use the tincture with caution and do not exceed recommended dosage. Because the oils in the plant are quite irritating, do not use arnica in any form on broken skin or allow it to make contact with delicate mucous membranes. Even chewing one little ray flower will tear up your mouth.

Future Harvests

Because the central flower and the side-shoot flowers emerge at different times, I feel comfortable gathering freely from a stand. Each plant I harvest from will have at least one flower that will have the opportunity to set seed.

In the past people harvested the whole plant for medicine, and in some areas arnica has become endangered. There is no need to take the life of the plant when the flowers alone make great medicine. By only harvesting the flowers, we can ensure arnica's long-term viability.

HERBAL PREPARATIONS

Flower Oil

Follow the directions for Fresh Herb Infused Oil on page 63.

Some folks prefer the dried flowers for medicine, but because the seeds will ripen and turn to white fluff even after they have been picked, I make mine with fresh flowers.

Flower Tincture

1 part fresh flowers
2 parts menstruum (100 percent alcohol)
Take 1–5 drops up to 3 times per day.

---

herb Robert

Geranium robertianum
Robert geranium, stinky Bob
PARTS USED root, leaf

Astringent leaves and roots reduce inflammation, soothe sore throats, and stop bleeding.

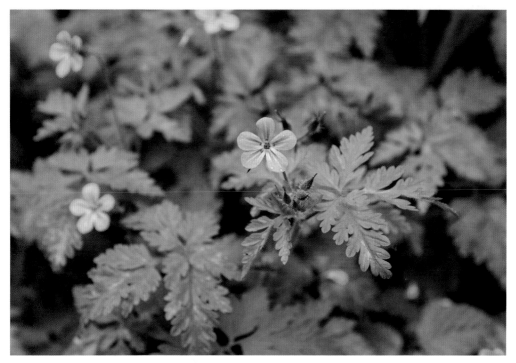

The root and the unpleasant-smelling leaves are helpful for a wide range of inflammatory conditions where the integrity of the tissues is compromised.

How to Identify

Light green, sometimes reddish leaves that smell like burnt rubber or plastic with 3–5 deeply dissected lobes and a triangular to pentagonal silhouette arise from a slender taproot. The 5-petalled, pink to reddish purple flowers, usually 2 per long flowering stalk, have 10 stamens and bristle-tipped sepals (the usually green segments of the floral envelope). At maturity, the 5-parted, beaked-capsule fruits peel open from the bottom to explosively release their seeds.

Where, When, and How to Wildcraft

This annual or biennial, introduced from Europe, has found a home in the western part of this region from southwestern British Columbia to California. It grows at low elevations in open to shaded forests, moist clearings, disturbed areas, and grassy meadows. Harvest the leaves when the plant is flowering. Dig the roots from early summer to late autumn.

Medicinal Uses

All parts of this plant are astringent and helpful for a wide range of inflammatory conditions where the tissues need tightening. An infusion or poultice of the roots or leaves applied externally relieves pain and inflammation from bites, stings, cuts, and abrasions. Gargle the root or leaf tea for a sore throat, or swish it around in the mouth to soothe inflamed gums.

Internally these same preparations reduce intestinal inflammation and temper the dehydrating effects of diarrhea. The powdered root applied topically stops bleeding.

Future Harvests

This plant needs no help establishing itself. In habitats where it thrives, herb Robert can take over and choke out native vegetation. It produces chemicals that prevent other plants from growing around it and uses a propulsive seed dispersal mechanism to colonize new areas. When harvesting this plant, avoid spreading the seeds to other places.

HERBAL PREPARATIONS

Leaf Tea
Standard infusion
Drink 2–4 fluid ounces up to 5 times per day.

Root Tea
Standard decoction
Drink 2–4 fluid ounces up to 5 times per day.

highbush cranberry

Viburnum edule
cramp bark, mooseberry, squashberry
PARTS USED bark

Astringent and somewhat pungent bark relaxes both smooth and
skeletal muscles to relieve cramps, spasms, and asthmatic constriction.

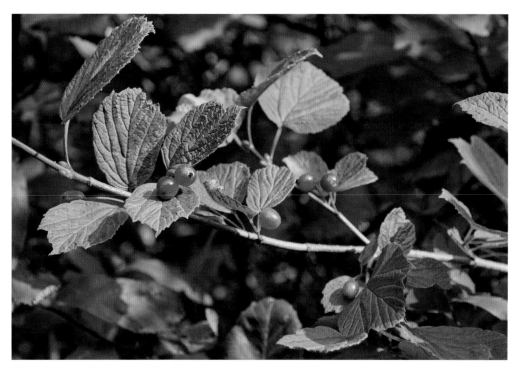

The red, sour-tasting berries ripen from late to summer to early autumn.

How to Identify

New, smooth- and reddish barked stems, reaching heights of 3–10 feet but rarely growing larger than 1½ inches in diameter, emerge from spreading rhizomes to sprawl or stand erect as their bark grays with age and becomes warty. Where the oppositely arranged, sharply toothed, and shallowly 3-lobed leaves, 1–4 inches long, emerge from the stem, a pair of persistent bud scales flare out. Sometimes hairy underneath, the

stalked, elliptical leaves turn bright red in the autumn before they fall to the ground. Short stalks bearing a single pair of leaves carry flat or rounded clusters of fewer than 50 white flowers that bloom from late spring to mid summer with inconspicuous stamens and petals that fuse to form 5-lobed tubes. Red to orange, sour, edible berry-like drupes, ⅜ to ⅝ inch long and containing a single flattened pit, sweeten after a frost and often remain on the plant through winter. Some leaves may lack lobes, and a pair of glands may be present where the leaf stalk meets the blade.

Where, When, and How to Wildcraft

This many-branched, moisture-loving shrub tolerates low temperatures and grows throughout this region on both sides of the Cascades from Alaska to northern Oregon where higher temperatures and lower precipitation restrict its range. Find highbush cranberry from the coast to upper-middle elevations in gravelly or rocky, nitrogen-rich soils along streams, at the edges of lakes and wet forests, or in swampy areas. In drier areas, it inhabits the wettest places. It becomes more abundant farther from the sea and, though shade-tolerant, does best in full sunlight.

Harvest mature stems after the leaves emerge in spring. Strip the bark promptly and dry on screens or in bags.

Medicinal Uses

Highbush cranberry bark is antispasmodic and astringent, and it reduces inflammation. The tea or tincture aids both smooth and skeletal muscle cramping. Use it to relieve menstrual and leg cramps, to stop intestinal and bladder spasms, to prevent threatened miscarriage, and to relax asthmatic constriction and bronchial inflammation. It may also provide some relief of pain from endometriosis, the abnormal growth of the uterine lining outside of the uterus.

Future Harvests

Harvest a few branches per plant from large stands, and propagate whenever possible. The seed is difficult to sprout, but stem cuttings can be rooted by placing them in a bucket or jar of water. After the roots develop, plant the cuttings in wet, nutrient-rich soil.

HERBAL PREPARATIONS

Bark Tea
Standard decoction
Drink 4–6 fluid ounces up to 3 times per day.

Bark Tincture
1 part dried bark
5 parts menstruum (50 percent alcohol, 50 percent distilled water)
Take 30–60 drops up to 5 times per day.

Himalayan blackberry

Rubus armeniacus

PARTS USED leaf, root bark

Astringent leaves and root bark allay the effects of diarrhea, soothe inflammatory skin conditions, and heal bleeding hemorrhoids.

How to Identify

Hooked prickles, stout and flattened, arm clambering 5-angled stems that sprawl 20 feet or more from a deep-growing, woody root system. Alternately arranged, palm-shaped compound leaves with sharply toothed, pointy-tipped, egg-shaped leaflets, 5 on first-year canes and usually 3 on the flowering second-year canes, are green and hairless above and grayish white and woolly with prickly midveins below. Clusters of 5–20 white to pinkish, 5-petalled flowers bloom from mid spring to early summer and ripen into black or dark purple, sweet, juicy, globe-shaped aggregations of small, fleshy fruits with stony seeds. The biennial stems grow erect and tend to arch over and root in or trail along the ground.

Where, When, and How to Wildcraft

Introduced from Eurasia in the late 1800s, this thicket-forming perennial shrub has adapted well to the Pacific Northwest climate. Himalayan blackberry thrives almost everywhere in areas wet or dry. Find it in gardens, disturbed lands, abandoned farms, open sites, and riparian areas at low elevations from British Columbia to California.

Harvest the leaves when the plant is flowering and the roots throughout the year. Remove the bark from the roots and process fresh or dried.

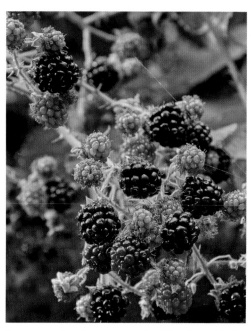

Ever-present and ever-expanding Himalayan blackberry bushes offer more than just delicious berries.

Medicinal Uses

The leaves and root bark of blackberry resolve mucus, dry tissues, and stop bleeding. Gargle a tea of either for throat inflammation, mouth sores, or bleeding gums. Drink the tea for diarrhea or to reduce inflammation and tone and dry mucous membranes of the digestive tract. If diarrhea is from an intestinal infection, it is wise to let it run its course, but if the diarrhea lasts for more than 2 days, it can lead to dehydration and weakness. Identify and treat the root cause, and drink

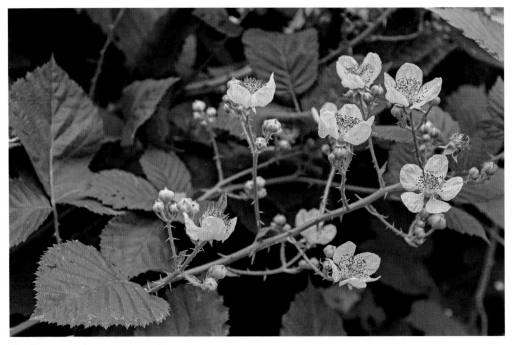

The flowers are borne on second-year canes.

a cup of tea every hour until the diarrhea stops. If the condition persists for more than a few days and the herbs aren't helping to resolve the issue, consult a qualified health care professional.

For damp, white discharges of the female genitourinary system, apply a vaginal douche. An external wash speeds the healing of wounds, soothes inflammatory skin conditions, and heals bleeding hemorrhoids. The root bark contains higher levels of tannins and is more astringent than the leaf.

Future Harvests

We've all seen old barns consumed and completely overtaken by blackberry brambles. Because it grows so vigorously, spreads through layering, and has seeds that are well dispersed by animals, Himalayan blackberry will also overrun gardens, stream banks, and natural areas. We need not worry about its future availability.

HERBAL PREPARATIONS

Leaf Tea
Standard infusion
Drink 4–6 fluid ounces up to 3 times per day.

Root Bark Tea
Standard decoction
Drink 3–4 fluid ounces up to 3 times per day.

Root Bark Tincture
1 part fresh root bark
2 parts menstruum (75 percent alcohol, 15 percent distilled water, 10 percent glycerin)
or
1 part dried root bark
5 parts menstruum (50 percent alcohol, 40 percent distilled water, 10 percent glycerin)
Take 30–60 drops up to 4 times per day.

hookedspur violet

Viola adunca
early blue violet, western dog violet
PARTS USED herb

Cooling and moistening leaves and flowers bring relief to dry and inflamed mucous membranes, restore lymphatic flow, and soothe sore throats.

How to Identify

Branched stems from slender, hairy rhizomes produce short- to long-stalked, round to egg-shaped, hairless to minutely hairy leaves with finely blunt-toothed edges. During the spring, single, blue to dark violet flowers flare out 5-petaled at the end of curved-topped stalks. Bee-guiding white patches with purple veins mark the bases of the 3 lower petals. Short, frilly white hairs beard the hook-spur-tipped lateral pair, and a slender spur extends over half the petal's length from the rear of the central petal. The upper pair of petals stands erect or reflexes strongly backward. Smooth, 3-valved pods explosively eject dark brown seeds far into the forest. This highly variable species produces petaled flowers in spring and self-pollinating, seed-producing flowers that remain budded later in the season. This type of flower, called cleistogamous from the Greek "closed marriage," forms underground and lays its ant-attracting seeds on the earth's surface or deposits them directly into the soil.

Where, When, and How to Wildcraft

Reaching heights up to 4 inches tall, these shade-loving spring beauties inhabit dry to moist meadows, open woods, grasslands, and disturbed sites from sea level to near timberline throughout this region. Widely distributed across North America, their occurrence decreases with elevation and in places with higher levels of precipitation.

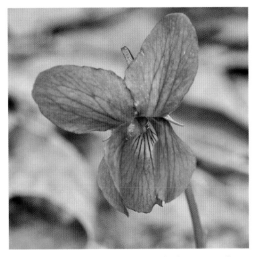

Purple-veined white patches on the lower petals guide pollinating bees to the flower's nectar.

All species of violet possess healing virtues, but the blue species are preferred for medicine. Collect the aerial parts while the plants are blooming. Process fresh for tincture or dry on screens for tea.

Medicinal Uses

Containing flavonoids, saponins, and salicylates, violet herb cools and moistens dry inflamed tissues, clears lymphatic stagnation, and relieves pain. Take the tea or tincture to soothe dry, raw, and inflamed digestive or respiratory tract tissue or to reduce dry, bloodshot eye soreness. Use these same preparations for dry asthma, bronchitis, or whooping cough.

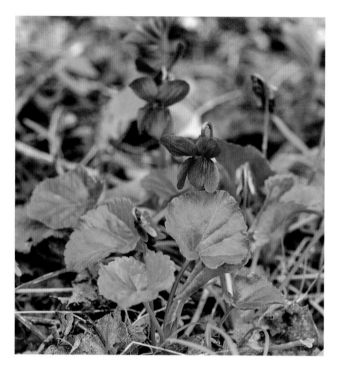

Delightful patches of low-growing violets enliven the forest floor in spring.

Future Harvests

Violets are plentiful throughout their range, but if you'd like to help them out you can propagate them from seed. As their stems uncurl, the almost mature seedpods start to face upward and turn from green to a yellowish or purple color. You'll need to collect the capsules before they explode. Test a few likely candidates for ripe, brown seeds (immature seeds will still be white). Once you've determined which capsules contain ripened seeds, pick similar looking pods, place them in a closed paper bag, and wait for them to eject their seeds. Store the seeds in plastic bags in a cool, dry place, and sow them in autumn. Violets are not amenable to root division.

Take the tea or tincture to restore lymphatic flow and reduce glandular swelling, especially in the throat and ears, or to speed the removal of waste products to alleviate eczema and other dry, itchy skin conditions.

Violet herb tea or tincture also relieves constipation, increases urine output to remove deposits, and soothes urinary tract irritation. When poulticed fresh and taken internally as tea, violet herb relieves joint and muscle pain and has been used traditionally to reduce the size of cancerous tumors in the breasts or lymphatic system. The syrup is especially indicated for sore throats made raw from coughing.

⚠ Caution

Violet seeds are considered somewhat toxic, and the roots reportedly provoke vomiting.

HERBAL PREPARATIONS

Herb Tea
Long or cold infusion
Drink 4–6 fluid ounces up to 5 times per day.

Herb Tincture
1 part fresh herb
2 parts menstruum (75 percent alcohol, 25 percent distilled water)
Take 30–60 drops up to 5 times per day.

horehound

Marrubium vulgare
white horehound
PARTS USED leaf

Bitter leaves relieve coughs, expel mucus from the lungs, stimulate digestion, and promote menstruation.

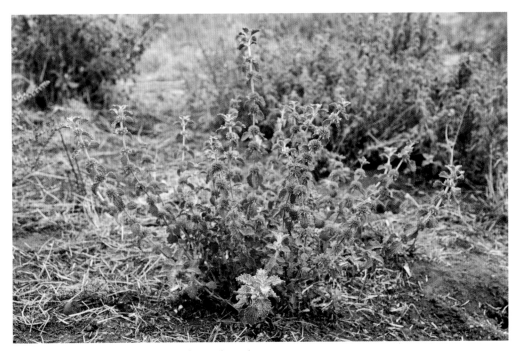

Scruffy-looking horehound thrives in dry, rocky soils.

How to Identify

From a thick taproot several square stems covered with long, interwoven white hairs spread out horizontally or curve upward. Becoming shorter-stalked but only slightly smaller as they near the top, oppositely arranged pairs of round to broadly egg-shaped, round-toothed leaves, green and fur-rowed above and blanketed with white wooly hairs below, line the 1- to 3-foot-tall branching stems. Whitish, tubular, 2-lipped flowers bloom from early summer to mid autumn in dense whorls in the leaf axils. The 2-toothed upper lip stands erect, and the 3-lobed lower lip flares out with a wide, creased central lobe. Persistent calyces with 10 spiny-tipped teeth house clusters of 4 smooth ovoid nutlets. After the calyces have dried, they cling to passersby, who unwittingly aid the dispersal of the seeds.

Where, When, and How to Wildcraft

Introduced from Eurasia and common throughout North America, this herbaceous perennial mint inhabits dry and disturbed soils from British Columbia to California. Find horehound along roadsides and in fields and pasturelands at low to middle elevations mostly east of the Cascades in Washington and Oregon. In southern Oregon and northern California, its range extends westward to the coast.

Clip stems at the base as they begin to flower. Process fresh for tincture, or dry in bundles or on screens.

Medicinal Uses

The leaf syrup especially, but the tea or tincture as well, eases coughing and soothes hoarse, inflamed throats. Take any of these preparations for bronchitis or just about any type of cough, including whooping cough and moist, dry, raspy, chronic, or asthmatic coughs.

The hot tea or the tincture or syrup in hot water promotes sweating to break the fever of a cold or flu and stimulates the expulsion of mucus to clear congested lungs. The tincture or the cooled tea improves digestion, stimulates appetite, and relieves indigestion. The hot tea stimulates uterine secretions to bring on delayed menses.

 Caution

Do not use during pregnancy. Long-term use may raise blood pressure. Ingesting large quantities is laxative and may cause nausea or vomiting.

Future Harvests

Collect seeds in autumn and sow in early spring.

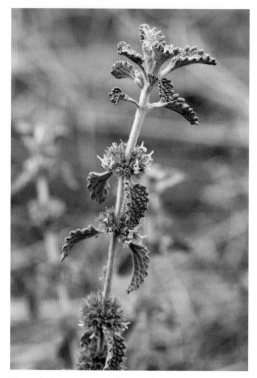

Densely interwoven, white, and wooly hairs cover the leaves, and spiny teeth help the seed-bearing calyces attach to the clothing or fur of passersby.

HERBAL PREPARATIONS

Leaf Tea

Standard infusion, neat or sweetened with honey

Drink 2–4 fluid ounces up to 5 times per day.

Leaf Tincture

1 part fresh leaf

2 parts menstruum (75 percent alcohol, 25 percent distilled water)

or

1 part dried leaf

5 parts menstruum (50 percent alcohol, 50 percent distilled water)

Take 15–45 drops up to 5 times per day.

Equisetum arvense
field horsetail, scouring rush
PARTS USED vegetative stalk

Mineral-rich stalks provide the building blocks for connective tissue, bones, hair, and nails; support the kidneys; and clear urinary tract infections.

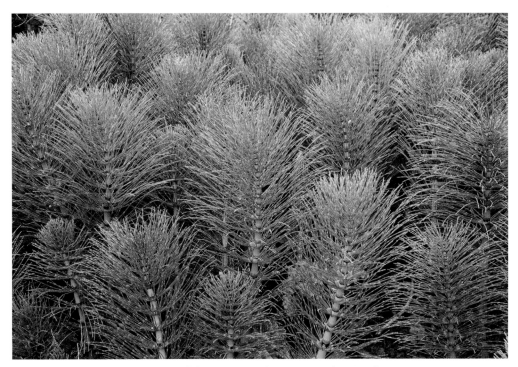

During the Paleozoic era, ancestors of these ancient plants grew to the size of trees.

How to Identify

From creeping rhizomes in early spring, whitish or brownish, non-photosynthesizing reproductive stalks rise to the surface. Topped with a cone that carries whorled rows of spore-bearing dots, these fleshy, fertile stems, growing up to 12 inches tall, are followed by hollow and ridged, 6- to 24-inch tall green vegetative stems. Small leaves fuse into toothed sheaths around the stalks, and whorls of branches radiate out from the nodes. Emerging upright, the branches elongate and hang down as the season progresses. The rhizomes, which look similar to the stems but are not hollow, produce storage tubers.

Except for the potentially toxic marsh horsetail (*Equisetum palustre*), all other species of *Equisetum* found in the Pacific Northwest may be used interchangeably with *E. arvense*.

Where, When, and How to Wildcraft

Horsetail prefers wet soils and grows at all elevations throughout this region. Harvest the sterile green shoots from early spring to early summer before the branches droop below horizontal.

Medicinal Uses

The stalks of this fern ally supply the body with minerals crucial to maintaining healthy structures. With its ridged stems and whorled branches, the plant itself is a model of structural integrity. As one of the few plants high in bio-available silica, drinking the tea helps repair and strengthen damaged connective tissue, mend broken bones, and

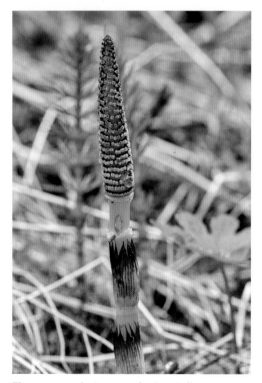

The spore-producing reproductive stalks emerge before the vegetative stalks but are not used for medicine.

promote strong hair and nail growth. In addition, the tea nourishes and strengthens the kidneys and bladder.

Diuretic horsetail stalk tea or tincture lowers urine pH to clear urinary tract infections and helps dissolve urinary stones and deposits. These same preparations stop internal bleeding or excessive menstrual flow, and an external wash helps poorly healing sores, stanches bleeding wounds, and reduces gum inflammation when gargled.

⚠ Caution

Consumption of horsetail for long periods may lead to thiamine deficiency. Also, the concentration of silica becomes too high at a certain point in the plant's life cycle and may cause gastrointestinal upset when consumed. To avoid this, herbalists harvest the stems before the branches droop down below horizontal. Avoid ingesting preparations of the closely related marsh horsetail (*Equisetum palustre*) as it may contain toxic compounds.

Future Harvests

You would be hard pressed to hinder the growth of this tough plant, which is considered an invasive weed by some. However, harvest respectfully.

HERBAL PREPARATIONS

Stalk Tea
Long infusion or standard decoction
Drink 2–4 fluid ounces up to 4 times per day.

Stalk Tincture
1 part fresh stalk
2 parts menstruum (100 percent alcohol)
Take 15–45 drops up to 4 times per day.

king's gentian

Gentiana sceptrum
king's scepter gentian
PARTS USED herb

Gentian, the bitter by which all other bitters are measured,
gets the digestive juices flowing and stimulates liver metabolism.

How to Identify

From a clump of fleshy roots, 1- to 2-foot-tall hairless stems bear several pairs of oppositely arranged, oblong leaves that increase in size from bottom to top. During summer, striking, often green-spotted, bluish purple flowers, solitary to several, emerge atop slightly nodding stems and from the upper leaf axils. The flowers, encased in a cup of 5 fused sepals, are pointy-tipped when closed and slowly unfurl to display 5 rounded lobes that top the tubular corolla. The space between these lobes is pleated.

When tasted on the tongue, the bitter flavor sends a cascade of signals through the entire digestive tract to prepare it for digestion.

Where, When, and How to Wildcraft

This regal gentian resides in wet areas throughout the western part of this region. Find it along lake edges and in low- to middle-elevation bogs, fens, and meadows.

The Pacific Northwest is rich in gentians. If you are unable to find king's gentian in your area, consult a more comprehensive field guide or flora to find other species, but do not harvest species listed as sensitive on the U.S. Forest Service's Special Status Species List.

In the summer months, harvest one or two flowering stalks from each plant. Snip the stems at the base and discard

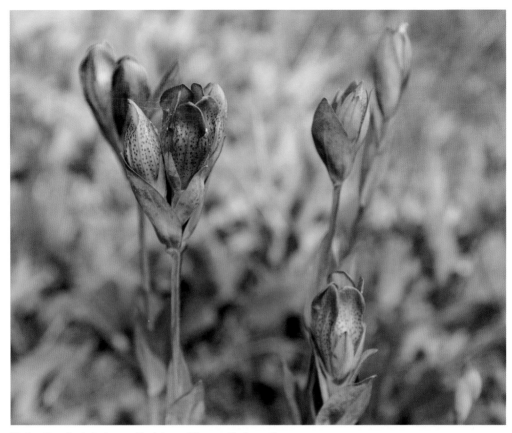

Notice the pleats between the lobes of the spotted corolla.

brown or damaged leaves. Use all of the aerial parts for medicine. When harvesting in meadows stay on the trail. One or two errant boot stomps can kill the sensitive plants that reside there and leave long-lasting impressions in the soil. Please be mindful of your impact on these ecosystems.

Medicinal Uses

Bitter glycosides found in all species of gentian stimulate the secretion of digestive juices and enzymes that help the body break down food and absorb nutrients. If you experience bloating, gas, a feeling of fullness after meals, or undigested food in the stools, take the tea or tincture 10–15 minutes before meals to support digestive function.

Beyond its effect on the digestive system, gentian herb also stimulates liver metabolism to help remove impurities from the blood, and because it affects nerves that interface with the gut, taking the herb tea or tincture aids those prone to nervousness or anxiety. If you are wondering about the connection, think about the feeling of butterflies in your stomach that comes when you are nervous.

Taking the tea or tincture also helps those who obsessively ruminate and get caught in patterns of circular thinking learn to properly digest their experiences.

Future Harvests

Traditionally herbalists preferred the roots of this popular medicinal plant, but harvesting pressure has virtually wiped out the main European species, *Gentiana lutea*, from the wild. Although the leaves aren't nearly as bitter as the roots, they get the job done and leave the plant intact to live another day.

Harvest conservatively and take only one or two stalks per plant. This is especially important for plants growing at higher elevations that need to do all of their photosynthesizing in a very short period of time.

HERBAL PREPARATIONS

Herb Tea
Standard infusion
Drink 2–4 fluid ounces up to 3 times per day.

Herb Tincture
1 part fresh herb
2 parts menstruum (75 percent alcohol, 25 percent distilled water)
Take 15–20 drops up to 3 times per day.

Make Your Own Local Bitter Tonic

Gentians are a favored ingredient in bitter tonic formulas worldwide. Generally, these formulas are made up of intense bitters like gentian or buckbean with aromatic bitters like mugwort or wormwood and pungent carminatives like sweetroot or angelica.

To make your own local formula, combine these ingredients.

3 parts gentian herb tincture
3 parts Oregon grape root tincture
2 parts sweetroot tincture
1 part angelica root tincture
1 part mugwort leaf tincture

Labrador tea

Ledum palustre subsp. *groenlandicum*
bog Labrador tea
PARTS USED leaf

*Spicy and aromatic leaves speed the healing of colds and flus and clear mucus
from the lungs and sinuses. Externally the leaves kill lice and help resolve
external fungal infections.*

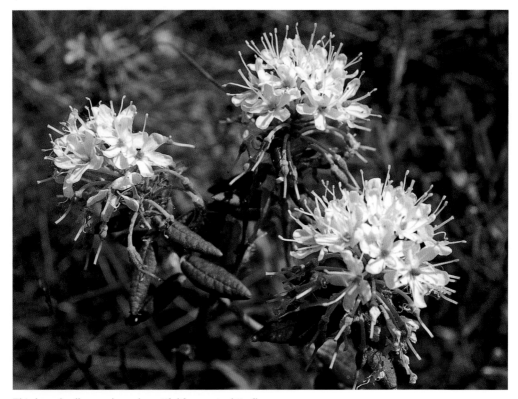

This bog-dweller produces beautiful fragrant white flowers.

How to Identify

Multiple, spreading, 2- to 5-foot-long branches form rounded evergreen shrubs. Densely curly-haired new-growth stems become smooth as they age. Resinous and aromatic, 1- to 3-inch-long, narrowly elliptic leaves, leathery, hairless, dark green, and semi-wrinkly above and densely covered with felt-like orange-brown hairs below, roll under at the edges and droop downward as they mature. The alternately arranged leaves are blunt-tipped. Many fragrant white flowers with 5 spreading petals and protruding stamens bloom from late spring to late summer in short clusters at the ends of branches. Somewhat egg-shaped, fuzzy,

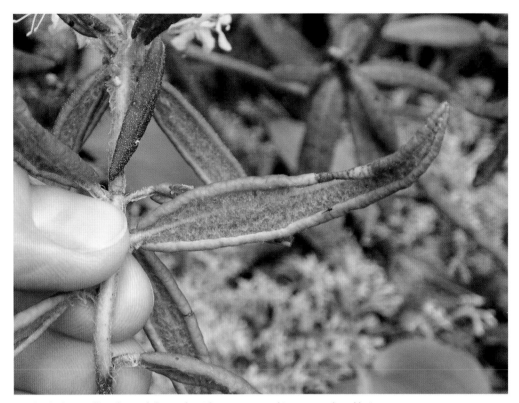

The leaf edges roll under and the undersides are covered in rusty-colored hairs.

5-parted capsules, ⅛ to ⅜ inch long and each tipped with a persistent style, open at the base to release many seeds in autumn. Empty capsules may remain attached to the plant for years.

The closely related trapper's tea (*Ledum glandulosum*) is distinguished by leaves with usually white-haired undersides. Use it in the same way you would use Labrador tea.

Where, When, and How to Wildcraft

Labrador tea (formerly *Ledum groenlandicum*) resides in bogs, fens, muskegs, swamps, and peatlands in wet, coniferous forests throughout the upper reaches of North America. In the Pacific Northwest, it grows at low to middle elevations across Alaska and British Columbia and can be found west of the Cascades in Washington and northern Oregon.

Cut branch ends above an outward-facing node from mid summer to mid autumn after the plants set seed. Dry in bags or on screens.

Medicinal Uses

The spicy-aromatic leaves make a nice beverage tea that speeds the healing of colds and flus, clears mucus from the lungs and sinuses, relieves constipation, and soothes digestive upset. To get rid of lice, apply the fresh tincture externally, remove nits daily with a special lice comb, and wash all of your linens in hot water. The fresh tincture diluted in water and rubbed into the skin helps resolve fungal infections.

Caution

The leaves contain ledol, a toxic substance that may, in large doses, cause cramps, delirium, and paralysis. Do not ingest concentrated, long infusions or decoctions of the leaves. In normal doses the standard infusion is considered safe, but avoid drinking the tea during pregnancy or while nursing.

Future Harvests

Left alone, fire-tolerant Labrador tea becomes leggy and produces fewer leaves over time. Indigenous peoples intentionally set periodic fires in the areas where it grew not only to stimulate new growth but to prevent the surrounding forest from taking over the wetlands where the plants thrive. Today it is not feasible to set fires in the forest, but we can harvest and prune shrubs to stimulate new, bushy growth.

If you'd like to propagate this handsome shrub, collect seeds from dried capsules and sow them in autumn or spring in acidic, peaty soil. Rooted suckers can also be removed from the crowns and transplanted to appropriate sites.

HERBAL PREPARATIONS

Leaf Tea
Standard infusion
Drink 4–6 fluid ounces up to 3 times per day.

Leaf Tincture
1 part fresh leaf
2 parts menstruum (100 percent alcohol)
For external use only.

lemon balm

Melissa officinalis
common balm
PARTS USED leaf

Gentle but strong, lemon balm is a cooling digestive aid that both calms and uplifts the spirit, calms overactive thyroid, and speeds the healing of herpes lesions and flus.

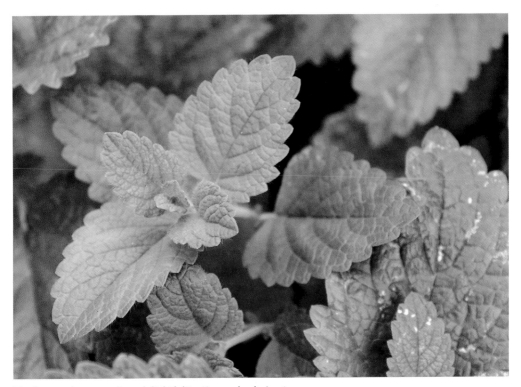

The lemony leaves make a delightful tasting and calming tea.

How to Identify

Lemon-scented, deeply veined, oppositely arranged leaves line often-branching square stems that rise up to 3 feet tall from fibrous-rooted, woody rhizomes. The vibrantly green, coarsely blunt-toothed, egg-shaped, 1½- to 3½-inch-long leaves gradually become smaller and shorter-stalked as they ascend the stem. Small, 2-lipped flowers, white to yellow to pinkish, bloom in whorls around the upper leaf axils from early to late summer. Four stamens hug the flat, notched upper lip. The hairy lower lip spreads outward in 3 lobes to guide bees and other pollinating insects to the flower's nectar. Pollinated flowers produce clusters of 4 smooth, egg-shaped seeds that nest in persistent green calyces with spiny-tipped teeth. The leaves are slightly

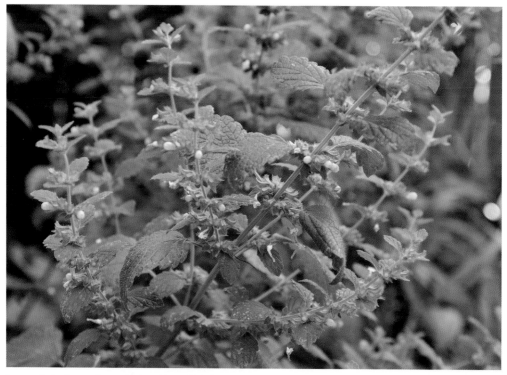

Lemon balm has a deep relationship with bees. Its Latin name, *Melissa*, comes from the same Greek root as that of the European honey bee, *Apis mellifera*.

hairy with a somewhat crinkled appearance. As the season progresses the lower part of the stalk becomes rigid while the upper new-growth portion remains pliable.

Where, When, and How to Wildcraft

A widespread garden escapee introduced from Eurasia, this perennial mint inhabits moist places, ditches, meadows, trail sides, and disturbed areas from Alaska to California. Lemon balm grows in full sun or partial shade and may show up in your garden unexpectedly.

Harvest from early to late summer just prior to or during the initial stage of flowering. Clip the stalks at the base and remove discolored leaves. For teas, bundle the stems at the base with rubber bands or string and hang to dry. Remove the leaves as soon as they are completely dry and store in airtight containers in a cool, dark place. Stored well, the delicate leaves of lemon balm will retain their medicinal properties for between 6 and 12 months after drying. For tincture, strip the leaves and flowers from the stalks and process them fresh. Include the flexible upper parts of the stem if they have the same lemony flavor as the leaves.

Medicinal Uses

The tea or tincture of lemon balm leaf is mildly antispasmodic and relieves nervous indigestion, nausea, and gas. These same preparations lift the spirit, dispel depression, calm anxiety, and cool an agitated heart. They are especially indicated for those with a rapid or fluttery heartbeat, restlessness, and/or elevated blood pressure. Use the tea or tincture for hyperthyroidism or Graves' disease, an autoimmune condition that causes an overproduction of thyroid hormones.

Apply the full-strength tincture topically and take it internally to lessen the severity of and speed the healing of herpes or shingles outbreaks. The tea drunk hot promotes sweating to break a fever and helps resolve colds and flus. Overstimulated children may relax and find focus after drinking a cup of the tasty tea.

Future Harvests

Lemon balm seeds readily, transplants easily, and, once established, thrives wherever it grows. Even if you cut it to the ground, lemon balm will continuously resprout and provide medicine year after year.

HERBAL PREPARATIONS

Leaf Tea
Standard infusion

A fresh-leaf solar infusion makes a delightfully cooling summer beverage.
Drink as needed or desired.

Leaf Tincture
1 part fresh leaf
2 parts menstruum (100 percent alcohol)
Take 15–60 drops up to 5 times per day.
High-quality tincture has a buttery flavor.

lungwort

Lobaria pulmonaria
lung lichen
PARTS USED thallus

This lichen of damp and shady forests soothes persistent, dry, wheezing coughs.

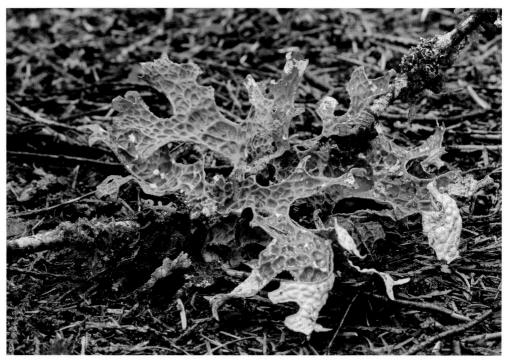

Lungwort, which according to some looks like lung tissue, concentrates air-borne nitrogen in its thallus and releases it into the soil as it decomposes.

How to Identify

Covered with lumps and ridges, the large, lobed, leaf-like thallus of this lichen, an organism made up of a symbiotic partnership between a fungus and an alga, grows lightly attached to rocks and tree bark. It looks like a thick, almost rubbery piece of lettuce. It is bright green when wet and dries to a pale bluish green. The underside is pale and sometimes covered with blue spots.

Where, When, and How to Wildcraft

Found on both coniferous and deciduous trees in humid and shady low-elevation forests throughout this region, lungwort (formerly *Sticta pulmonaria*), like many other lichens, will only grow in clean, healthy ecosystems because of its sensitivity to atmospheric contamination. Gather lungwort that has fallen to the ground during the wet season when it is actively growing from early spring to early summer.

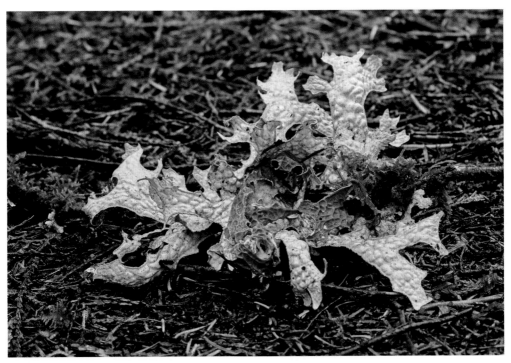

When you harvest lungwort, the underside of the thallus should be vibrantly white.

Medicinal Uses

Lungwort thallus was used by early American botanical doctors to treat various types of coughing. Drink the moistening and soothing tea to relieve dry persistent coughs accompanied by wheezing and irritation. It is also used to treat whooping cough and croup, a childhood viral infection that causes inflammation around the vocal cords, windpipe, and bronchial tubes. This swelling produces a harsh, rasping cough that sounds like the barking of seal.

Future Harvests

For the most sustainable harvest of this slow-growing lichen, only gather lungwort that has fallen to the ground.

HERBAL PREPARATIONS

Thallus Tea
Standard decoction
Traditionally lungwort was decocted in milk to treat coughs.
Drink 4–6 fluid ounces up to 5 times per day.

Arctostaphylos species
PARTS USED leaf

Astringent leaves help heal urinary tract infections, reduce postpartum inflammation and bleeding, and speed the healing of cuts and scrapes.

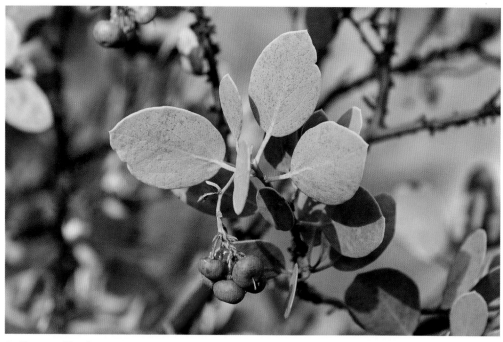

As illustrated by the ripe berries of this greenleaf manzanita, the name manzanita means "little apple" in Spanish.

How to Identify

At least sixteen species of manzanita are native to the Pacific Northwest. All have alternately arranged, smooth-edged, evergreen leaves that are often pointy-tipped and smooth to hairy; sometimes gland-covered twigs; trunks and branches covered with thin, reddish brown or purplish red bark that sheds to reveal smooth, polished skin; and white to pink, urn-shaped, 5-lobed flowers that ripen into small, reddish brown, apple-like, and mealy-textured berries. Leaf stalks often twist to hold leaves erect. Several less common species can be found in the southernmost portions of this region, but three common species are widely distributed throughout the Pacific Northwest.

The young grayish haired twigs of hairy manzanita (*Arctostaphylos columbiana*), a 3- to 10-foot-tall upright shrub lacking a burl, turn purplish red with age. Egg- to lance-shaped to elliptic, dull-surfaced leaves, 1½ to 2½ inches long, covered with white hairs narrow at the tip. Leaf-like bracts hold terminal clusters of

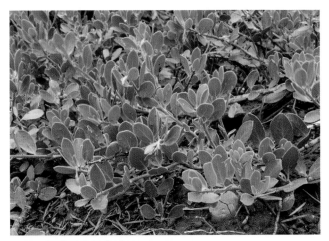

Low-growing pinemat manzanita has a growth habit similar to that of its cousin uva ursi.

white to pink flowers that bloom from late spring to mid summer and ripen into brownish red berries.

The short, mat-forming pinemat manzanita (*Arctostaphylos nevadensis*) sends brownish red–barked branches spreading over 3 feet long across the dry, rocky soils it inhabits. It can be distinguished from its cousin, uva ursi (*A. uva-ursi*), by its brownish red berries and pointy-tipped, lance- to egg-shaped leaves with same-colored sides. Small clusters of white to pinkish flowers bloom from late spring to mid summer.

Greenleaf manzanita (*Arctostaphylos patula*) spreads or stands upright 3–7 feet tall with reddish brown bark. Thick, bright yellow-green, mostly hairless, usually pointy-tipped leaves fan out roundish to egg-shaped and 1 to 2½ inches long. Scale-like bracts skirt the undersides of flower clusters that bloom from late spring to early summer to form dark reddish brown berries.

Where, When, and How to Wildcraft

All manzanita species inhabit dry, rocky or clay soils in sunny openings in oak woodlands, chaparral communities, or pine and mixed coniferous forests. Find hairy manzanita at low elevations west of the Cascades from British Columbia to California; pinemat manzanita from middle to high elevations on both sides of the Cascades from Washington to California; and greenleaf manzanita from low to high elevations east of the Cascades in Washington and on both sides of the Cascade Crest south through Oregon into California.

Collect leaves individually or clip off the ends of stems from mid spring to mid autumn. After drying on screens or in bags, strip the leaves and discard the stems. Store the dried leaves in a glass jar. Adding a tablespoon of grain alcohol to the jar softens the waxy coating on the leaves and makes the medicinal constituents more available.

Medicinal Uses

Manzanita leaf is astringent, reduces inflammation, increases urine output, and makes the urinary tract less hospitable to bacteria like *Escherichia coli*, the main cause of lower urinary tract infections. For acute urinary tract infections, drink the leaf tea along with 1 pint of unsweetened cranberry juice per day to alleviate pain and inflammation and prevent *E. coli* from adhering to the walls of the urethra. Avoid stimulants, alcohol, and sweets, including fruit.

Use a douche of the leaf tea to reduce vaginal inflammation and to speed the healing of yeast infections. Soaking the hips and groin area, known as a sitz bath, in tea-infused water reduces postpartum inflammation and bleeding, and as an external wash decreases redness and swelling, stops

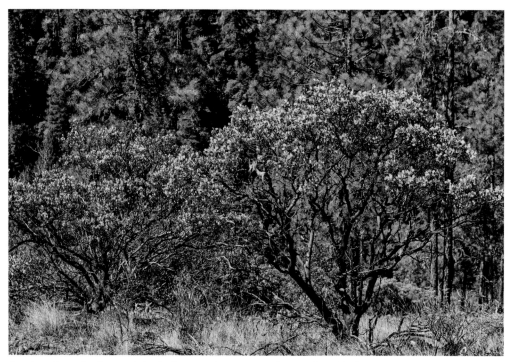

An attractive pair of smooth-barked manzanitas grow in their preferred habitat.

bleeding, and helps heal cuts, scrapes, and abrasions.

Add small amounts of the crushed leaf to herbal smoking blends.

Caution

Do not use during pregnancy. Because the astringent tannins can aggravate the gut, restrict internal use to 3–4 days.

Future Harvests

The extremely fire-tolerant manzanitas rely on periodic burns to maintain their habitat, stimulate growth, and encourage seed germination. After collecting ripe berries, separate and clean the seeds. In a wooden box with drainage holes, sow seeds ¼ inch deep in sandy potting soil, and cover with 4 inches of flammable plant material, such as leaves, pine needles, small sticks, and/or bark. Set it ablaze, and after the fire has died down, thoroughly water the soil. Alternatively, transplant rooted sections of pinemat manzanita into areas with dry, well-drained soil.

HERBAL PREPARATIONS

Leaf Tea
Standard infusion
Drink 3–4 fluid ounces up to 4 times per day.

Leaf Tincture
1 part dried leaf
5 parts menstruum (50 percent alcohol, 50 percent distilled water)
Take 30–60 drops up to 4 times per day; for urinary tract infections, add to 8 fluid ounces of water and sip throughout the day.

Menzies' larkspur

Delphinium menziesii

PARTS USED seed

When applied externally, these toxic seeds provide a reliable remedy to rid the body of scabies and head lice.

How to Identify

Thin, hairless to slightly hairy stems attach to small, tuber-like roots. The few dissected and long-stalked basal leaves divide into palmately cleft segments. The stem leaves are similarly shaped but have shorter stalks, becoming stalkless near the top. Loose clusters of 3–20 deep blue to purplish flowers bloom above the foliage from mid spring to mid summer. Each flower is made up of differently shaped and widely flaring sepals with 4 small petals in the center. The lower pair of petals are blue and lightly veined; the upper pair are white or light blue. A distinctive nectar-containing spur, ½ to ¾ inch long, protrudes from the back of the flower. The seeds are contained in dry, usually hairy, pointy-tipped, 3-parted capsules.

Where, When, and How to Wildcraft

This common larkspur grows on coastal bluffs and prairies and in grasslands, forest openings, and lower mountain meadows west of the Cascades from British Columbia to northern California. Gather the seedpods as they mature from late spring to late summer.

Medicinal Uses

Throughout human history and in many places around the world, larkspur seeds have been made into medicinal preparations to kill lice and scabies. Apply the rubbing alcohol or vinegar tincture of the seeds several days in a row to treat infestations of body or pubic lice and scabies. For head lice, use a shampoo of the seeds, flowers, and buds steeped in tincture of green soap (a liquid soap made from vegetable oils, glycerin, ethyl alcohol, and lavender essential oil that is available in drug stores and from online retailers). Leave it in the hair for 10 minutes before rinsing, being careful not to let it get in the eyes.

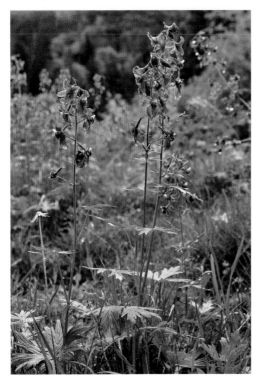

Large stands of vibrantly purple-flowered Menzies' larkspurs bring spring color to meadows and grasslands.

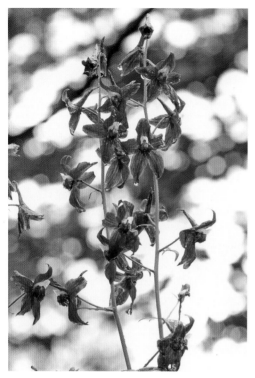

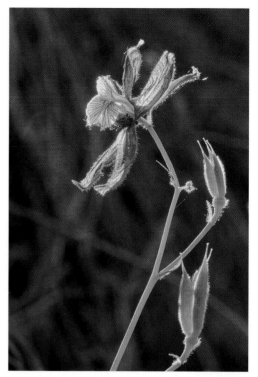

The budded flowers at the top of this flower cluster bear a resemblance to the tiny dolphins from which the delphiniums derive their name.

The pointy-tipped, three-chambered seedpods of this Menzies' larkspur are still ripening and not quite ready for medicine.

 Caution

This is a toxic plant. Do not take any of the preparations internally. Discontinue use if a rash develops, and don't use on open wounds or broken skin as the alkaloids can be absorbed into the bloodstream and cause nausea, vomiting, and other symptoms.

Future Harvests

The tubers are difficult to transplant. Never take more than half the seeds from any given plant, and sow fresh, ripe seeds as you harvest.

mountain monardella

Monardella odoratissima
coyote mint
PARTS USED leaf and flower

Pennyroyal-scented leaves and flowers relieve upset stomachs, promote sweating to break a fever, and stimulate uterine secretions to bring on delayed bleeding.

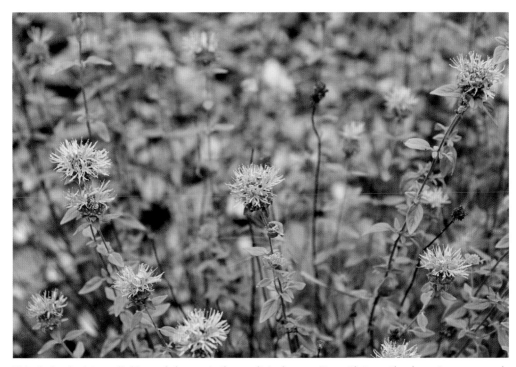

This dryland mint smells like and shares similar medicinal properties with its wetland cousin, pennyroyal.

How to Identify

From a woody base, several usually unbranching, square stems lined with very aromatic, green to gray, ovate to lance-shaped leaves rise up 4–20 inches. The oppositely arranged, ¼- to 1¾-inch-long leaves smell like pennyroyal and are often purple-tinged. Many white to lavender to purple, 2-lipped, tubular flowers bloom from late spring to late summer in dense, terminal, pincushion-like flower heads cupped by several leaf-like purplish bracts with long hairs on the edges. Each flower's upper 2-lobed lip stands erect, while its lower 3-lobed lip bends back. All aerial parts of this clump-forming perennial are hairy.

Where, When, and How to Wildcraft

In the southern part of this region, the distribution of this dryland mint extends from the coast to the eastern border of Oregon and beyond. As mountain monardella spreads northward, the width of its range tapers and moves east until it reaches the narrow tip of its northern limit in far eastern British Columbia. It prefers dry, rocky soils and open areas with full sun at low to middle elevations.

While the plants are flowering between late spring and late summer, snip the stalks just above the node of the lowest pair of healthy leaves. Process fresh for tincture. Include any portion of the stalk that tastes like the leaves. For teas, dry on screens or in bags. Once dried, remove the leaves and flowers, and discard the stalks.

Medicinal Uses

Take the leaf and flower tea or tincture for upset stomachs with gas and bloating, to relieve nausea, and to treat children with colic. Drink the tea hot or take the tincture in hot water to promote sweating to break the fever of a cold or flu. Larger doses of the tea, up to 3 times the normal dose, stimulate the uterus to bring on a delayed menses and resolve the bloating that comes with it.

Caution

Because of its uterine-stimulating properties, this plant is most definitely not for use during pregnancy.

Future Harvests

These plants are slow growing and often inhabit nutrient-lacking soils. Harvest with care, taking just a few stems from each plant.

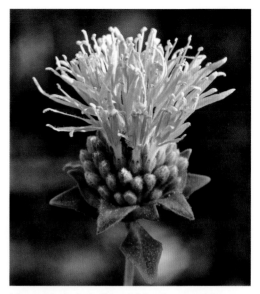

Like most plants in the mint family, mountain monardella produces tubular, two-lipped flowers with a two-lobed upper lip and a three-lobed lower lip.

HERBAL PREPARATIONS

Leaf and Flower Tea
Standard infusion
Drink 2–4 fluid ounces up to 5 times per day.

Leaf and Flower Tincture
1 part fresh leaf and flower
2 parts menstruum (100 percent alcohol)
Take 15–30 drops up to 5 times per day.

mullein

Verbascum thapsus
common or wooly mullein
PARTS USED leaf, flower, root

Famous for its leaves' beneficial effect on the lungs, various parts of mullein also aid the urinary tract, moisten the joints, and clear swollen and congested lymph glands.

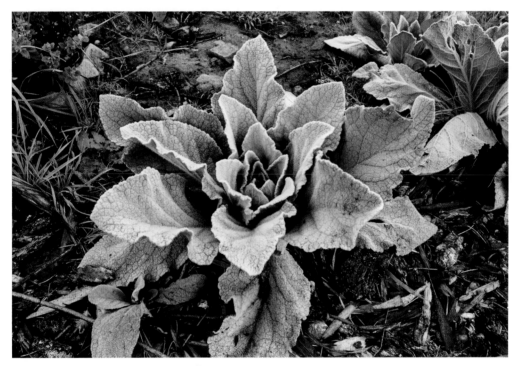

Harvest leaves before the flowering stalks shoot up.

How to Identify

During the first year, a rosette of densely hairy, 4- to 15-inch-long, lance-shaped basal leaves, smooth-edged to inconspicuously round-toothed, taper to broad, winged stalks and radiate out from a crown of thickly growing taproots anchored by fibrous side roots. In its second year of growth, the plant sends up a single, erect, 4- to 6-foot-tall, unbranched flowering stalk alternately lined with numerous leaves that steadily decrease in size as they ascend the stem. The upper leaves become stalkless with clasping bases that extend slightly down the stem from where they attach. Between early summer and early autumn, short-tubed yellow flowers with 5 slightly irregular-shaped lobes bloom for 1 day each on a 4- to 20-inch tall, densely bracted, spike-like cluster at the top of the stalk. Hairy, egg-shaped, 2-celled capsules

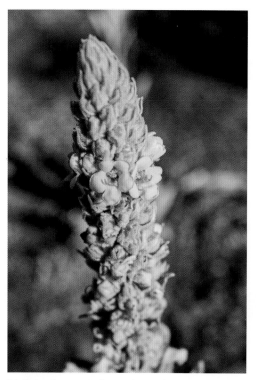

Mullein plants usually produce a few flowers at a time. It is best to gather from a large stand. Otherwise it may take many days to pick enough flowers to make medicine.

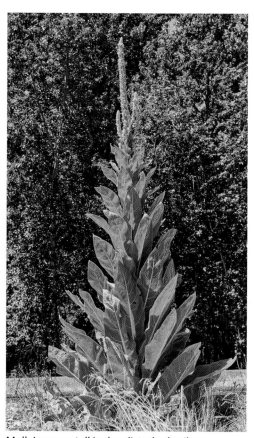

Mullein grows tall in dry, disturbed soils.

split at maturity to deposit many small ridged seeds near the base of the plant. The entire plant is densely covered in white wooly hairs that hinder water evaporation. Flowers that remain unfertilized at the end of their short bloom time—lasting from just before dawn to midafternoon—are able to self-pollinate. The dried fruiting spike often persists through winter.

Where, When, and How to Wildcraft

Introduced from Eurasia, mullein, a biennial widely distributed throughout North America, occupies disturbed areas, waste places, fields, and logged areas, and often stands sentinel-like along roadsides at low to middle elevations in this region. It rarely grows in undisturbed areas, but in open sunny locations with some type of soil disturbance, it can occupy almost any habitat including meadows, prairies, desert shrublands, chaparral, deciduous woodlands, and coniferous forests.

During the first year of growth, gather leaves from late summer to early spring and dig roots from early autumn to early spring. Pick flowers individually as they bloom. After the flowering stalks emerge, the roots become woody and the leaves dry up. At this point, neither are useful for medicine.

Medicinal Uses

Mullein leaf is useful for hot, dry respiratory conditions. The tea or tincture moistens the mucous membranes, reduces inflammation, and stimulates the flow of mucus to clear and open the lungs and sinuses. Take it for dry, raspy coughs that rack the body such as whooping cough; dry, scratchy sore throats with hoarseness; laryngitis; bronchitis; and asthma with wheezing and tightness in the chest and/or throat.

Mullein root and leaf moisten dry, stiff joints to improve flexibility and reduce pain. The tea or tincture of the root or leaves aligns the vertebrae and relieves pinched nerve pain and irritation.

The leaf smoke can be inhaled to relieve asthma and spasmodic coughing. To soothe an earache, gently blow the smoke into the ear canal or use a few drops of the flower oil.

Take the flower tincture to calm the nerves when you are agitated, irritable, or anxious. The tea or tincture of the root tightens and strengthens the bladder to relieve incontinence, reduces prostatic swelling and bladder inflammation, and relaxes spasms and soothes irritation of the urinary tract.

Apply the root tincture topically for Bell's palsy and other pain and trauma of the facial nerves. Apply a compress of the leaf tea to resolve swollen lymph glands.

Future Harvests

These hardy colonizers of disturbed ground get all the help they need from humans. Allow seeds to ripen on the stalk, and the mulleins will take care of themselves.

HERBAL PREPARATIONS

Leaf Tea
Standard infusion
Drink 3–4 fluid ounces up to 5 times per day.

Root Tea
Standard decoction
Drink 3–4 fluid ounces up to 4 times per day.

Leaf Tincture
1 part fresh leaf
2 parts menstruum (75 percent alcohol,
    25 percent distilled water)
Take 30–60 drops up to 5 times per day.

Root Tincture
1 part fresh root
2 parts menstruum (75 percent alcohol,
    25 percent distilled water)
Take 30–60 drops up to 5 times per day.

Flower Oil
Follow directions for Fresh Herb Infused Oil on page 63.

Plantago lanceolata
ribwort, white man's footsteps
PARTS USED leaf

The cooling and moistening leaves of plantain are soothing wound healers with the power to draw out splinters, infections, and insect venom.

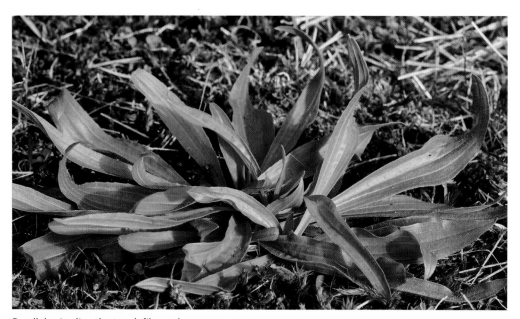

Parallel veins line the tough fibrous leaves.

How to Identify

A rosette of lance-shaped, finely and irregularly toothed basal leaves hugs the ground or stands erect attached to a tenacious taproot. Prominent parallel-ribbed veins on the 2- to 6-inch-long leaves reveal tough fibrous strings when torn. At the base where they attach to the root, the leaves are white with a purple tinge and sometimes wooly. Small green flowers with many long-extending yellow stamens form a dense, oblong, 1- to 3-inch spike at the top of leafless, 6- to 25-inch stalks that shoot up from the center of the plant. A blooming ring of flowers resembling orbiting satellites ascends the spike from bottom to top as the flowers open over time. Shiny black seeds, encased in a thin brown seed coat, form a mucilaginous gel when wet.

Common or broad-leaved plantain, *Plantago major*, with its wider, spoon-shaped leaves can be used interchangeably with *P. lanceolata*.

Where, When, and How to Wildcraft

Spreading far and wide across the globe, this introduced European perennial makes its home in all but the wildest and most remote

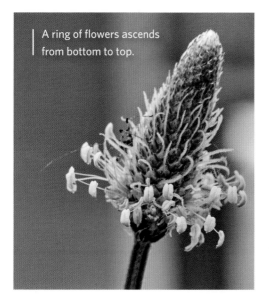
A ring of flowers ascends from bottom to top.

draw out the venom, and even for those who are severely allergic to bee stings, little or no swelling will occur.

Gargle the tincture alone or combined with a tincture of Oregon white oak bark, 30–60 drops in ½ fluid ounce of water, to tighten the gums or to draw out pus from abscessed teeth.

The tea or tincture taken internally is soothing to the digestive and urinary tracts. In the same way the plant breaks up hard, compacted soils and draws minerals to the surface, narrow-leaved plantain softens people with hard, emotionally protected exteriors.

⚠️ Caution

Always spit out any of the fluid or saliva from your mouth when drawing out infectious material from the teeth or gums. Swallowing it may spread infection to the blood and other areas of the body leading to serious and even life-threatening complications.

Future Harvests

Try as you might, this plant cannot be eradicated. Enjoy its presence wherever you find it.

places. Find it just about anywhere in this region from low to middle elevations thriving in compacted soil, disturbed areas, lawns, gardens, and growing from cracks in the sidewalk.

Gather anytime during the growing season that you can find green unblemished leaves. Avoid harvesting in areas where dogs frequently urinate.

Medicinal Uses

Cooling, moistening, astringent, and anti-microbial, narrow-leaved plantain leaves stop bleeding, seal wounds, soothe damaged tissue, and prevent infection. Apply the salve or a poultice of the fresh or dried leaves to skin abrasions, cuts, mouth sores, or infected wounds. Out in the field place a wad of the chewed leaves, affectionately known as a spit poultice, directly on the injured area.

The poulticed leaves also pull out splinters and infectious material and pus from boils and abscesses. The leaves of this humble plant can be a lifesaver for those who are allergic to the venom of bees or other insects. If applied immediately, the poulticed leaves

HERBAL PREPARATIONS

Leaf Tea
Standard infusion
Drink 4–8 fluid ounces up to 3 times per day.

Leaf Tincture
1 part fresh leaf
2 parts menstruum (75 percent alcohol, 25 percent distilled water)
Take 30–60 drops up to 5 times per day.

Leaf Oil and Salve
For leaf oil, follow directions for Fresh Herb Infused Oil on page 63. For the salve, follow directions on page 65.

Urtica dioica subsp. *gracilis*
stinging nettle
PARTS USED herb, root, seed

Abundantly useful nettle, sometimes feared for its sting, is nourishing to many body systems, relieves seasonal allergies, and is a specific remedy for gout.

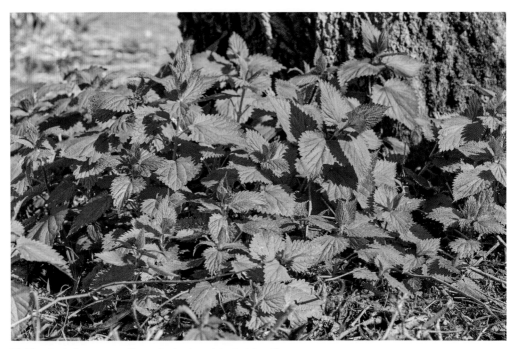

Nettle plants form spreading colonies in nutrient-rich soils.

How to Identify

Intertwining networks of spreading rhizomes form dense patches that give rise to 3- to 7-foot-tall plants whose leaves, stems, and flowers are covered with stinging hairs. The stout, squarish, and fibrous stems are unbranched with opposite, 2- to 3-inch-long, lance-shaped, oval, or heart-shaped leaves with serrated edges. Densely clustered, tiny greenish flowers hang down in strands from the upper leaf joints. Separate male and female flowers are found on the same plant; after pollination the female flowers, usually growing closer to the top, develop into tiny greenish seeds that ripen in the summer months.

Where, When, and How to Wildcraft

Nettle prefers deep, rich, and damp soils from sea level to high elevation. It grows in shady forest clearings, on mountain slopes, and on disturbed sites. In drier areas, find it along streams and drainage ditches.

Nettle begins to emerge from dormancy in

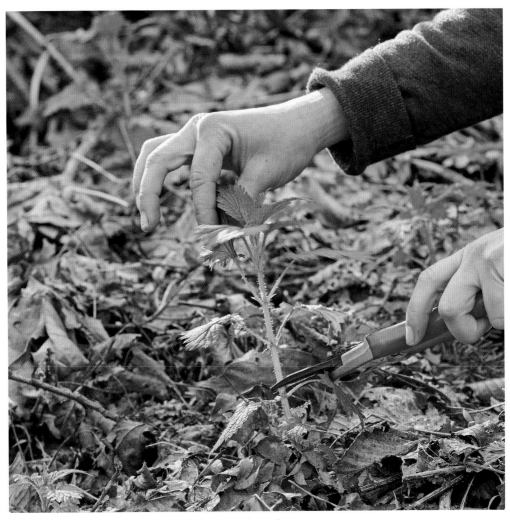

If you are careful, you can harvest nettle leaves without gloves.

late winter or early spring. Start harvesting the leaves along with the stems when the plants are just a few inches tall and continue until they begin to flower. As one of the first harvests of the year, I encourage using this experience as an opportunity to affirm careful and attentive harvesting practices in preparation for the wildcrafting season that will follow.

I find the sting of nettle to be invigorating and don't mind a sting or two while I'm harvesting, but if you pay close attention, you won't get stung. Although both sides of the leaves of some subspecies have stinging hairs, you will find that the tops of the leaves of most have few or no stinging hairs. Without gloves (if you dare), lightly grip the top of a leaf between your thumb and forefinger and cut the stalk just above one of the lower leaf nodes, then carefully guide it into your bag.

Gather the ripe, green seeds from late summer to early autumn. Dig the dormant roots and rhizomes after the tops die back.

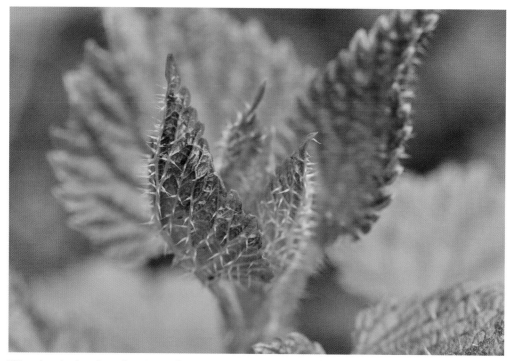

When brushed against, the stinging hairs inject a potent cocktail of beneficial compounds into the skin.

Medicinal Uses

Nettle is an abundant source of minerals like silica and calcium, is vitamin-rich, and contains more protein than just about any other plant. Drinking the herb tea or eating the cooked fresh leaves builds the blood; strengthens the lungs, hair, nails, and connective tissue; and increases the production of breast milk. It is highly recommended to drink the tea regularly during all phases of pregnancy to support the growing fetus.

Drink nettle herb tea to remedy gout, a suddenly arriving, intensely painful inflammation of the joints most often occurring at the base of the big toe. The fresh herb tincture or a meal of the cooked leaves can alter the body's histamine response to relieve seasonal allergies.

The juice in the stinging hairs contains acetylcholine, a neurotransmitter also found in the human body, and formic acid, found in the

venom of ants. Repeatedly stinging oneself with the fresh leaves helps restore communication between the nerves, aids the repair of old injuries to the joints, and has even been reported to reverse cases of paralysis.

Nettle herb and seed tonify and nourish the kidneys and adrenals to renew vigor in cases of adrenal burnout and can restore function to failing kidneys. Drink the seed tea, eat 1 teaspoon of the dried seeds daily, or mix the seeds into smoothies.

The root is a specific remedy for enlarged prostate, also known as benign prostatic hyperplasia, which affects most men to one degree or another as they age.

⚠ Caution

Harvest nettle far from conventional farms and other places that use chemical fertilizers. Nettle will uptake and concentrate these compounds just as it concentrates minerals.

Future Harvests

The rhizomes are easily transferred to appropriate sites. To establish new colonies, dig them up for transplanting in autumn or winter when they are dormant.

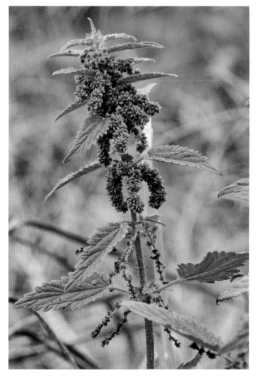

Hoary nettle (*Urtica dioica* subsp. *holosericea*), which grows in the eastern parts of this region, has larger clusters and bigger seeds than its western counterpart.

HERBAL PREPARATIONS

Herb or Seed Tea
Standard infusion
Drink 4-6 fluid ounces up to 5 times per day.

Root Tea
Standard decoction
Drink 4-6 fluid ounces up to 3 times per day.

Root or Herb Tincture
1 part fresh root or herb
2 parts menstruum (75 percent alcohol,
    25 percent distilled water)
Take 30-60 drops up to 5 times per day.

Seed Tincture
1 part fresh seed
2 parts menstruum (75 percent alcohol,
    25 percent distilled water)
or
1 part dried seed
5 parts menstruum (50 percent alcohol,
    50 percent distilled water)
Take 30-60 drops up to 3 times per day.

Agastache urticifolia
butterfly mint, nettleleaf horsemint
PARTS USED leaf

Richly fragrant leaves calm an upset stomach, promote sweating, and stimulate vividly colored dreams.

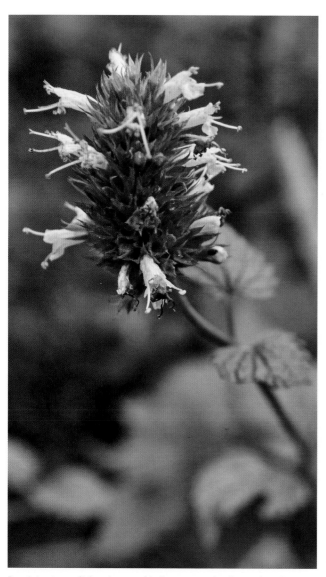

Persistent purplish calyces add vibrancy to the flower heads.

How to Identify

From a thin, branching root system and woody-stemmed base, many usually branching stems, square and finely hairy to smooth, stand erect 2–6 feet tall. Aromatic, oppositely arranged, egg- to heart-shaped leaves with round-toothed edges extend 1–4 inches. Smooth-textured or rough-haired above and below, the leaf undersides are a paler shade of green than the tops. Stalkless, tubular, 2-lipped flowers, white to pink to purple, bloom from late spring to late summer in 1- to 6-inch-long many-flowered, terminal spikes. Clusters of 4 brown, hairy-tipped nutlets ripen in purplish tinged, 5-toothed, and prominently veined calyces.

Where, When, and How to Wildcraft

Occurring throughout much of the American west, the range of this perennial mint, a relative of anise-hyssop (*Agastache foeniculum*), cuts an ever-widening swath from the extreme southeastern corner of British

Columbia through the eastern half of Washington and northern Oregon. From there it heads progressively westward to cover most of the southern portion of Oregon and all of northern California. Nettleleaf giant hyssop prefers moist to dry meadows and open hillsides and woodlands from low to high elevations.

Just before or while the plants are flowering, clip stalks at the base just above a leaf node and hang to dry in a shaded area with ample airflow. After drying, strip the leaves and discard the stems. Process the leaves fresh for tincture.

Medicinal Uses

Take the leaf tea or tincture to soothe the digestive tract and relieve indigestion, nausea, and gas pain; to promote sweating to break a fever; to speed the healing of colds and flus; or for their somewhat calming influence on the nerves. These same preparations also bring vividly colored and sometimes zany dreams. Externally a poultice reduces joint inflammation.

Future Harvests

Refrain from harvesting nettleleaf giant hyssop in British Columbia, where it is rare and has been blue-listed by the Canadian government because it is "sensitive or vulnerable to human activities or natural events."

Collect seed heads 3–4 weeks after flowering or after the seeds have darkened. After drying the heads in a paper bag, shake vigorously to release the seeds. Sow in spring.

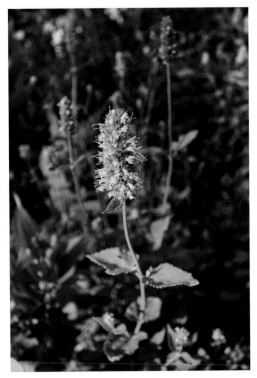

Nettleleaf giant hyssop forms large stands that attract nectar-seeking butterflies.

HERBAL PREPARATIONS

Leaf Tea
Standard infusion
Drink 4–6 fluid ounces up to 5 times per day.

Leaf Tincture
1 part fresh leaf
2 parts menstruum (75 percent alcohol,
   25 percent distilled water)
Take 15–45 drops up to 5 times per day.

Lycopus uniflorus
northern water horehound
PARTS USED leaf

Bitter leaves slow overactive thyroid activity, calm the nerves, support digestive function, and halt excessive bleeding.

How to Identify

Thin rhizomes, thickened tuber-like at the distal end, give rise to single or sometimes branched, 4-sided stems that curve upward or stand erect 4–22 inches tall. Scentless, short-stalked, and oppositely arranged leaves, smooth to minutely hairy, ¾ to 3 inches long and lance-shaped with coarsely and irregularly toothed edges, line the square, finely haired stems and become only slightly smaller as they near the top. Blooming from mid summer to early autumn, small, white to pale pink, 4-lobed, tubular flowers form tight whorls in the leaf axils and produce clusters of 4 slightly flattened and finely toothed nutlets. The corolla of fused petals is longer than the 5-toothed calyx.

American bugleweed (*Lycopus americanus*) is hairy only at the leaf nodes and has more deeply cleft leaves. Its calyces are nearly as long as the corollas. Rough bugleweed (*L. asper*) is hairy on the edges of the stem, has evenly toothed leaf edges, and may have rough-textured upper leaf surfaces. All of these species have similar medicinal properties.

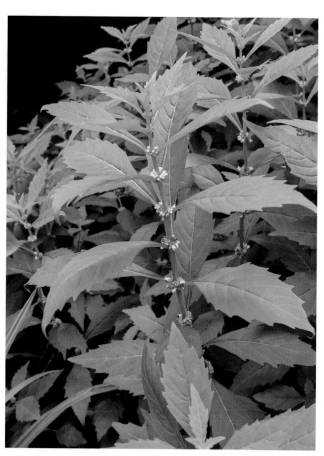

A calming, scentless mint, northern bugleweed prefers to grow in wet, boggy areas.

Where, When, and How to Wildcraft

Found throughout much of North America as well as in Japan and Siberia, this herbaceous perennial forms colonies in wet areas at low to middle elevations. Find northern bugleweed in this region along the edges of lakes and streams and in marshes and bogs from Alaska to the northwestern corner of California. While the plants are flowering, clip stalks at the base just above a leaf node, discard damaged leaves, and process fresh for tincture or hang to dry in a shaded area with ample airflow for teas.

Medicinal Uses

Early American botanical doctors used bugleweed as a sedative and pain reliever for acute fevers with rapid pulse and general irritability, for acute and chronic pulmonary conditions with irritating and debilitating coughs with excessive mucus flow, and for heart conditions with difficulty breathing and tightness in the chest. For those with insomnia caused by fear of dying from disease, they used it to promote sleep, and they report it as being beneficial for stopping frequent hemorrhaging of small amounts of blood from the lungs, nose, stomach, kidneys, or uterus.

Herbalists today employ bugleweed for hyperthyroidism and other excess conditions, to improve stress-affected digestive function, and to stop bleeding. Take the tea or tincture to lower the production of thyroid hormone from an overactive thyroid gland, to relieve hot flashes, to resolve fevers with a rapid and irregular pulse, or to calm agitated and overstimulated nerves with skittishness, fear, anxiety, or insomnia.

As a bitter tonic, northern bugleweed strengthens digestion and calms a nervous, irritated stomach. Take frequent doses of the tincture to stop excessive uterine bleeding or to stanch nosebleeds.

Caution

This plant is not suitable for use with low functioning thyroid.

Future Harvests

Divide roots in spring or autumn and transplant small pieces to suitable sites.

HERBAL PREPARATIONS

Leaf Tea
Standard infusion
Drink 2–3 fluid ounces up to 4 times per day.

Leaf Tincture
1 part fresh leaf
2 parts menstruum (75 percent alcohol, 25 percent distilled water)
Take 15–45 drops up to 4 times per day; for hot flashes take 1 teaspoon.

---

oceanspray

Holodiscus discolor
PARTS USED leaf, bark

Astringent bark and leaves stanch bleeding and bring tone to lax tissues.

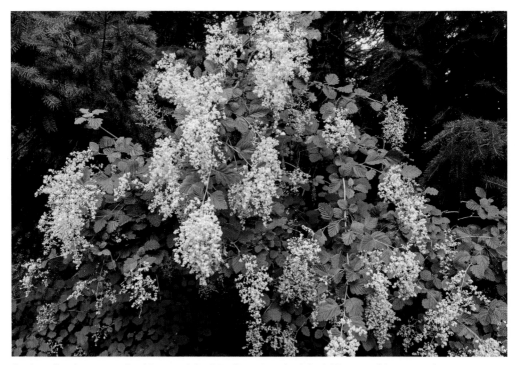

Copious floral sprays make this graceful, white-flowering shrub look like a crashing coastal wave.

How to Identify
Ridged, new-growth stems develop a reddish gray, peeling bark as they age and grow up to 10 feet tall. Soft and plush, finely haired, light green leaves, shallowly lobed with several secondary teeth, alternately line the stems and drop to the ground in autumn. Blooming from late spring to mid summer, very small, white to cream-colored, 5-petaled flowers, arranged in terminal clusters droop down from the ends of the long arching stems, turn brown after pollination, and often remain on the plant through winter. Dry, 1-seeded fruits ripen from mid to late summer.

Where, When, and How to Wildcraft
A highly adaptable plant, oceanspray is moderately drought and salt tolerant and thrives in both sunny and shaded forested areas across western North America. Find it growing in dry to wet soils at low to middle elevations from the coast to the mountains on both sides of the Cascades from British Columbia to California. Harvest leaves and stem bark from mid spring to early autumn.

Medicinal Uses

Like many plants in the rose family, oceanspray has been used traditionally for its astringent and diuretic properties. A wash of the bark or leaves applied externally stops bleeding from cuts and scrapes. Drink the leaf or bark tea to tone the uterus postpartum or to tighten the bowels in cases of diarrhea.

There is little written information about this plant, but the peppery and fruity flavor of its leaves is intriguing and may point to other uses. It deserves further investigation.

Future Harvests

Although these plants are hardy and abundant, harvest respectfully.

HERBAL PREPARATIONS

Leaf Tea
Standard infusion
Drink 4–8 fluid ounces up to 5 times per day.

Bark Tea
Standard decoction
Drink 4–6 fluid ounces up to 5 times per day.

oneseed hawthorn

Crataegus monogyna
English or common hawthorn, mayblossom
PARTS USED leaf and flower, berry

Spring-harvested leaves and flowers and autumn-harvested berries strengthen the heart, lower cholesterol levels, and open the chest to relieve asthma.

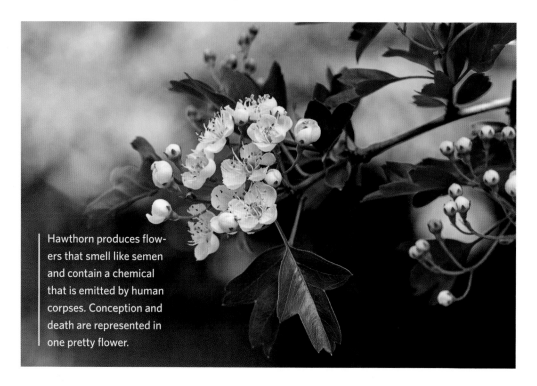

Hawthorn produces flowers that smell like semen and contain a chemical that is emitted by human corpses. Conception and death are represented in one pretty flower.

How to Identify

From mid spring to early summer, flat-topped clusters of white, 5-petaled and many-stamened flowers blanket trees that have scaly, grayish brown trunk bark. Smelling fishy or semen-like, the flowers attract pollinating insects and in autumn ripen into roundish, red, 1-seeded berries. Behind the inviting floral display, protective thorns up to ½ inch long line branches covered with alternately arranged, few-toothed, and 1- to 2-inch-long, oval leaves with 3–7 lobes. The lobes cut more than halfway to the midrib of the leaves.

The less common but widespread native black hawthorn (*Crataegus douglasii*) has leaves with less deeply cut lobes and blackish purple berries. The medicinal properties of its leaf, flower, and berries are the same as those of oneseed hawthorn.

Where, When, and How to Wildcraft

At low elevations west of the Cascades from Alaska to California, these 7- to 30-foot-tall,

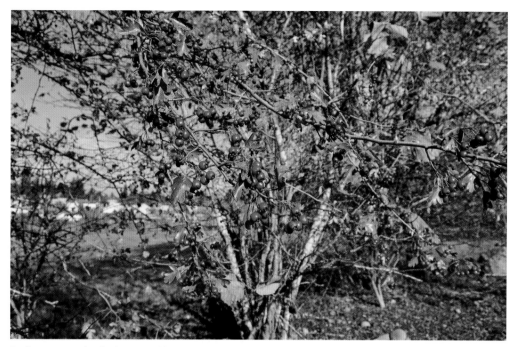

Each year an individual oneseed hawthorn tree can produce as many as two thousand berries.

introduced European deciduous trees or small shrubs grow along fence lines and the edges of forests and in clearings, open fields, waste places, and disturbed areas.

Snip off the little bundles of leaf and flower when the tree is in full bloom from mid spring to early summer. The berries are best gathered in autumn after the first frost, which sweetens them up. Dry the berries on screens or in a dehydrator on the lowest setting.

Medicinal Uses

Astringent, sweet, and somewhat sour, hawthorn is this region's most important heart medicine. Rich in antioxidant and nourishing flavonoids that lessen inflammation, the leaf and flower or the berries, alone or combined, open blood vessels in the heart, lower blood pressure, and nourish and strengthen the heart muscle. The tea or tincture eases many heart-related problems including high or low blood pressure, chest pain caused by lack of blood to the heart muscle known as angina, irregular heartbeat, hardening of the arteries (arteriosclerosis), and pitting edema from congestive heart failure. Hawthorn also reduces cholesterol levels and opens the chest and lungs to ease the effects of asthma.

Hawthorn's cooling nature clears heat and calms the nervous system to reduce anxiety, agitation, excitability, and hypersensitivity that may lead to insomnia and difficulty focusing. It has been used by some for attention deficit disorder.

Heart disease, the leading cause of mortality in the United States, is responsible for one in every four deaths. While this can be attributed to various hereditary and lifestyle issues, don't underestimate the importance of love, joy, and happiness because when it comes to living a physically healthy life, the emotional health of the heart cannot be ignored. Hawthorn teaches us how to give and receive more love. Take it tonically or in

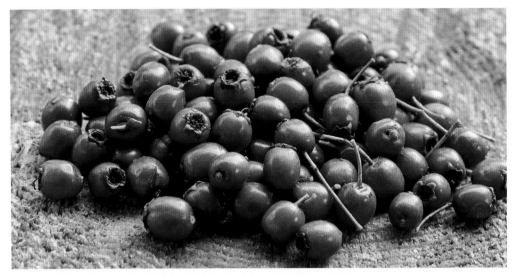

These hawthorn berries are ready for drying. Each berry contains a single large seed and is marked by a five-pointed star on its bottom.

times of distress to open and soothe the emotional heart, to connect with unexpressed grief or other feelings, or to find compassion for yourself and others.

Caution

Although hawthorn is considered nontoxic and safe to use for extended periods, 10–15 drops as an everyday tonic may be more effective than higher doses, which may cause some agitation. Except for possibly potentiating the effects of *Digitalis*, there appear to be no adverse interactions with other heart medications. In any case, consult with a doctor before taking hawthorn with prescription drugs.

Future Harvests

The birds do a fantastic job of distributing the seeds of this tree. Because hawthorn is considered invasive, all of the trees in a small urban wilderness in Portland, Oregon, where many herbalists had been harvesting hawthorn for years, were futilely cut down, but seeds that were deposited in the soil by birds continue to sprout.

HERBAL PREPARATIONS

Leaf and Flower Tea
Standard infusion
Drink 4–6 fluid ounces up to 3 times per day.

Berry Tea
Standard decoction
Drink 4–6 fluid ounces up to 3 times per day.

Leaf and Flower Tincture
1 part fresh leaf and flower
2 parts menstruum (75 percent alcohol, 15 percent distilled water, 10 percent glycerin)
Take 10–15 drops 3 times per day.

Berry Tincture
1 part dried berries
5 parts menstruum (50 percent alcohol, 40 percent distilled water, 10 percent glycerin)
Take 10–15 drops 3 times per day.

Oregon figwort

Scrophularia californica var. *oregana*
PARTS USED leaf and flower

Blood cleansing and lymphatic stimulating, figwort leaf and flower reduce swelling and congestion and clear infection.

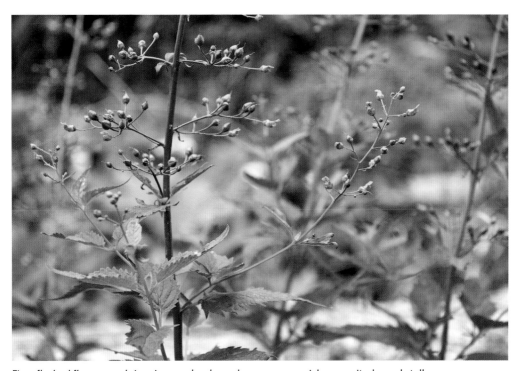

Firm-fleshed flowers and ripening seedpods are borne on squarish, opposite-leaved stalks.

How to Identify

From thickened roots, clusters of squarish stems stand straight and reach 20–48 inches tall. Pairs of triangular to egg-shaped, pointy-tipped leaves, gradually growing smaller as they ascend the stem, line the stalks opposite each other with roughly single- or double-toothed edges. Rigid-fleshed, tubular flowers, open-mouthed like baby birds awaiting a meal, bloom from late spring to mid summer in tall, narrow, leafless, opposite-branching clusters at the ends of the stalks. Brownish to maroon above and paler or yellowish green below, each of the stalked, 2-lipped, ¼- to ½-inch-long flowers features a flat, 2-lobed upper lip that juts forward and a shorter, 3-lobed lower lip whose middle lobe angles downward. Pear-shaped capsules contain many angular, ridged seeds, and small glandular hairs usually cover the leaves and stalks.

Oregon figwort, with its club-shaped, longer-than-wide fifth sterile stamen, is distinguished from lance-leaved figwort

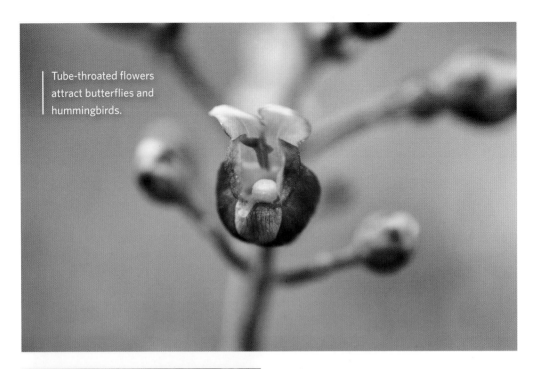

Tube-throated flowers attract butterflies and hummingbirds.

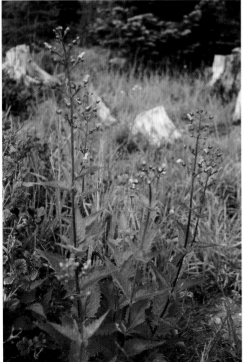

With its distinctly shaped flowers, this plant it easy to spot while driving along forest roads.

(*Scrophularia lanceolata*) by the latter's fan-shaped and wider-than-long sterile stamen. Lance-leaved figwort has the same medicinal properties as Oregon figwort.

Where, When, and How to Wildcraft

Growing throughout Oregon at low to middle elevations in meadows, clearings, and along roadsides and streambanks, this handsome perennial is mainly found in the coastal counties of Washington and British Columbia and on both sides of the Cascades in Oregon.

While it is flowering, collect the aerial portions of the plant. Process fresh for tincture using the pliable part of the stem along with the leaf and flower, or dry on screens, in bags, or in upside-down hanging bundles for tea. Once dry, remove the leaf and flower and discard the stems.

Medicinal Uses

Oregon figwort cleans the blood and stimulates lymphatic flow to relieve congestion, reduce swelling, and clear infection. Take the leaf and flower tea or tincture for swollen, congested lymph nodes; infected lymph nodes in the neck with oozing sores; red, itchy, and scaly skin conditions like eczema; allergic rashes; or chronic infections and sores of the skin or mucous membranes. These same preparations reduce arthritic inflammation, relieve constipation, soothe and tone the urinary tract, and promote the flow of urine.

Apply a poultice of the fresh leaves, the oil, or the salve to alleviate discomfort and speed the healing of bruises, burns, hemorrhoids, rashes, eczema, fungal infections, swollen glands, or infected sores, or to soothe sore nipples.

Early American botanical doctors employed the related carpenter's square (*Scrophularia marilandica*), native to eastern North America, for cancer with lumps in the neck and upper back. Oregon figwort is commonly combined with other blood-cleansing and lymphatic herbs such as burdock, yellow dock, dandelion, and cleavers.

⚠ Caution

Although it is unclear whether our native *Scrophularia* species contain the same cardiovascular-affecting constituents as the European species *S. nodosa,* avoid ingesting this plant in any form during pregnancy, with ventricular tachycardia, or when taking pharmaceutical heart medications.

Future Harvests

Directly sow the easy-to-germinate seeds on the surface of the soil or in containers.

HERBAL PREPARATIONS

Leaf and Flower Tea
Standard infusion
Drink 2–4 fluid ounces up to 3 times per day.

Leaf and Flower Tincture
1 part fresh leaf and flower
2 parts menstruum (75 percent alcohol,
  25 percent distilled water)
Take 20–45 drops up to 3 times per day.

Leaf and Flower Oil and Salve
For leaf and flower oil follow directions for Fresh Herb Infused Oil on page 63. For the salve, follow directions on page 65.

Oregon white oak

Quercus garryana
Garry oak
PARTS USED bark

Astringent bark benefits sore throats and inflamed gums and speeds the healing of cuts, abrasions, and burns.

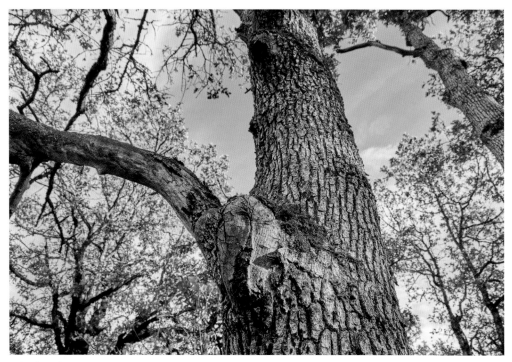

Whether they grow tall and stately like this tree or short and scrubby, Oregon white oaks have distinctively fissured, light-colored bark.

How to Identify

Heavily fissured, thick, light gray bark encases the heavy, dense, fine-grained wood of these stout deciduous trees. Hairy, new-growth twigs become smooth as they age, and leathery, dark green leaves, light green and hairy below, have 5–7 rounded lobes. On the same tree, separate male and female flowers emerge with the leaves from early to late spring. Tiny male flowers are borne in drooping, green-tinged, pale yellow catkins, and small, deep red female flowers bloom solitary or in small clusters in the axils of developing leaves. The acorns, ¾ to 1¼ inches long, sit in warty-scaled cups and mature in their first year. On richer soils these broad-crowned trees can reach heights up to 100 feet. On drier soils they may be small, gnarled shrubs.

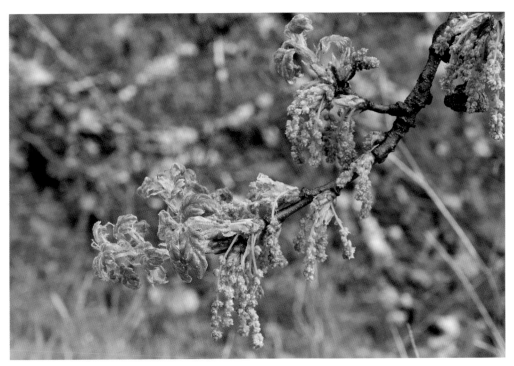

The flowers emerge with the leaves in spring.

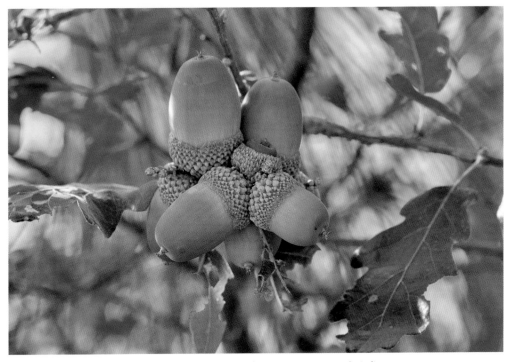

Acorns, edible after processing in water to remove the tannins, ripen in their first year.

Where, When, and How to Wildcraft

Oregon white oak grows in open woodlands on dry, rocky soils at low elevations. It attains its highest concentration in Oregon's Willamette Valley. From there it grows east and north into Washington's Yakima Valley via the Columbia River Gorge and can be found as far north as Vancouver Island in British Columbia.

Cut branches thumb-sized or bigger after the leaves emerge. Strip the tough and stringy bark promptly and dry on screens or in bags.

Medicinal Uses

The highly astringent tannins in the bark tone and tighten tissues. The diluted bark tincture (30 drops in 1 fluid ounce of water) or a tea of the bark used as a mouth rinse helps receding and inflamed gums and can be gargled for a boggy sore throat.

For diarrhea, drink the bark tea. Externally a powder or decoction of the bark will aid the healing of cuts, abrasions, and burns.

Drop doses of the tincture may help willful people who persistently struggle yet are never satisfied with what they achieve.

Caution

Due to its high tannin content, frequent internal use may cause gastric upset.

Future Harvests

Sow fresh acorns ½ inch deep from early to late autumn. It will take many years for these acorns to become oaks large enough to produce harvestable bark, but it is vital that we look far into the future to ensure that succeeding generations of humans and other creatures have access to this valuable food and medicine plant.

HERBAL PREPARATIONS

Bark Tea
Standard decoction
Drink 2–4 fluid ounces up to 3 times per day.

Bark Tincture
1 part dried bark
5 parts menstruum (50 percent alcohol, 40 percent distilled water, 10 percent glycerin)
Take 30–45 drops up to 3 times per day.

---

oxeye daisy

Leucanthemum vulgare
PARTS USED herb

Aromatic leaves and flowers ease respiratory tract inflammation, dry excessive mucus discharge, and resolve fungal infections.

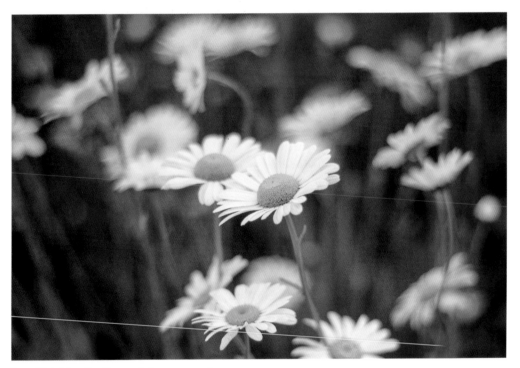

Beautiful daisy-like flowers bring summer joy.

How to Identify

In spring, creeping rhizomes produce single to several moderately branching stems. Long-stalked, egg- to spoon-shaped basal leaves emerge with rounded teeth and lobes. As the leaves alternately ascend the hairless stems they diminish in size, vary in shape, become stalkless, and may or may not remain toothed. Blooming from late spring to mid autumn, white ray female flowers, fertile, and fewer than 22 in number and many yellow, hermaphroditic disk flowers comprising 4- or 5-lobed tubes make up 1- to 1¼-inch composite flower heads. The daisy-like flower heads are cupped by narrowly lance-shaped, brown-edged bracts. Pollinated flowers produce black, nearly cylindrical, 10-ribbed seeds that lack a crown of bristly hairs.

Where, When, and How to Wildcraft

Found across North America and throughout this region at low to middle elevations, this 1- to 3-foot-tall, introduced Eurasian perennial (formerly *Chrysanthemum leucanthemum*) thrives in many different types of soil. Oxeye daisy grows in disturbed areas, such as roadsides, clearings, and pastures, as well as in meadows, prairies, and grasslands and prefers sun but tolerates partial shade.

Gather the aerial parts including the stalks while the flowers are blooming. Clip the stems at the base, remove dead or damaged leaves, and bundle or lay on screens to dry.

Medicinal Uses

Cooling and drying, oxeye daisy herb reduces inflammation and checks excessive secretions from the lungs, sinuses, and stomach. Take the tea or tincture to alleviate seasonal allergies, to clear mucus and relieve respiratory tract congestion, to ease damp asthmatic conditions, or to cool stomach irritation and ulcers.

A vaginal douche speeds the healing of yeast infections. An external wash stanches bleeding, prevents wounds from becoming infected, and soothes and speeds the healing of fungal infections such as ringworm, athlete's foot, or jock itch.

The tea soothes the urinary tract, the fresh young leaves make a nice addition to salads, and the powdered flowers ward off and kill fleas.

Future Harvests

Considered an invasive weed by some, this drought-tolerant plant attracts bees and butterflies. In autumn divide and replant the roots or directly sow seeds in areas where they won't hinder the growth of native plants.

HERBAL PREPARATIONS

Herb Tea
Standard infusion
Drink 2–4 fluid ounces up to 3 times per day.

Herb Tincture
1 part dried herb
5 parts menstruum (50 percent alcohol, 50 percent distilled water)
Take 40–60 drops up to 3 times per day.

Pacific bleeding heart

Dicentra formosa
PARTS USED whole plant

All parts of this bitter-tasting plant provide relief from pain and bring calmness and grounding to those who have experienced traumatic events.

How to Identify

Succulent, scaly, and brittle rhizomes run just under the soil's surface and give rise to many basal, deeply dissected, and long-stalked 3- or 4-times divided leaves. Beginning in early spring, leafless flowering stalks arise from ground level producing 3–15 pink to purplish pink, 4-petaled, nodding flowers that bloom heart-shaped at the base. Short spurs flare out at the end of the 2 sac-forming, outer petals; the inner pair of petals fuse to form a wing-crested tip. Oblong, pod-like capsules, carrying shiny black seeds with an oil-bearing appendage, poke out ¾ to 1⅜ inches long from between the petals. The foliage of this 6- to 18-inch tall perennial is hairless, juicy, and somewhat waxy coated.

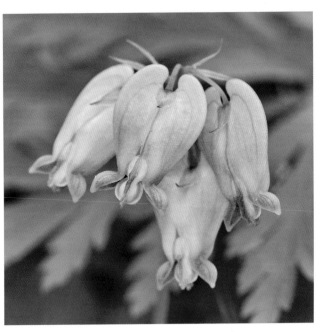

The uniquely shaped flowers of Pacific bleeding heart are a favorite of hummingbirds.

Where, When, and How to Wildcraft

Occurring less frequently as the elevation rises, Pacific bleeding heart is mainly found west of the Cascades in the understory of wet, shady forests with nitrogen-rich soils from the coast to higher elevations in the mountains from British Columbia south to California. Harvest the whole plant when in flower or gather the roots by themselves after the seeds ripen.

Medicinal Uses

Bleeding heart contains opiate-like alkaloids that numb and deaden pain. Take the whole-plant tea or tincture internally as a general analgesic. In addition to their numbing effect, the alkaloids restore the flow of knotted and blocked energy at sites of physical trauma. The tea or tincture works just like acupuncture in this regard and may be applied externally to aching teeth, sore

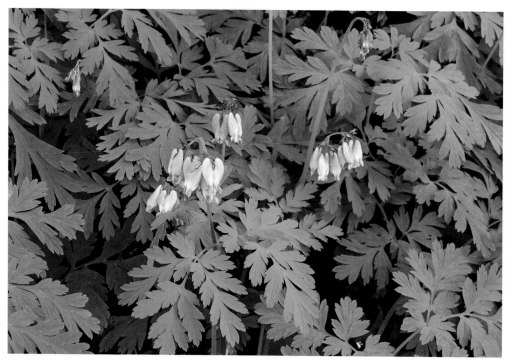
The delicate leaves of Pacific bleeding heart promise relief from pain and anxiety.

gums, bruises, sprains, strains, and joint or nerve pain.

The tincture of the root by itself, which can be used for all of the previously mentioned maladies, is a more potent pain reliever than the whole-plant preparations, which are well suited to relieve acute anxiety or shock after a traumatic event. The aboveground parts of the plant, in addition to their analgesic effect, are nourishing to the nervous system.

⚠️ Caution

Do not use during pregnancy, combine with prescription medications, or exceed recommended dosage. The presence of bleeding heart's narcotic alkaloids in your urine may trigger a false positive result for drug tests screening for opiates.

Future Harvests

Respectfully harvest a few plants from each large healthy stand. The seeds do not store well. Sow them fresh after they ripen from later summer to early autumn. Divide or transplant the rhizomes during the dormant season.

HERBAL PREPARATIONS

Root, Whole Plant, or Herb Tea
Standard infusion
Drink 2–4 fluid ounces up to 3 times per day.

Root or Whole Plant Tincture
1 part fresh root or whole plant
2 parts menstruum (75 percent alcohol,
  25 percent distilled water)
Take 10–20 drops up to 3 times per day.

Pacific dogwood

Cornus nuttallii
mountain dogwood, western flowering dogwood
PARTS USED bark, flower

Bitter bark and flower heads aid digestion and relieve pain and inflammation.

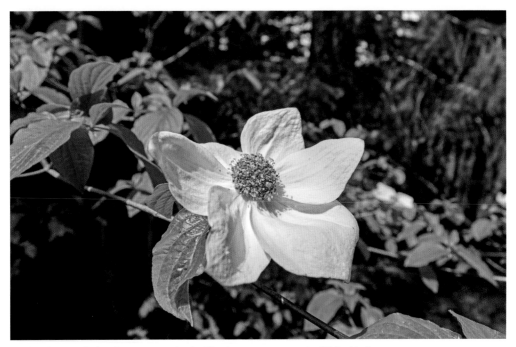

Pacific dogwood, the showiest tree in the Northwest, grows up to 50 feet tall.

How to Identify

Smooth, gray, white-patched bark becomes finely ridged with age on trunks that divide into branches and grayish purple twigs that hold themselves like antlers. Distinct veins run parallel to the edges of 1½- to 4-inch-long, oppositely arranged, oval, and pointy-tipped leaves that turn bright red or orange in autumn. Surrounded by 4–7 white to pale green, petal-like, ¾- to 2¾-inch-long modified leaf bracts, several small purple-tinged, whitish green, 4-petalled flowers bloom from mid spring to early summer in densely clustered buttons in the centers of showy flower heads. Intensely bitter, red-clustered fruits ripen in autumn. If you carefully tear one of the deciduous leaves crosswise, you will see thin, cottony threads running along the major veins.

Where, When, and How to Wildcraft

On both sides of the Cascade Crest from northern California to British Columbia, Pacific dogwood inhabits damp, low- to middle-elevation mixed coniferous forests. It thrives under the canopy of large conifers

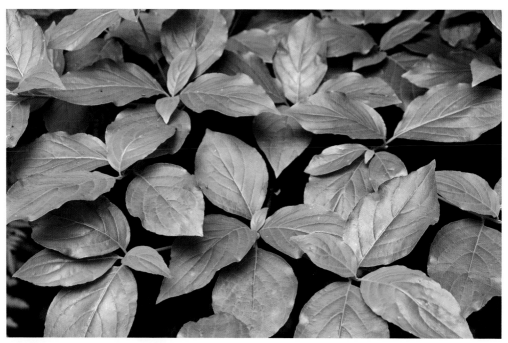

Dogwood leaves are specially equipped to make use of whatever sunlight is available in the understory of the shaded coniferous forests they inhabit.

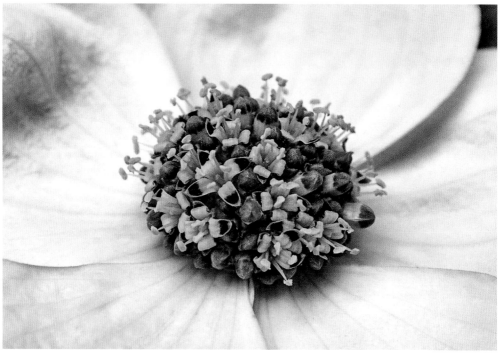

Purple-tipped flowers bloom in the center of capitate flower heads that illuminate the forest during spring.

Disease-Afflicted Dogwoods

A fungal disease called dogwood anthracnose is afflicting all types of ornamental and forest-dwelling dogwoods. At the onset of the disease, small spots form on the leaves before they shrivel up and turn brown. Infected leaves remain on the tree after normal leaf fall. The disease spreads from leaves to twigs to branches to trunk, greatly weakening the trees and eventually killing them. If you or your tools come in contact with an infected tree, steer clear of other trees to prevent the spread of infection. Sanitize your tools by cleaning them with rubbing alcohol or by soaking them for 30 seconds in a 10 percent bleach solution.

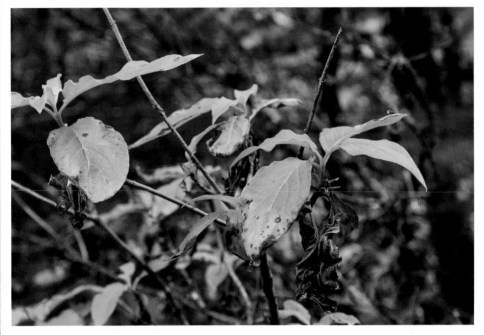

This tree has been infected with dogwood anthracnose.

where other hardwood trees struggle because it is able to achieve maximum photosynthesis with only one-third of full sunlight. Harvest the bark after the sap begins to run as the leaves emerge in mid spring, and gather flowers when they are in full bloom from mid spring to early summer.

Medicinal Uses

The bitter bark and flowers help regulate the release of bile into the stomach to aid digestion. Take the tincture of the bark or flowers 15 minutes before meals if you experience bloating, gas, discomfort after eating, and/or undigested food in the stools.

Aspirin-like salicylates in the bark and flowers relieve pain, lessen inflammation, and reduce fever. In general, it is best to let fevers run their course, but in some cases, like for small children who may experience seizures when their temperature rises above 104°F, temperature-cooling remedies like Pacific dogwood bark or flower may be necessary. For other instances of fever, use herbs like yarrow, blue elder flower, or feverfew that support the body's natural response to infection and promote sweating to break the fever.

Traditionally the dogwoods have been used as a substitute for quinine to treat malaria; a tea or tincture of the bark or flowers is useful for any condition characterized by alternating fever and chills.

These same preparations relieve headache pain and are especially indicated for chronic headaches focused in the middle of the forehead. In some cases these types of headache result from a blocked or constricted capacity to see visions.

Work with this plant to illuminate the depths of your being, to bring light to the dark places, and to open the third eye and activate your ability to see visions. While we may be confronted with things we'd rather not see, if we go through this process, Pacific dogwood helps us to see and appreciate the inherent beauty that we all possess. Smoke the dried leaves alone or mixed with other herbs for their mildly euphoric effect.

Caution

For those who are sensitive to aspirin, preparations of Pacific dogwood may cause stomach irritation.

Future Harvests

Harvest from downed trees that are still rooted and alive. Cut the tree at the base and it will resprout from the crown. Also look for broken branches that are still attached and alive, or cut branches that are crossing or growing into the center of the tree.

HERBAL PREPARATIONS

Bark Tea
Standard decoction
Drink 2–4 fluid ounces up to 5 times per day.

Flower Tea
Standard infusion
Drink 2–4 fluid ounces up to 5 times per day.

Bark or Flower Tincture
1 part fresh bark or flowers
2 parts menstruum (75 percent alcohol, 25 percent distilled water)
or
1 part dried bark or flowers
5 parts menstruum (50 percent alcohol, 50 percent distilled water)
Take 15–30 drops up to 5 times per day.

Pacific madrone

Arbutus menziesii

madrona

PARTS USED leaf

Thick, leathery leaves help heal urinary tract infections, decrease skin inflammation, and stanch the bleeding of cuts, scrapes, and abrasions.

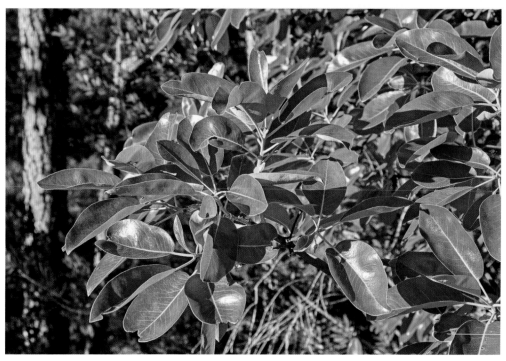

The glossy leaves remain on the tree for 2 years before falling to the ground.

How to Identify

Papery thin, pale yellow-green bark ages to a reddish orange and then a deep brownish red. It sheds in strips during the summer months to reveal smooth-skinned, curved trunks that divide into thick-limbed branches. Branches taper into forking twigs that spread to form a wide canopy of broad evergreen leaves. In early summer, second-year leaves fade to orange and begin falling to the ground as the glossy green, new-growth leaves mature.

These hairless, alternately arranged, egg-shaped to elliptic leaves spread 3–6 inches long with whitish green undersides and smooth edges. From mid spring to early summer, large terminal clusters of white to pinkish, urn-shaped, and 5-lobed flowers bloom with a sweet aroma that attracts pollinating insects. Orange to red berry-like fruits, ⅜ inch wide, rough-textured and mealy-fleshed, ripen in autumn and remain on the tree through the early winter or until

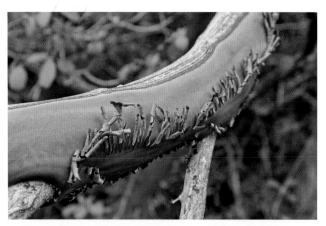

With its peeling skin and smooth, multi-hued bark, Pacific madrone is one of the most sensually pleasing trees of the Pacific Northwest bioregion.

they are gobbled up by birds who disseminate their small seeds. Trees growing in areas with richer soil and mild weather may live for 200 years and reach heights of between 50 and 80 feet with trunks 2 feet in diameter, but their size and age may be drastically limited in nutrient-poor, stressful environments. Younger leaves may be finely toothed, and older trunks may form gray-scaled bark. After burns, the trees resprout from the base.

Where, When, and How to Wildcraft

Though it occupies both high-and low-rainfall areas, this generally shade-intolerant tree, one of the few non-coniferous evergreen trees in this region, grows only west of the Cascades in places with mild winters and dry conditions during summer. Pacific madrone inhabits dry, well-drained soils from British Columbia to California including the driest sites on southeastern Vancouver Island in British Columbia and the San Juan Islands in Washington. It is more common at lower elevations, nearer to the coast, and in the southern latitudes of this region.

Clip leaf clusters from the branch ends between mid spring and mid autumn, and dry on screens or in bags. Store crushed leaves in a glass jar with an added tablespoon of grain alcohol or vodka to make the medicinal constituents more available when you make tea.

Medicinal Uses

Astringent and diuretic, madrone leaf reduces pain, soothes inflammation, and accelerates the healing of acute urinary tract infections. Like its cousins manzanita and uva ursi, it contains arbutin, which makes the urethra less hospitable to bacteria like *Escherichia coli*, the main cause of lower urinary tract infections. While avoiding stimulants, sweets, and alcohol, drink the leaf tea along with 1 pint of unsweetened cranberry juice per day to alleviate pain and inflammation and prevent *E. coli* from adhering to the walls of the urethra.

Use a douche of the leaf tea to reduce vaginal inflammation and to speed the healing of yeast infections. Soaking the hips and groin area, known as a sitz bath, in tea-infused water reduces postpartum inflammation and bleeding. As an external wash, the tea decreases redness and swelling, stops bleeding, and helps heal cuts, scrapes, and abrasions. Small amounts of the crushed leaf will add body to herbal smoking blends containing mullein or other light fluffy herbs.

Caution

Do not use during pregnancy. Because the astringent tannins can aggravate the gut, restrict internal use to no more than 4–6 days.

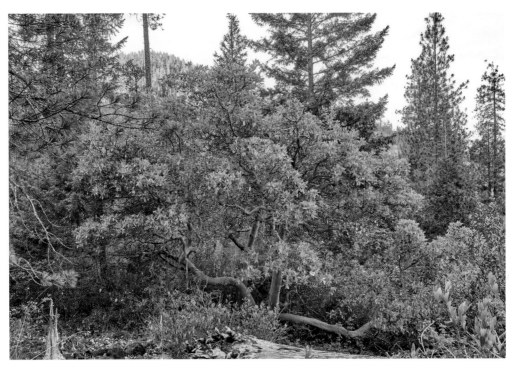

This smooth-barked tree depends on very specific mycorrhizal relationships for its sustenance.

Future Harvests

Pacific madrone, with its very specific water and soil requirements, is an indicator species whose populations throughout this region are decreasing. We can help by propagating and planting Pacific madrone trees. Remove the seeds by soaking the ripe fruit in water. Prior to sowing, cold stratify the seeds for at least 1 month in a mixture of peat and sand. This stimulates germination by mimicking the seasonal cycle that helps break the seed's dormancy. Before transplanting, add soil that you've collected from around an established, healthy madrone tree to the ground where you will plant your seedling. This will inoculate the site with symbiotic, soil-dwelling fungi known as mycorrhizae that increase the tree's ability to receive nutrients.

HERBAL PREPARATIONS

Leaf Tea
Standard infusion
Drink 3–4 fluid ounces up to 4 times per day.

Leaf Tincture
1 part fresh leaf
2 parts menstruum (75 percent alcohol, 25 percent distilled water)
or
1 part dried leaf
5 parts menstruum (50 percent alcohol, 50 percent distilled water)
Take 30–60 drops up to 4 times per day; for urinary tract infections add to 8 fluid ounces of water and drink throughout the day.

Pedicularis racemosa
betony, sickletop lousewort
PARTS USED herb

Leaves and flowers bring relief from tense muscle pain, relaxation to cramping muscles, and restful sleep to those with fear-induced insomnia.

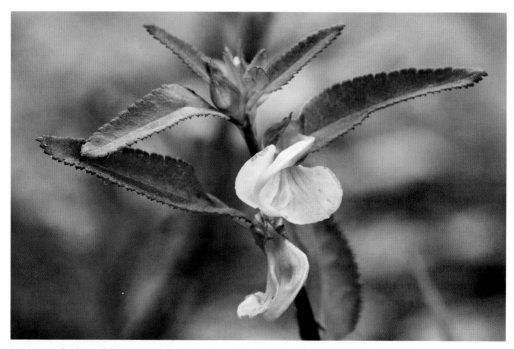

Interestingly shaped flowers are a common trait of plants in the genus *Pedicularis*.

How to Identify

From a thick woody base anchored by coarse fibrous roots with appendages, known as haustoria, that penetrate the roots of other plants to gain extra nutrients, several hairless stems extend outward or trail along the ground. Narrowly lance-shaped, slightly curving, short-stalked to stalkless leaves, 1½ to 4 inches long, with finely toothed edges alternate along 8- to 20-inch-long stems. Loose, elongated clusters of purplish pink to white, 2-lipped flowers interspersed with leaf-like bracts bloom at the branch ends from early summer to early autumn. The hooded upper lip of the flower curves downward and tapers to a beak-like tip that rests on the spreading and shallowly 3-lobed lower lip. Seeds ripen in flattened, asymmetrical, ⅜- to ⅝-inch-long capsules. Basal leaves are very small or absent. Some flowers emerge from the leaf axils, and the bracts on the flowering stalks grow progressively smaller and less leaf-like as they approach the tip.

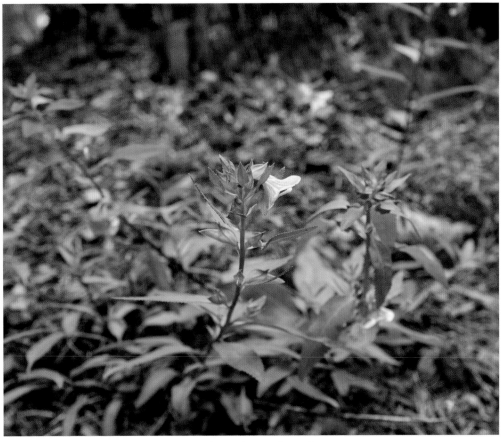

Parrot's beak usually forms hemiparasitic relationships with coniferous trees.

Several other medicinally active and commonly occurring relatives inhabit the region, including the 1- to 4-foot-tall, yellow-flowered bracted lousewort (*Pedicularis bracteosa*); the 6- to 24-inch-tall Indian warrior (*P. densiflora*), with deep red to reddish purple flowers; and the 8- to 32-inch-tall elephant's head (*P. groenlandica*), with its spikes of light pink to red-purple, elephant head–shaped flowers.

Where, When, and How to Wildcraft

Occurring more frequently as their range extends eastward, these hemiparasitic plants—they can photosynthesize as well as extract nutrients from surrounding plants—can be found adjacent to subalpine meadows and in open-canopied, mid- to high-elevation, coniferous forests from British Columbia to California.

From large patches, clip no more than two or three stems from each plant just before or while the flowers are in full bloom. Process fresh for tincture, or dry on screens for teas or smoking.

Medicinal Uses

All species of *Pedicularis* relax skeletal muscles, those muscles that we can consciously control. Take the herb tea or tincture to relieve back, neck, or shoulder pain caused by muscle tension. It doesn't deaden the pain but alleviates it by releasing the tension causing the pain.

Massage therapists, Rolfers, or other bodyworkers can offer the tincture during sessions to make adjustments easier and recommend that their clients take it post-session to prevent muscles from reverting to ingrained patterns of tension. In this same way, parrot's beak helps clear traumas stored in the musculature that cause armoring and chronic muscle tension and pain.

The tea or tincture relieves muscle pain and cramping from overexertion and insomnia when fear or traumatic events prevent sleep. Smoke the dried herb alone or mixed with other plants to enjoy its relaxing and sometimes giddiness-inducing effects.

Caution

Pedicularis species may tap into and take up constituents from toxic plants. Avoid harvesting from plants growing in close proximity to monkshoods (*Aconitum* species), senecios, or lupines.

Future Harvests

Sow ripe seeds in autumn near non-toxic, potential host plants like ponderosa pine and white fir (*Abies concolor*).

HERBAL PREPARATIONS

Herb Tea
Standard infusion
Drink 4–8 fluid ounces up to 3 times per day.

Herb Tincture
1 part fresh herb
2 parts menstruum (75 percent alcohol,
   25 percent distilled water)
or
1 part dried herb
5 parts menstruum (50 percent alcohol,
   50 percent distilled water)
Take 30–60 drops up to 5 times per day.

pearly everlasting

Anaphalis margaritacea
western pearly everlasting
PARTS USED leaf and flower

Cooling leaves and flowers tighten tissue to reduce mucous membrane swelling and inflammation.

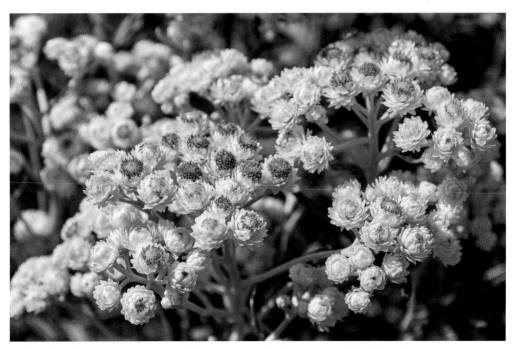

It is hard to tell when the long-lasting flowers are actively blooming. Look for the yellow, pollen-dusted stamens.

How to Identify

Loose clumps of unbranched stems from spreading rhizomes stand 8–40 inches tall. Wooly white hairs thickly cover the undersides of stalkless, lance-shaped to linear leaves. The alternately arranged leaves, green and sparsely haired above with thick midveins, roll under at the edges and maintain their size as they ascend the stem. Forming spherical, composite flower heads, several rows of dry, papery, pearly white bracts overlap to surround small yellowish flowers that bloom from mid summer to early autumn. These flower heads, up to ⅜ inch wide and lacking ray flowers, bunch together to form dense, flat-topped, terminal clusters. Pollinated flowers produce small rough-textured seeds with crowns of white bristly hairs. Dried flower heads persist intact for long periods of time, and mature plants usually lack basal leaves.

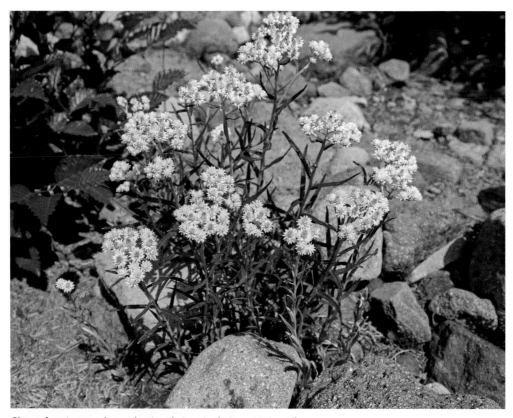

Clump-forming pearly everlasting thrives in dry mountain soils.

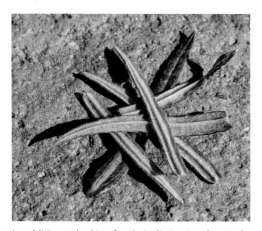

In addition to looking for their distinctive, bracted flower heads, these plants are easily identifiable by their leaves: the edges roll under, and the light-colored undersides are covered with interwoven, wooly hairs.

Where, When, and How to Wildcraft

A widely distributed, sun-loving perennial, pearly everlasting occupies dry to somewhat wet sites throughout this region and across most of North America. It prefers the mountains, but can be found growing at all elevations in forest openings, drier meadows, fields, logged areas, and along roadsides.

While the flowers are blooming, clip the stems at the base, remove dead or damaged leaves, and bundle or lay on screens to dry. After the plant material is fully dry, remove the leaves and flowers and discard the stems.

Medicinal Uses

Cooling and astringent, pearly everlasting has an affinity for the respiratory and digestive tracts and reduces mucous membrane swelling and inflammation. Drink the leaf and flower tea to soothe lung or stomach irritation, to gently clear mucus from the lungs, to relieve seasonal allergies, or to dry a runny nose. The tea also alleviates the effects of diarrhea and the stomach flu.

Gargle or swish the tea for sore throats or to heal mouth sores. Externally a wash or poultice of the leaves speeds the healing and lessens the swelling of bruises, wounds, and sunburns.

Added to smoking blends, the dried leaves and flowers add a pleasant, cooling flavor and stimulate the flow of mucus to help cleanse the lungs.

Future Harvests

Gather a few stalks per clumping plant. Divide root masses in spring and autumn or shallowly sow seed in spring to create new stands.

HERBAL PREPARATIONS

Leaf and Flower Tea
Standard infusion
Drink 4-6 fluid ounces as needed.

pipsissewa

Chimaphila umbellata
western prince's pine
PARTS USED leaf

Astringent and somewhat warming leaves clear urinary tract infections, strengthen the bladder and kidneys, and resolve swollen and inflamed lymph glands.

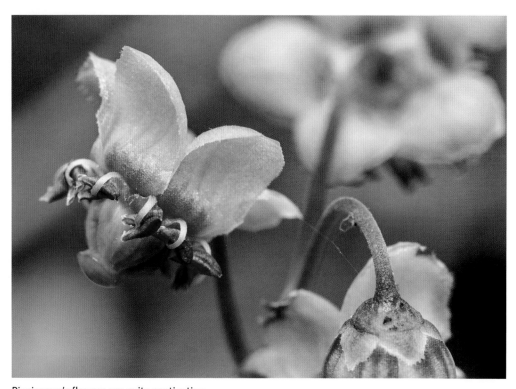

Pipsissewa's flowers are quite captivating.

How to Identify

Slender rhizomes creep slowly through deep forest duff. False whorls of 3–5 shiny green, sharply toothed, lance-shaped leaves ring 6- to 14-inch tall, sometimes branching stems supported by slightly woody bases. The thick, 1- to 3-inch-long, evergreen leaves taper at the base and are more prominently toothed near their abruptly pointed tips.

From early to late summer, small clusters of 3–10 flowers nod at the end of 1½- to 4-inch-long, slightly hairy stalks. Waxy, pink to red, concave petals reflex backward to display bulbous green ovaries surrounded by 10 purplish, swollen, 2-tipped stamens. Almost round 5-chambered capsules dry and crack open to release recently matured seeds.

Where, When, and How to Wildcraft

Shade-tolerant pipsissewa, a member of the pyrola family, prefers loamy, uncompacted, well-drained soils and can be found growing in deep forest duff throughout North America. In the Pacific Northwest, it inhabits the understory of mostly coniferous forests at low to middle elevations from Alaska to California.

Snip the upper pseudo-whorl of leaves from plants that are not flowering or actively maturing seeds. The leathery leaves are difficult to dry and turn brown easily. Dry them quickly and thoroughly on well-ventilated screens or use a dehydrator on the lowest setting to ensure they retain their green color and medicinal properties.

Medicinal Uses

Warming and stimulating pipsissewa leaf, most often used for urinary tract infections, also remedies cold stagnant conditions characterized by water retention and accompanied by discharges of pus or mucus. To speed the healing of urinary tract infections and reduce the incidence of their occurrence, drink the leaf tea or tincture in water while avoiding stimulants and sweets. Include 1 pint of unsweetened cranberry juice per day. Pipsissewa leaf has constituents similar to those of uva ursi and manzanita but is less astringent and can be used for longer duration to relieve urinary tract infections.

The tea or tincture strengthens the bladder to resolve incontinence and painful or frequent urination in cases where the muscles of the bladder are weak or lack tone. It stimulates and strengthens the kidneys and increases urine output to resolve pitting edema. This diuretic action also lessens arthritic pain worsened by swelling from excess water retention.

Pipsissewa leaf tea or tincture resolves swollen glands and skin eruptions by stimulating the removal of waste products via the lymphatics. Take it for swollen prostate, leukorrhea, or mucus discharges of the vagina or urethra.

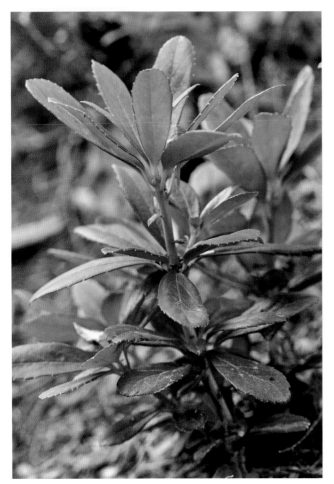

When harvesting pipsissewa, take only one pseudo-whorl per plant.

Apply hot compresses of the leaf as a counterirritant to relieve the pain of swollen, arthritic joints.

 Caution

Fresh leaves applied to the skin may cause blistering.

Future Harvests

Avoid stepping too close to the plants, as the roots are sensitive to soil compaction. Cultivation is challenging because pipsissewa needs soil mycorrhizae to thrive. To sustain healthy populations of this slow-growing forest perennial, respect its wildness and harvest conservatively. Take only one pseudo-whorl of leaves per plant, and for urinary tract infections consider using pipsissewa's more commonly found and similarly acting relatives, heart-leaved pyrola (*Pyrola asarifolia*) and white-veined pyrola (*P. picta*).

HERBAL PREPARATIONS

Leaf Tea
Standard infusion
Drink 4–8 fluid ounces up to 3 times per day.

Leaf Tincture
1 part fresh leaf
2 parts menstruum (75 percent alcohol,
 25 percent distilled water)
or
1 part dried leaf
5 parts menstruum (50 percent alcohol,
 50 percent distilled water)
Take 20–40 drops up to 4 times per day; for treating urinary tract infections, add to 8 fluid ounces of water.

ponderosa pine

Pinus ponderosa
bull pine, western yellow pine
PARTS USED bark, needle, pitch, pollen

The many uses of the bark, needles, and other parts of this majestic pine include clearing the lungs and sinuses, healing wounds, preventing infection, and increasing endurance.

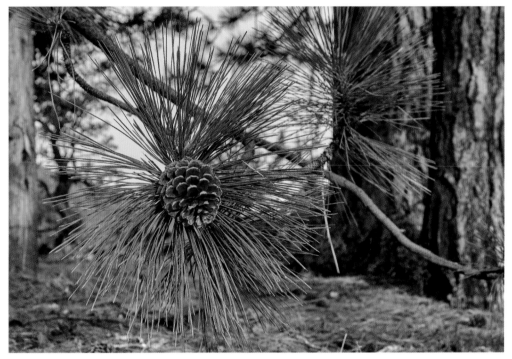

Three-needled bundles form tufts at the ends of branches.

How to Identify

Straight trunks, clear of lower branches at maturity, covered with thick, deeply furrowed, reddish brown, and black-fissured bark rise 90–200 feet in height with conical crowns of thick, heavy branches. At the ends of stout branches bundles of 3 yellowish green, pointy-tipped evergreen needles, 4–10 inches long, fan out in spherical clumps. Yellow to purplish pollen cones cluster tightly at the base of the new-growth shoots. Broadly egg-shaped, 3- to 5½-inch-long seed cones form at the ends of branches. They start out deep reddish purple, turn reddish brown, and as they mature late in their second year, end up a flat brown. Each cone scale thickens yellowish brown at its tip and terminates in a sharp outward-facing prickle. The bark of older trees is divided into large, broadly rectangular, orange-brown plates comprising

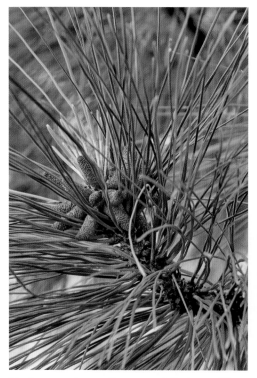

The trees produce pollen cones at the base of the new-growth shoots.

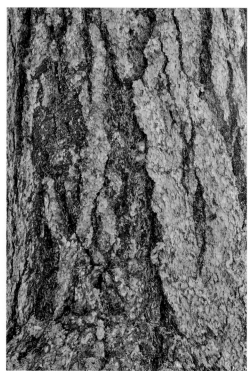

Globs of pitch ooze from bark that flakes off like jigsaw puzzle pieces.

irregularly shaped scales that flake off like jigsaw puzzle pieces. Occasionally the needles form bundles of 2–5. Trees can attain ages of 300–600 years and grow to be 4–5 feet in diameter.

Where, When, and How to Wildcraft

Shade-intolerant and able to grow on sites receiving as little as 12 inches of rain per year, ponderosa pine forms stands on the borders of grasslands and on open, dry slopes at low to middle elevations. It grows mainly east of the Cascade Crest from southern British Columbia to California, but isolated stands west of the Cascades can be found in Oregon's Willamette Valley and in the upper Skagit Valley and Puget Trough of Washington.

Gather new-growth needles in spring and summer and dry for teas or process fresh as a tincture. This is also a good time to harvest branch bark. Remove thick lower branches, and strip the bark promptly to dry in bags or on screens. Remove chunks of pitch year-round from below wounded portions of trunk. Don't gather it directly from an active wound because the trees use this protective resin to seal injuries to the bark. Collect the male cones when they are actively producing pollen from early to late spring and tincture them fresh.

Medicinal Uses

The needles, bark, and pitch are warming, drying, and stimulating. The tea, tincture, or steam of the needles or bark opens the sinuses; breaks up hard, stuck phlegm; and increases secretions to clear the lungs of mucus. The same preparations will also dry

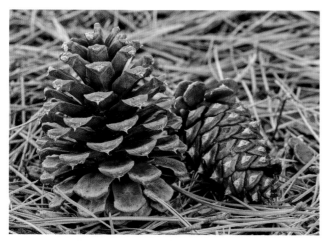

Future Harvests

Unfortunately, modern-day fire-suppression policies have contributed to a reduction in the number of ponderosa pines in this region. Without periodic fires, ponderosa pine habitat is overrun by less fire-tolerant conifer species like Douglas-fir. Please contact your local government agencies to bring awareness of the ecological threat of these policies.

The cones of ponderosa pine, smaller than those of the similar-looking Jeffrey pines found in the southern part of this region, have sharp, outward-facing prickles.

excessive and copiously flowing mucus, resolve respiratory infections and coughing, and soothe sore throats. Chewing on a chunk of pitch releases warming aromatic resins into the lungs for use in all of the above conditions. It takes some practice to find the right consistency: too hard and it cracks and sticks; too soft and it fills in the cracks of your teeth, where it stays for days and makes everything you eat taste bitter.

The needle or bark tea helps heal urinary tract infections. The needles are high in vitamin C. Pine pitch salve speeds the healing of wounds and prevents infection. Warmed pitch placed directly on the skin pulls out splinters and other foreign objects. Ingest a pollen-laden tincture of the male cones to boost the immune system, strengthen vital organs, increase endurance, and raise levels of free testosterone.

HERBAL PREPARATIONS

Needle or Bark Tea
Standard decoction
Drink 6–8 fluid ounces 3 times per day.

Needle Tincture
1 part fresh needles
2 parts menstruum (100 percent alcohol)
Take 20–60 drops up to 4 times per day.

Tincture of Male Cones (Pollen)
1 part fresh pollen-bearing cones
2 parts menstruum (75 percent alcohol,
    25 percent distilled water)
Take 30 drops 3 times per day.

Pitch Oil and Salve
For pitch oil, follow directions for Dry Herb Infused Oil (page 64) but use 1 part pitch by weight to 10 parts oil by volume. For the salve, follow directions on page 65.

quaking aspen

Populus tremuloides

PARTS USED bark

Bitter bark stimulates digestion, reduces fever, and relieves anxiety by connecting the mind with the emotions.

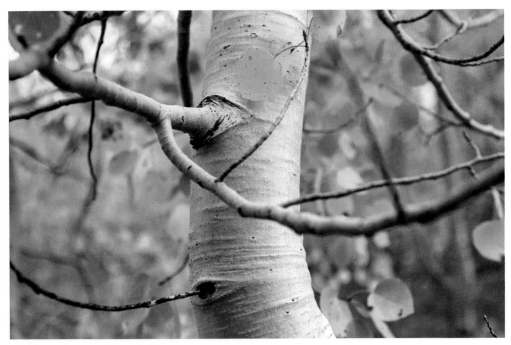

A layer of photosynthetic green bark lying just below the thin outer bark produces food for the trees during winter dormancy, allowing them to grow year-round.

How to Identify

Clonal root systems spread underground to form large, genetically identical stands. Dark horizontal lines and black, eye-like scars left by self-pruned branches mark smooth, greenish white, powder-coated bark that covers trunks ranging from short and twisting to tall and straight. Borne on long, flattened stalks that enable them to tremble in the slightest wind, round to egg-shaped, pointy-tipped, and alternately arranged leaves, green on top and silver-white below, emerge in spring from dark, shiny, non-resinous buds. Drooping catkins, male and female on separate trees, bloom from mid spring to early summer. The wind disseminates seeds coated in white fluff. In autumn, the leaves of each tree in an interconnected grove simultaneously turn brilliant orange and golden yellow before they fall to the ground. Bark at the base of very old trees, which may attain heights of 40–60 feet, becomes dark and heavily fissured.

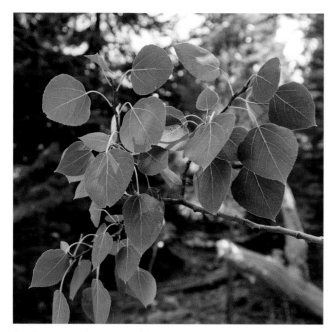
Quaking aspen leaves tremble in even the slightest breeze.

gas, discomfort after eating, and/or undigested food in the stools. It is especially helpful as a digestive tonic for nervous system–dominant people who have trouble putting on weight and is commonly used to cool the metabolism in cases of hyperthyroidism.

Aspirin-like salicylates in the bark and flowers relieve pain, lessen inflammation, and reduce fever. Quaking aspen bark was used traditionally as a substitute for quinine to treat malaria. Take the tea or tincture for any condition characterized by alternating fever and chills.

Quaking aspen bark relieves anxiety and is especially appropriate for people with anxiety stemming from a dissonance between the heart and mind. Just as the leaves of the tree quake in the slightest breeze, the person needing quaking aspen is set aflutter by the slightest external influence.

When our internal danger response system is out of whack, we may experience excess sympathetic nervous system activity that is characterized by anxiety, heart palpitations, tremors, high blood pressure, excessive sweating, a dry mouth, abdominal cramps, diarrhea, and/or frequent urination. Small doses of quaking aspen bark restore balance to the autonomic nervous system and relieve anxiety and worry by grounding the electricity of the mental sphere in the waters of the emotions. Continuing along this spectrum of healing, we may see that connecting the mind with the depths of the emotional being not only relieves anxiety but inspires creative and artistic expression.

Where, When, and How to Wildcraft

Quaking aspen, the most widely distributed tree in North America, grows in wet canyons, meadows, wetlands, and along watercourses from Alaska to California. In Washington and Oregon, it most often resides east of the Cascades. The presence of aspens in a dry area is a tell-tale sign that there is underground water nearby.

In spring, after the leaves emerge, remove branches that are thumb-sized or bigger. Strip the bark promptly and process fresh or dry on screens or loosely in bags.

Medicinal Uses

Quaking aspen bark is bitter and astringent with a slightly resinous flavor reminiscent of its cousin, black cottonwood. The tea or tincture of the bark helps regulate the release of bile into the stomach to aid digestion. Take either preparation 15 minutes before meals if you experience bloating,

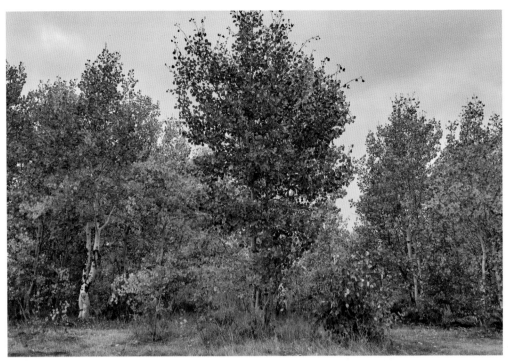

Quaking aspen is a clonal tree. An 80,000-year-old quaking aspen colony in Utah, known as Pando, is considered by some to be the oldest and largest living organism in the world.

 Caution

Do not use with hypothyroid conditions.

Future Harvests

Cutting branches stimulates growth. Respectfully harvest single branches from trees in large, healthy stands.

red alder

Alnus rubra

PARTS USED bark

The bark of red alder, whose motto is "give more to receive more," speeds the removal of waste products and increases the body's ability to absorb nutrients. It also heals wounds and reduces pain and inflammation.

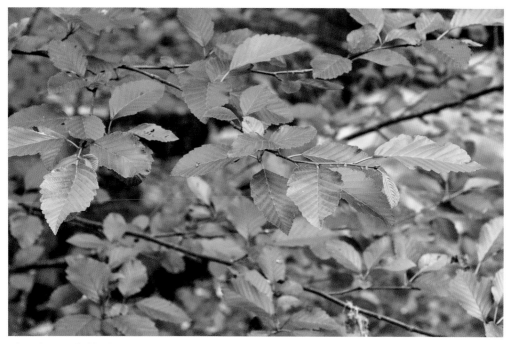

After these red alder leaves fall, they will decompose into the soil to provide root-nodule-captured nitrogen and other nutrients for nearby trees and plants.

How to Identify

Smooth, gray, white-mottled bark, often covered with greenish or gray lichens, covers trunk wood that turns red when cut. Before the leaves emerge in spring, clusters of pendulous male and woody cone-like female catkins sprout from the previous year's new-twig growth. Male catkins borne on stalks, surprisingly rose flavored and scented when fresh and blooming, dangle 2–4¾ inches long; ½- to ¾-inch-long female catkins remain on the tree throughout the year. From brown, short-stalked buds, alternately arranged, pointy-tipped, elliptic leaves unfurl with doubly round-toothed and rolled-under edges. Their upper surfaces are smooth and dark green, and their undersides are a paler grayish green and covered with short rusty hairs. Small nutlets with narrowly winged margins are spread by the wind.

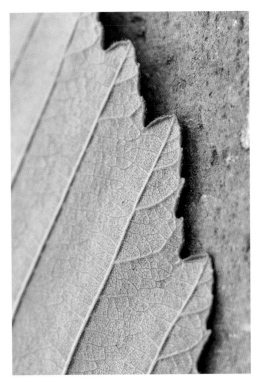

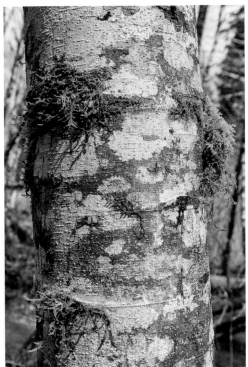

The rolled-under leaf edges make for easy identification.

Red alder's beautiful white-mottled bark is often home to mosses and lichens.

Where, When, and How to Wildcraft

Rapidly growing, short-lived, and shade intolerant, the broad-leaved red alder grows up to 80 feet tall with 10- to 20-inch-diameter trunks and colonizes disturbed lands to prepare the way for longer-lived conifers. With a range extending from Alaska to California and eastward into Idaho and Montana, it forms extensive stands in wet forests, along waterways, and on disturbed sites such as floodplains and clear cuts from sea level to middle elevations. Find it growing mainly west of the Cascade Crest, on the Olympic Peninsula, and in a few isolated stands in northeastern Washington.

Unlike other trees that yield good medicine from thumb-sized or bigger branches, in red alder I've found that the thicker trunk bark makes the best medicine. After the leaves emerge in spring, peel the bark off of downed but living trees or remove thin vertical strips from standing trees.

Medicinal Uses

Stagnant lymph or "dirty" blood may lead to a buildup of toxins in the body that can result in skin eruptions or chronic infections. Red alder bark cleans and purifies the blood by increasing the flow of lymphatic fluids to speed the removal of waste products. Take the tea or tincture to alter the internal terrain that gives rise to eczema or other red, itchy skin eruptions. Applied externally as a wash, a tea of the bark soothes acute episodes of these conditions.

Bitter red alder bark also gets the digestive juices flowing to prepare the body to receive nourishment, while its astringent tannins improve tissue tone throughout the digestive tract. Tightening permeable and lax tissues and strengthening digestive function increases the body's ability to absorb nutrients.

Salicin, a constituent similar to aspirin found in red alder bark, reduces pain and inflammation both externally and throughout the digestive tract. Preparations of the bark also stop bleeding, seal gaping wounds, and heal damage to the mouth, stomach, and intestines.

 Caution

The fresh bark ingested as a tea is reported to be emetic.

Future Harvests

Red alder, which rehabilitates disturbed forestlands, often grows in unstable places where you are sure to find individuals that have been knocked over by the wind, by other trees, or by waters that have eroded the banks upon which they grow. Search for a fallen tree that is still rooted, and cut the trunk at its base. Remove as much bark as you can use. The tree will re-sprout from its intact root system and form a new trunk or trunks. If the root system is exposed, test the bark to be sure it is living: if you are harvesting while the sap is running, the bark should easily separate from the trunk wood.

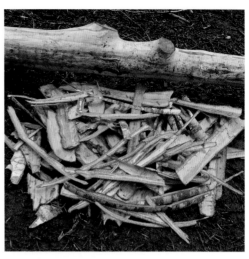

Soon after it is stripped, the inner bark turns red.

HERBAL PREPARATIONS

Bark Tea
Standard decoction
Drink 2–4 fluid ounces up to 4 times per day.

Bark Tincture
1 part dried bark
5 parts menstruum (50 percent alcohol, 50 percent distilled water)
or
1 part fresh bark
2 parts menstruum (75 percent alcohol, 25 percent distilled water)
Take 15–45 drops up to 4 times per day.

Actaea rubra

red cohosh

PARTS USED root

Although the enticingly red and shiny berries are toxic and should be avoided, the roots of red baneberry make an effective medicine for dull achy muscles, menstrual cramps, hypertension, and insomnia.

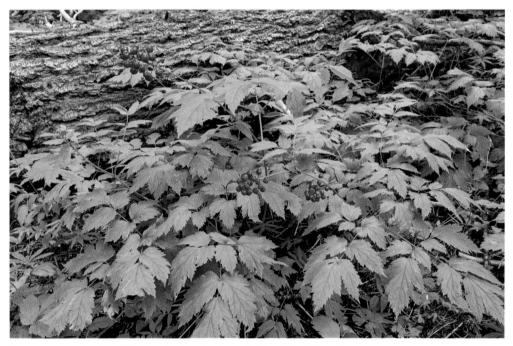

The berries are toxic, but they make the plants easily identifiable in autumn.

How to Identify

One or more stems ascend from thinly dark-barked, woody rhizomes anchored into the soil by many fleshy side roots. Alternately arranged, long-stalked compound leaves divide 2 or 3 times into groups of 3 irregularly toothed, sharply cleft, egg-shaped leaflets with deeply impressed veins. The primary leaf extends out from near the bottom of the 1- to 3-foot-tall, slightly hairy, branched stem, and 1 or 2 leaves form on the middle and upper parts of the stem. From mid spring to mid summer, white flowers on long thin stalks bloom from bottom to top in compact, terminal clusters as 3–5 whitish to purplish green, petal-like sepals open to reveal 5–10 slender, white, egg- to spoon-shaped petals. Numerous stamens, longer than the petals, radiate out from 1-pistiled centers whose ovaries ripen into toxic, oval-shaped, shiny red berries with many cone-shaped, brown seeds inside. Some plants

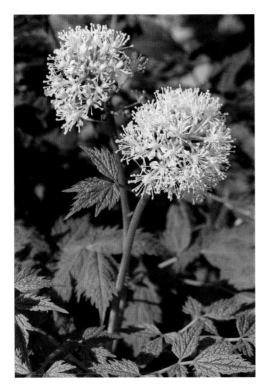

Long white stamens protrude from each flower to form a bushy inflorescence.

produce white berries, each marked with a single black dot, and older rhizomes may have reddish tinged interiors.

Unless you see it flowering or fruiting, it is difficult to distinguish red baneberry from the much less common and increasingly rare native black cohoshes, tall bugbane (*Actaea elata*) and Mount Hood bugbane (*A. laciniata*), whose much longer flowering stalks produce seed pods rather than berries.

Where, When, and How to Wildcraft

Widely distributed in forests on both sides of the Cascade Crest and throughout much of North America, this shade-tolerant perennial prefers moist, nitrogen-rich soils in mixed-evergreen or coniferous forests. In this region, red baneberry grows from Alaska to California at low to high elevations in the shade of the forest understory but can occasionally be found in open, sunny locations. Harvest the roots and rhizomes from late summer through autumn after the berries ripen and the tops begin to die back.

Medicinal Uses

Red baneberry's sweet and saponaceous roots relax the blood vessels to promote cardiovascular circulation and open the energetic channels to aid the smooth flow of energy through the muscles. Take the tea or tincture for dull muscular pain characterized by feelings of congestion and heaviness, to ease fibromyalgic pain, for uterine cramping with thick heavy menstrual flow, or for other smooth muscle spasms.

Preparations of the root relax the blood vessels to evenly disperse blood throughout the system. This slows the heart rate and respiration, reduces hypertension, and opens the surface vasculature to vent heat and toxins through the skin, which may help speed the healing of eruptive and feverish conditions like the measles. The tea or tincture also sends waves of relaxation throughout the body and calms the nervous system to promote deep, restful sleep.

Unlike its sister plant, black cohosh, which asks you to wrestle with your inner demons, red baneberry brings light-hearted joy and provides distance from the darkness of your psychological processes. If you are trying too hard to figure out the answers, take some red baneberry tincture. It may provide an opening that allows you to step back from the stresses of your life and find the resolution you seek.

⚠ Caution

Many field guides insist that all parts of red baneberry are highly poisonous, and some claim that the roots are violently purgative.

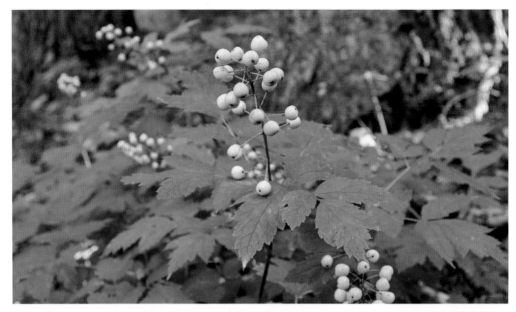
Some plants produce white berries known as doll's eyes.

The berries are toxic, but in my experience and that of many other herbalists the roots are quite safe to use and not at all purgative. However, do not exceed the recommended dosage or use during pregnancy. High doses may cause frontal headaches. Because red baneberry root may lower blood pressure, use with caution for those with bradycardia, a slow heart rate of less than 60 beats per minute.

Future Harvests

After digging up roots, trim off and discard the aerial parts, and replant a 3- to 4-inch chunk of the front portion of the rhizome with attached side roots. The rhizomes of older individuals may branch off into several crowning sections. Carefully pull them apart and replant one of the sections in the hole from which it came. Alternatively, you can remove seeds from freshly ripened berries and sow immediately in moist, nutrient-rich soil. Some of the seeds will sprout in the following spring; others will emerge a year later.

Stands of the related black cohoshes *Actaea elata* and *A. laciniata* are disappearing or diminishing in size. Admire the elegance of these beautiful medicinal plants, but do not harvest them from the wild. Instead grow these plants in the shady parts of a garden or sow their seeds in the forest to reestablish healthy populations.

HERBAL PREPARATIONS

Root Tea
Standard decoction
Drink 4 fluid ounces 3 times per day.

Root Tincture
1 part fresh root
2 parts menstruum (75 percent alcohol, 25 percent distilled water)
The roots are best tinctured fresh because they lose their sweetness after drying.
Take 10–20 drops up to 3 times per day.

red-belted conk

Fomitopsis pinicola
PARTS USED fruiting body

Tree-decaying conks provide medicine to boost the immune system,
inhibit the growth of tumors, and reduce digestive tract inflammation.

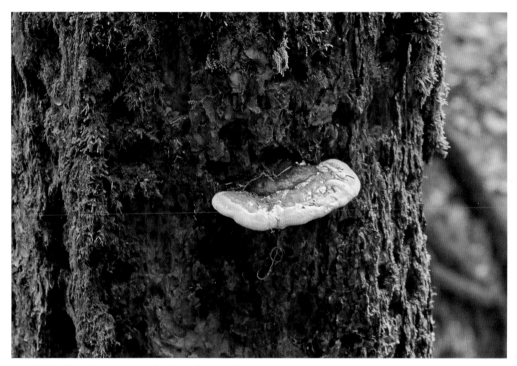

A red-belted conk grows on a dead conifer in a forest in Oregon.

How to Identify

White sheets of mycelium that break down the wood of dead or dying trees produce stalkless, knob-like conks that emerge smooth, varnished, and yellowish to orange-brown. The woody fruiting body becomes semicircular, convex to hoof-shaped, dull, and dark to blackish brown with a reddish to orange-brown belt just behind the thickened, rounded, whitish to yellow growing edge. As the fruiting body ages, concentric grooves form on its cap while the front portion near the growing edge often remains varnished. Cream-colored to pale yellow undersides with tiny spore tubes bruise a barely perceptible yellowish or pinkish color, often exude drops of clear nectar, and emit a slightly sweet and fruity aroma. Each year a new tube layer is formed, up to ⅓ inch wide, below the corky and woody, whitish to yellowish brown flesh. The color of the caps is highly variable, and it should be noted that the undersides do not bruise brown like the *Ganoderma* species with which they may be confused.

Where, When, and How to Wildcraft

Widely distributed throughout the coniferous forests of North America, these perennial, shelf-like fungi are the most prevalent polypores in the Pacific Northwest. Decomposing wood to enrich the soil of the forest floor, red-belted conks grow up to 16 inches across, 8 inches deep, and 6 inches thick, alone or in small groups, on the stumps, fallen logs, and standing trunks of dead conifers, and they are occasionally found on living trees.

Gather them when they are actively producing spores during the autumn rainy season by applying strong downward pressure to the cap. If they persist, they'll need to be pried off with a knife or digging tool. Cut them into 1-inch cubes as soon as possible. If you wait too long they become incredibly hard, and you'll need a saw to chop them up.

Medicinal Uses

Containing long carbohydrate molecules, known as polysaccharides, that stimulate the production of white blood cells, red-belted conk boosts immune system function, inhibits the growth of cancerous tumors, and lessens gastrointestinal inflammation. Drink the tea alone or with the tincture added as a daily tonic for several months to prevent, reduce, or eliminate cancerous tumors; to support general immune system function in cases of frequent colds or flus; to help autoimmune conditions such as rheumatoid arthritis; or to allay the effects of chemotherapy.

Powdered red-belted conk was traditionally used to stanch bleeding wounds. Early American botanical doctors used this fungus for intermittent fevers, enlarged spleen, chronic diarrhea and dysentery, nervous headaches, nerve pain associated with malaria, jaundice, and tubercular fevers and chills.

Future Harvests

Even though these conks are very common in our forests, harvest conservatively. Two to four ought to supply family and friends with medicine for the year.

HERBAL PREPARATIONS

Fruiting Body Tea
Long decoction
Add 1 tablespoon of coconut or olive oil per quart of water to increase the extraction of the inflammation-reducing and tumor-inhibiting constituents known as triterpenes. Simmer over very low heat for at least 2 hours.
Drink 4–6 fluid ounces twice daily.

Fruiting Body Tincture
1 part dried fruiting body
12 parts menstruum (50 percent alcohol, 50 percent distilled water)
To get the full medicinal spectrum of this fungus, add the tincture to the tea.
Take 30–60 drops up to 3 times per day.

red clover

Trifolium pratense
PARTS USED flowering top

Pink-flowered, mineral-rich red clover nourishes the nervous system,
brings balance to the female hormonal system, and cleanses the blood.

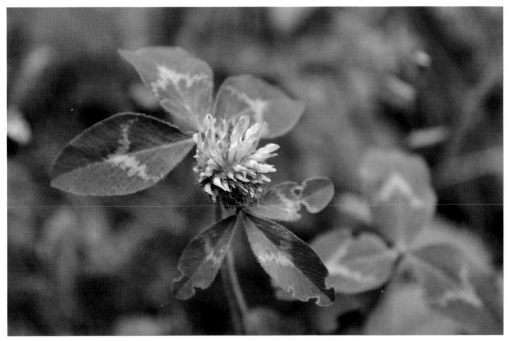

With white chevrons on its leaves and pink-flowered terminal clusters, red clover is easy to identify.

How to Identify

Several hollow, hairy stems ascend from a taproot. Widely lance- to egg-shaped, ½- to 1½-inch-long leaflets, each minutely serrated or smooth-edged and emblazoned with a whitish chevron near its base, make up 3-parted, softly fuzzy leaves that are arranged alternately along the stems. Membranaceous, prominently green-veined, ⅜- to 1⅛-inch-long, sheathing stipules (a pair of short, leaf-like appendages sometimes found at the base of a leaf stalk) taper to wispy, bristled tips. At the top of the stems, dense, conical to globe-shaped, more or less unstalked flower heads made up of 50–200 pale to purplish pink, pea-like flowers bloom from early to late summer above a pair of reduced, subtending leaves. From each flower, 2 kidney-shaped seeds, ranging in color from yellow to deep purple, ripen in egg-shaped pods.

Where, When, and How to Wildcraft

An escaped forage crop introduced from Eurasia, this 6- to 24-inch-tall, biennial or short-lived perennial commonly grows at low to middle elevations throughout the United States and Canada but is less commonly found in the upper reaches of British Columbia. Red clover occupies disturbed lands, roadsides, fields, meadows, and grassy areas.

Pick the flowering tops—the flower head and the pair of leaves below it—as they begin blooming. This is one of the more difficult plants to dry properly for tea. In order to maintain the rich color of the flowers, which can be thought of as an indicator of their medicinal activity, the tops must be dried carefully. Place them in a dry environment with plenty of airflow, and turn them over frequently.

Medicinal Uses

Mineral-rich red clover is moistening, nourishing, and high in amino acids. The tea of the flowering tops supplies essential nutrients for those recovering from major illnesses and nourishes the nervous system to mitigate the effects of stress and impart calmness.

Red clover helps balance the female hormonal system to improve fertility, relieve chronic painful menstruation, harmonize uneven menstrual cycles, and prepare for and support menopausal transitions.

The tea or tincture is a gentle, but effective, slow-acting alterative that alkalinizes the blood, aids in the assimilation of nutrients, and supports the elimination of waste products. Use it for skin rashes including eczema and to support the lymphatic system in general or to clear congested, swollen glands and lymph nodes. Apply a poultice externally for breast lumps or mastitis, a condition characterized by pain and inflammation of the breast caused by a bacterial infection or a clogged milk duct.

Caution

Because red clover contains blood-thinning coumarins, don't use it in conjunction with pharmaceutical blood thinners. Ingesting large quantities prior to surgery may lead to excessive bleeding.

Future Harvests

To ensure future harvests, leave many flowers in a patch. Insects will get nourishing nectar, flowers will get pollinated, and seeds for succeeding years' crops will be produced.

HERBAL PREPARATIONS

Flowering Top Tea
Standard infusion
Drink 4–6 fluid ounces up to 3 times per day.

Flowering Top Tincture
1 part fresh flowering top
2 parts menstruum (75 percent alcohol, 25 percent distilled water)
The herb material tends to float to the top and turn brown. Fill your jar to the top to reduce oxidation and check back in a day or two to add more menstruum if necessary.
Take 30–60 drops up to 5 times per day.

---

red root

Ceanothus velutinus
snowbrush, snowbrush ceanothus
PARTS USED root bark

*Astringent and saponaceous root bark resolves damp stagnation,
clears mucus, and improves the flow of blood and lymph.*

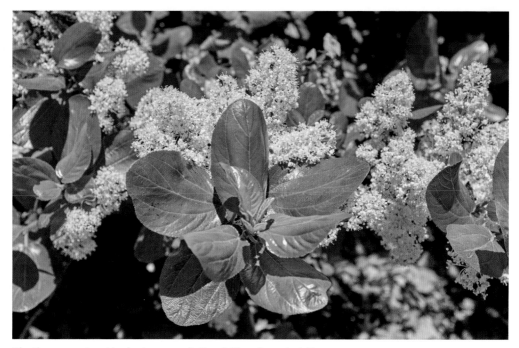

The three prominent leaf veins are a distinguishing characteristic.

How to Identify

From a very large and dense root mass, thick branches extend outward and upward up to 10 feet. The central root dives into the earth and sends out thick-as-your-arm branches that can extend horizontally as far as their aerial counterparts spread above. The outer root bark looks as if the hard and dense inner wood is expanding to stretch its skin. The inner bark is pink to dark blood red, giving this plant its name, and has a chalky, tannic, and saponaceous taste. At the end of some rootlets you may find nitrogen-fixing nodules. Shiny, aromatic, prominently 3-veined leaves, sticky with resins, fill the air with their sweet, spicy smell, and small, white flowers form dense clusters that ripen into shiny 3-chambered capsules.

In the Pacific Northwest, there are many different species worthy of the name red root. Each can be used interchangeably with *Ceanothus velutinus*. The most common are deerbrush (*C. integerrimus*), with smaller leaves, a narrower growth habit, and flowers

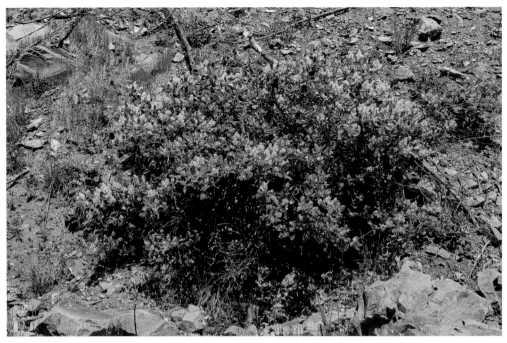

If you are driving through the mountains on a hot summer day and smell a sweet, spicy aroma, look for this lymphatic-cleansing evergreen shrub.

ranging from white to light blue to violet, and buckbrush (*C. cuneatus*), with small, ¼- to ¾-inch leaves with very short petioles, rigid branches, spines, and white flowers.

Where, When, and How to Wildcraft

Red root thrives in full sun on both sides of the Cascades in dry, mid-elevation mountains from southern British Columbia to northern California. The seeds, fire-dependent germinators, sprout in clear cuts where slash piles have been burned and in areas touched by wildfire. The roots have nodules—a signature for lymph nodes—that fix nitrogen in the soil to prepare the way for trees and other plants to re-inhabit the forest after a fire.

Harvest the root bark from mid summer to late autumn and the leaves from mid summer to early autumn. If you are harvesting a larger specimen, set aside a good chunk of time to dig the roots and to strip the root bark. Start by removing some branches to create space to dig an exploratory hole around the root crown to see which direction the side roots travel. Continue to dig around the crown and follow the spreading roots to their ends. It's easier to extract the side roots if you saw them off where they connect to the crown. When you are done, fill in the hole and mulch with the cut branches and leaves.

Medicinal Uses

I love plants that have two seemingly opposite properties. The tannins in the root bark tighten and tone tissues, whereas the saponins open and restore flow, making red root an excellent remedy for damp stagnation of all sorts. Red root has a neutral temperature, so you can add other herbs to bring warmth or cooling as necessary.

Use red root tea or tincture for boggy sore throats, swollen lymph glands, mumps, tonsillitis, lymphedema, or general lymphatic cleansing. It is a specific remedy for mononucleosis and other conditions resulting in an enlarged spleen.

It improves the flow of blood to relieve headaches after eating a high-fat meal; clears mucus in the head, lungs, and digestive tract; and as a tonic aids damp stagnation in the gut indicated by post-meal digestive sluggishness, poorly digested food, a swollen, scalloped tongue, and/or melancholy mood.

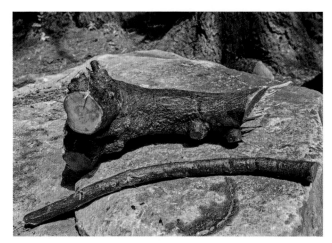

The bark of this red root crown and a small side branch was stripped soon after it was harvested.

This melancholic stagnation may also block creativity. Digesting and assimilating what we take in intellectually and energetically is an important part of the creative process. Work with red root to resolve artistic blocks and inspire creativity. Include the root bark in formulas that stir things up to speed the removal of waste products. The leaves can be added to smoking blends and make a nice beverage tea.

⚠ Caution

Don't use in conjunction with medications that thin or coagulate the blood.

Future Harvests

Find a branch that has layered and rooted in. If the root bark is pink or red, it will make good medicine. You can dig this up without disturbing the roots. When harvesting from larger shrubs, dig up one side of a plant and take a side root or two, leaving the rest. Trim off an equal-sized portion of the corresponding aerial parts to avoid stressing the plant.

HERBAL PREPARATIONS

Root Bark Tea
Standard decoction or cold infusion
Drink 4–6 fluid ounces up to 3 times per day.

Root Bark Tincture
1 part dried root bark
5 parts menstruum (50 percent alcohol, 40 percent distilled water, 10 percent glycerin)
or
1 part fresh root bark
2 parts menstruum (65 percent alcohol, 25 percent distilled water, 10 percent glycerin)
Take 30–60 drops up to 5 times per day.

sagebrush

Artemisia tridentata
big sagebrush
PARTS USED leaf, flower

Pungent and bitter leaves promote sweating, help clear lung infections, and stimulate digestive function.

How to Identify

Strips of shredding, gray to light brown bark cover 2- to 6½-foot-tall solitary stems that sometimes branch at the base. Highly aromatic, ½- to 2-inch-long leaves, silvery to grayish green, linear, and wedge shaped, widen to a usually 3-toothed tip and remain on the plant through winter. Many hairy-bracted, disc-shaped, and rayless composite flower heads usually made up of 3–6 tiny, tubular, yellowish flowers, form erect or spreading spike-like clusters with shortened leaves at their base. Blooming between mid summer and early autumn, the flowers ripen into dry seeds lacking a hairy crown. The seeds as well as the leaves are an important winter food source for wildlife, tiny hairs cover the leaves and new-growth branches, and the roots spread laterally along the surface and dive deep into the ground to make the best use of limited water resources.

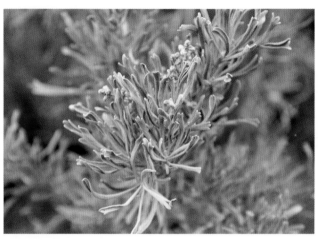

True to its specific epithet *tridentata,* the leaves of this omnipresent, high desert shrub have three-toothed tips.

Where, When, and How to Wildcraft

Growing from low to high elevations in fertile, well-drained soils throughout western North America, this woody perennial, characteristic of shrub-steppe ecosystems, inhabits valley bottoms, dry plains, and rocky slopes east of the Cascades from British Columbia to California. It is the most common high desert shrub in this region and grows very densely in the places it inhabits. Harvest branch tips when they are flowering from mid summer to early autumn.

Medicinal Uses

Sagebrush leaves make very strong medicine: it doesn't take much to get the desired effect. Drink a few ounces of the hot infusion or small doses of the tincture in hot water to promote sweating to aid the body's recovery from feverish colds and flus, to clear mucus from the lungs, or to stimulate secretions to bring on a delayed menses.

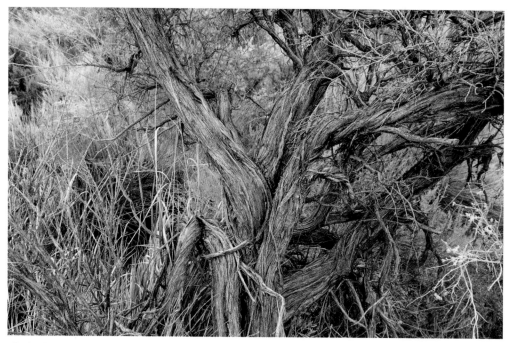
The bark on older individuals shreds in strips from the sometimes gnarled and twisting stems.

Externally, the oil rubbed on the chest or the inhaled steam clears lung congestion and speeds the healing of respiratory infections. The cold infusion stimulates digestive function and resolves dryness in the gut.

Add small amounts of the tincture (less than 10 percent) to formulas for gut infections or parasites. Smoke from the leaves has traditionally been used as a smudge to clear rooms of infection or negative energies.

⚠ Caution

Do not use during pregnancy or for extended periods of time.

Future Harvests

Because sagebrush prefers rich soils, European settlers used its presence as a guide in choosing farmland sites. Though it would seem difficult to have an impact on this widespread plant, all of the high desert land cleared for farming has greatly reduced the historical range of sagebrush. Respectfully harvest a few branches from many different plants and leave the rest for the sage grouse, elk, deer, antelope, rabbits, and other animals that rely on it for their winter sustenance.

HERBAL PREPARATIONS

Leaf Tea
Hot or cold infusion; infuse a small pinch of leaf in 4 fluid ounces of water.
Drink 1–3 fluid ounces up to 3 times per day.

Leaf Tincture
1 part dried leaf
5 parts menstruum (50 percent alcohol, 50 percent distilled water)
Take 5–10 drops up to 3 times per day.

Leaf Oil
Follow directions for Dry Herb Infused Oil (page 64).

Saint John's wort

Hypericum perforatum
Klamath weed
PARTS USED flowering top

Most famous for treating depression, Saint John's wort also resolves viral infections, relieves pain in sore muscles, and is a specific remedy for sciatica.

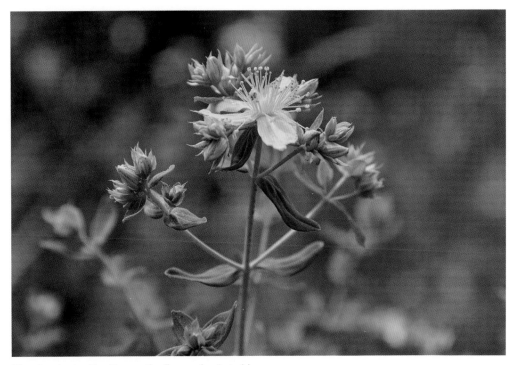

It's prime harvesting time as the flowers begin to bloom.

How to Identify

From a spreading taproot, straight green stalks with branches arranged at 45 degree angles stand erect, 2–3 feet tall. Black glands and tiny translucent holes that are visible when held up to the light dot the surface of oppositely arranged, linear to oblong leaves whose edges roll under. Clusters of bright yellow, 5-petalled, and many-stamened flowers bloom from early to late summer at the ends of the branches. The petals, lined with dark red or black glands, twist after being pollinated. The flowers and buds release a deep red to purple oil when crushed between the fingers, and the 3-parted seed capsules contain a multitude of very tiny, light to dark brown seeds.

Where, When, and How to Wildcraft

Inhabiting roadsides, clear cuts, pasture land, gardens, and waste places throughout North America, this introduced European perennial

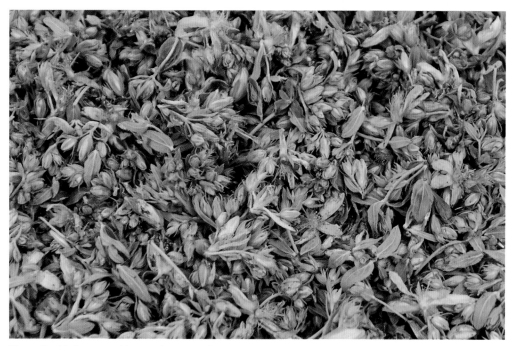

These freshly harvested Saint John's wort flowering tops are ready to be made into medicine.

grows in this region at elevations below 5000 feet from central British Columbia south into California.

Pick the flowering tops—buds, flowers, and leaves—just prior to or a bit after the flowers open but before they are pollinated. The continuously blooming flowers start to open from around the summer solstice in the lowlands to late summer in the mountains. Grasp the flowering twig ends between your fingers and give a gentle tug. Pollinated flowers will remain on the stem, but the parts you want will break free. I prefer to harvest when most of the flowers are in the budding stage because the buds contain more of the dark purple oil. Confirm this for yourself by squeezing a bud and then a flower between your fingers.

Medicinal Uses

This plant, strongly associated with the sun, brings light to dark situations, relieves seasonal affective disorder, and resolves depression especially as it relates to frustration. You may have instant results, but taking the tincture regularly for several weeks will recalibrate the brain's chemistry and help elevate the mood.

Saint John's wort flowering tops soothe and invigorate the nerves. Apply the oil externally and take the tincture internally to reduce the pain and inflammation of sciatica, a condition caused by the pinching of the sciatic nerve that starts in the lower back and travels down the leg. The tincture also harmonizes digestion by stimulating the solar plexus.

Saint John's wort is a wound healer that is especially good for deep puncture wounds because it heals wounds from the bottom up. Include Saint John's wort in formulas for herpes outbreaks including shingles. European doctors recommend taking 1 tablespoon of the oil in the morning on an empty stomach to relieve gastric ulcers. The oil applied externally relieves muscle soreness and helps sprains, strains, and bruises.

⚠ Caution

Large doses may cause photosensitivity in fair-skinned folk. Stop taking the medicine if this occurs. Clinical studies show that Saint John's wort speeds up the liver's ability to break down certain medications, thereby reducing their effectiveness. Some of the medications in question include HIV medications and drugs to reduce the rejection of organ transplants. If you are taking any pharmaceutical medication, check for possible adverse interactions. Results conflict and opinions differ on whether this action also interferes with the use of oral contraceptives. You'll have to do some research and decide for yourself.

Future Harvests

Pick freely, as new flowers will soon bloom to replace the ones you've picked. As far as propagation goes, this tough little plant does pretty well on its own. Saint John's wort is considered a noxious weed by some governmental agencies who aggressively try to eradicate it, and in Washington and California it is illegal to distribute or sell the seeds.

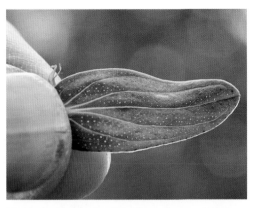

Tiny holes that let the light through are a signature for Saint John's wort's ability to relieve the darkness of depression.

HERBAL PREPARATIONS

Flowering Top Tea
Standard infusion
The effectiveness of dried Saint John's wort declines rapidly as it ages. For a medicinally active preparation, use fresh flowering tops or recently dried herb that is less than 3 months old.
Drink 4–6 fluid ounces up to 3 times per day.

Flowering Top Tincture
1 part fresh flowering top
2 parts menstruum (100 percent alcohol)
Take 15–45 drops up to 3 times per day.

Flowering Top Oil and Salve
For flowering top oil, follow directions for Fresh Herb Infused Oil on page 63. For the salve, follow directions on page 65. To make a deep red oil with more of the active constituents, crush the buds and flowers between your fingers before placing them in the oil.

salal

Gaultheria shallon
PARTS USED leaf, berry

Astringent leaves soothe intestinal inflammation, relieve diarrhea, and speed the healing of wounds. Flavonoid-rich berries can help prevent cancer and coronary disease.

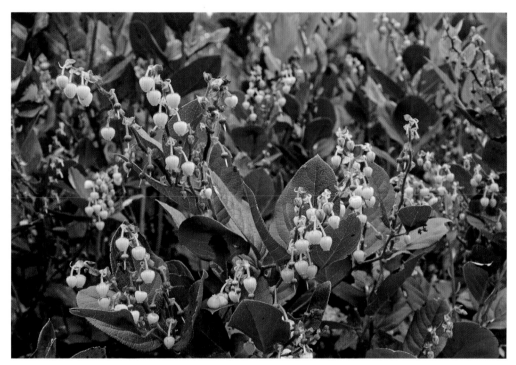

Urn-shaped flowers like these are common in members of the heath family.

How to Identify

An extensive and shallow network of roots and rhizomes spreads to form sometimes dense and almost impenetrable thickets. Thick leathery leaves, shiny, dark green, and finely serrated, are arranged alternately on hairy branched stems that extend up to 10 feet in length. White or pink-tinged, urn-shaped flowers, 5–15 per bracted raceme, hang downward covered with sticky glands and bloom from mid spring to early summer.

Covered in tiny hairs, the outer portion of the edible, berry-like capsules is made up of fleshy, modified sepals. The fleshy, round, reddish blue or dark purple pseudo-berries, filled with many seeds, ripen from late summer through mid autumn and may remain on the stem until early winter. The 2- to 4-inch-long, oval to egg-shaped evergreen leaves persist for 2–4 years, and individual plants that spread by layering and suckering may survive for hundreds of years.

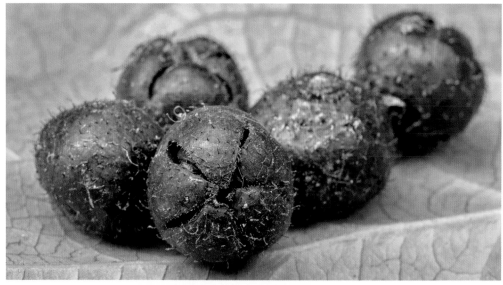

The purple berries are quite tasty if you harvest them when they are fully ripe.

Where, When, and How to Wildcraft

A common understory plant of coniferous forests, this shade-tolerant evergreen shrub forms extensive stands from southeastern Alaska southward into California. It grows from the coast to the western slopes of the Cascades at low to mid elevations.

Gather new-growth leaves from late spring to mid autumn. Cut the twig ends and bundle them for drying. Pick plump, semi-sweet berries from late summer to mid autumn after they have ripened to a dark, blackish purple color. Eat them fresh or dry them for later use.

Medicinal Uses

Drink the leaf tea to soothe intestinal and urinary tract inflammation with painful urination or to relieve diarrhea. Gargle the leaf tea to relieve sore throats or heal mouth sores. Externally a wash or poultice of the leaves stops bleeding wounds, soothes burns, and relieves irritation caused by insect bites.

As a regular part of the diet, flavonoid-rich salal berries help prevent coronary disease by lessening inflammation in the heart and blood vessels and may reduce the risk of cancer by protecting cells from free radical damage. The berries can be consumed fresh, dried into cakes, or processed into jams and jellies.

Future Harvests

Salal continues to be an important food and medicine plant for the native peoples of the Pacific Northwest. Some groups have reported illegal or inadvertent picking on ancestral harvesting grounds or a decline in berry production from plants that have been over-picked by the floral industry, which uses salal branches in flower arrangements. Do your part as a respectful herbalist. Gather leaves and berries from large healthy stands, and don't harvest on tribal lands or in places that look like they have been tended like gardens.

HERBAL PREPARATIONS

Leaf Tea
Standard infusion
Drink 4–8 fluid ounces up to 3 times per day.

Scouler's corydalis

Corydalis scouleri
Scouler's fumewort
PARTS USED whole plant, root

All parts of this bitter-tasting plant contain opiate-like, pain-relieving alkaloids.

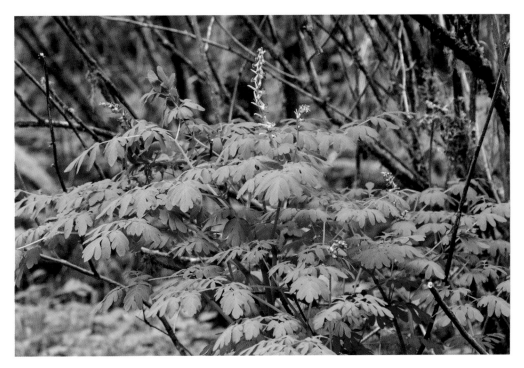

This handsome, forest-dwelling plant is a potent, low-dose pain reliever that is best used in formulas with other analgesic herbs.

How to Identify

Thick, colony-forming rhizomes produce erect hollow stems that rise 20–50 inches and sometimes branch near their tops. Bluish green, several times divided, and alternately arranged leaves, usually 2–3 growing on the upper half of the stem, grow 8–30 inches long covered with a bluish waxy powder. The ultimate leaflet segments are oblong to elliptic with round or sometimes pointy tips. Beginning in mid to late spring, 15–35 pink 4-petalled flowers, arranged in a crisscross fashion along a tall, spike-like inflorescence, bloom from bottom to top. Each ¾- to 1-inch-long thin, tubular flower is made up of a pair of outer petals with hooded crests. The upper petal has a backward-facing spur about twice as long as the rest of the flower. The tips of the inner petals fuse to form a hood that protects the flower's reproductive parts. Oval-shaped capsules, ⅜ to ⅔ inch long, forcefully explode when touched to propel shiny black seeds as

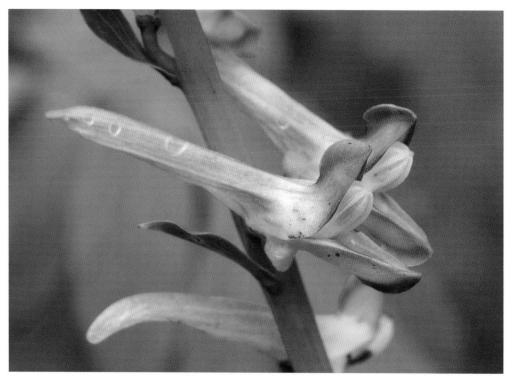

The epithet *corydalis* is Greek for "crested lark" and refers to the appearance of the flowers.

far as 3–6 feet into the forest. Oily appendages on the seeds encourage dispersal by ants.

Where, When, and How to Wildcraft

Scouler's corydalis often forms extensive patches in the understory of wet, nutrient-rich forests and along waterways in shaded riparian areas. Generally found at low elevations west of the Cascades from British Columbia to northwestern Oregon, its range extends as far north as southwestern Vancouver Island, where it is considered a somewhat rare plant. Gather the whole plant—roots, leaves, and flowers—while the plant is blooming from early to mid spring or the roots alone after the plant has set seed.

Medicinal Uses

As a member of the fumitory family, which is closely related to the poppy family,

Scouler's corydalis contains many potent, sedating, and pain-relieving opiate-like alkaloids. Combine a small amount of this low-dose plant with other plants to make a pain-relieving formula for traumatic physical injuries. Take the whole plant or root tincture internally as a general analgesic or apply externally to aching teeth, sore gums, bruises, sprains, strains, or to alleviate joint and nerve pain. The tincture of the root by itself is more potent than the whole-plant preparation.

Caution

Do not use Scouler's corydalis during pregnancy, combine with prescription medications, or exceed recommended dosage. The presence of its narcotic alkaloids in your urine may trigger a false positive result for drug tests screening for opiates.

Future Harvests

Scouler's corydalis is designated as threatened in British Columbia where road building, logging, and recreational activities have impacted the shady habitats it prefers and may threaten the continued existence of stands. Do not gather plants growing in British Columbia. Harvest only from large healthy stands in Washington and Oregon, and take just a few plants from each.

The germination rate of the seeds declines rapidly in storage. Sow the seeds immediately after they mature. Divide or transplant rhizomes to appropriate sites during the dormant season.

Pain-Relieving Formula

Combine these tinctures of local herbs for a potent pain-relieving formula.

5 parts tincture of Pacific bleeding heart root
4 parts tincture of California poppy whole plant
2 parts tincture of snapdragon skullcap herb
1 part tincture of Scouler's corydalis root

selfheal

Prunella vulgaris
common selfheal, heal all
PARTS USED herb

A supreme wound healer, this oft-overlooked plant soothes sore eyes,
clears infections, and relieves inflammation.

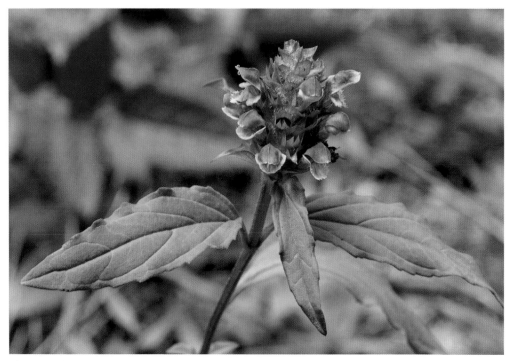

Like most plants in the mint family, selfheal has oppositely arranged leaves, square stems, and two-lipped tubular flowers.

How to Identify

Lance- to egg-shaped leaves, smooth-edged or slightly toothed, unfurl opposite each other on hairless or minutely hairy, unbranched, square-stemmed stalks that emerge from short, fibrous-rooted rhizomes. The stalked lower leaves grow up to 3½ inches long; the upper leaves, becoming shorter and narrower as they ascend, attach directly to the stem. Compact whorls of 2-lipped tubular flowers bloom blue-violet (or occasionally purplish pink or white) in terminal spikes with sharply pointed and hairy- and reddish edged bracts. The upper, smooth-edged, hood-like lips arch over 4 paired stamens, and the longer, 3-parted lower lips sport a fringed middle lobe. Each flower produces smooth, egg-shaped seeds clustered together in groups of 4 within persistent dark green to purplish calyces with wide, 3-toothed upper lips and deeply cleft lower lips with spine-tipped teeth. The flowers, minutely hairy inside, bloom from late spring to early autumn. Basal leaves are sometimes present, the lower leaf bases are more rounded than the upper, and a pair of pointed bracts tops the ¾- to 2-inch-tall flower spikes.

Where, When, and How to Wildcraft

This 4- to 16-inch-tall perennial prefers moist soils from sea level to middle elevations. Self-heal grows throughout this region and across most of the upper portions of the northern hemisphere in disturbed areas, forest edges, meadows, lawns, and gardens. Harvest the aerial parts—leaf, stem, and flower—while in full bloom from late spring to early autumn.

Medicinal Uses

Selfheal is an astringent and mucilaginous wound healer. Apply a poultice of the fresh or dried herb to stop bleeding, reduce inflammation, promote skin cell regeneration, or to draw out infection. Taken as a tea or tincture, it is a cooling fever reducer that clears infections, relieves lymphatic stagnation, and lowers elevated blood pressure. Gargle the tea to soothe inflammations of the mouth, gums, and throat including tonsillitis. Apply the tea as a wash to red inflamed eyes or to alleviate conjunctivitis, also known as pink eye.

Future Harvests

Pick away. This tough, weedy mint will keep coming back.

HERBAL PREPARATIONS

Herb Tea
Standard infusion
Drink 6–8 fluid ounces up to 4 times per day.

Herb Tincture
1 part fresh herb
2 parts menstruum (75 percent alcohol, 25 percent distilled water)
or
1 part dried herb
5 parts menstruum (50 percent alcohol, 50 percent distilled water)
Take 30–60 drops up to 5 times per day.

---

sharptooth angelica

Angelica arguta
Lyall's angelica
PARTS USED root, seed

Pungent roots warm and dry the lungs, break up mucus, aid digestive function, and stimulate the uterus to promote blood flow.

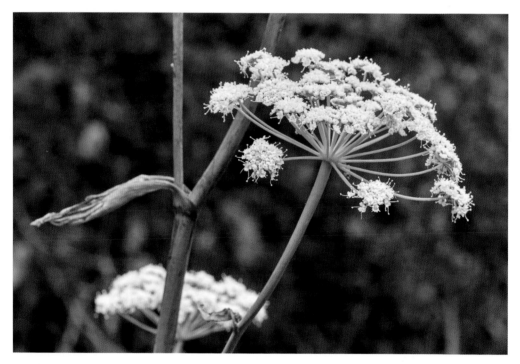

Angelica's flowering head of compound umbels is a signature for the opening of the crown that facilitates journeying.

How to Identify

Hollow, usually hairless, and sometimes purplish stems, 3 to 6½ feet tall, attach to thick, oily, big-branching taproots whose pungent smell is reminiscent of soapy perfume. Sharply toothed and irregularly cleft leaflets, narrowly oval to elliptic, pointy-tipped, and 1½ to 5½ inches long, make up thick, pale green, generally hairless compound leaves whose stalks clasp the stem with boat-like sheaths. The 3-parted leaves are further divided with leaflets arranged opposite each other along the leaf axis. Many white, 5-petalled flowers that mature into ⅓-inch-long winged, hairless seeds sit atop 1- to 4-inch-long, unequal stalks to form 2 or more flowering heads of 20–60 umbels each. The stems are occasionally very slightly hairy near the flower head, the flowers bloom from early to late summer,

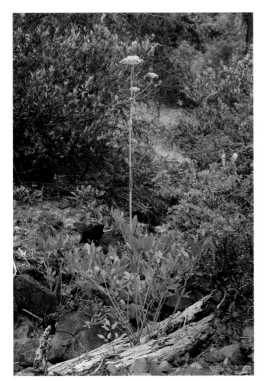

Standing tall, this sharptooth angelica grows along a dry stream bed in the Siskiyou Mountains of southern Oregon.

and mature plants are thick-foliaged at the base.

Kneeling angelica (*Angelica genuflexa*) with its angled central leaf axis is less widely distributed than sharptooth angelica. Seawatch (*A. lucida*) and Henderson's angelica (*A. hendersonii*) are stouter plants that grow along the coast. Each of these angelicas can be used for medicine; the coastal species are very bitter and pungent.

Make positive identification before harvesting this plant or any other in the parsley or Apiaceae family. Consult a botanical key to distinguish this plant from potentially deadly parsley family look-a-likes such as water hemlock (*Cicuta douglasii*), and check the "Toxic Plants" section (page 32) for tips on identifying these poisonous umbels.

Where, When, and How to Wildcraft

Find this regal, herbaceous perennial growing along waterways, in meadows, and on wet open-forested slopes from low to high elevations on both sides of the Cascades from southern British Columbia to California. In drier areas, sharptooth angelica grows only in the wettest places: roadside ditches, gullies, and below seeps and springs.

The immature seeds are greenish yellow. If left to mature on the plant, they dry to a light brown color. The optimum time to gather them is when they are just turning from yellow to brown. If they are too young their flavor will be overly sharp and pungent; too old and they will have lost much of their aromatic quality. When just right, the seeds present a roundly pungent sensation that expands throughout the mouth and head. Harvest the roots from late summer to mid autumn after the seeds mature and the leaves begin to die back.

Medicinal Uses

Warming and drying to the midsection and chest, angelica prevents chronic dampness-induced lung infections in autumn and winter. Drink the hot tea or take the tincture in hot water to improve circulation to the lungs, to break up thick mucus, and at the onset of colds or flus to open the exterior to promote sweating and drive off infection.

Bitter compounds and stimulating oils in the seeds and roots aid digestive function and relieve gas, bloating, nausea, and intestinal cramping. In cases of cold stagnation in the digestive or respiratory systems, take the tea or tincture of the root or seed to resolve dampness in and warm the gut or lungs. For delayed menstruation from cold stagnation in the womb, angelica root tea or tincture stimulates and warms the uterus to promote blood flow and relieve pain and cramping.

Angelica was used by the Saami and Laplanders of northern Europe to facilitate shamanic journeying. Sharptooth angelica opens the crown and teaches the importance of good grounding before leaving the body to travel in the angelic realms.

⚠ Caution

Because they contain an oil that can irritate the mucous membranes, do not ingest preparations made from the fresh roots. Angelica root and seed stimulate the uterus, so don't use either during pregnancy. Ingesting angelica in any form may cause skin photosensitivity.

Future Harvests

Replant the crowns and sow seeds after harvesting.

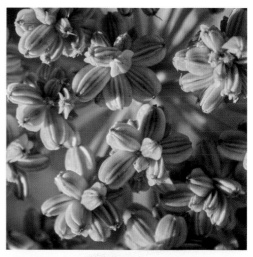

These sharptooth angelica seeds are entering the perfect stage for making good medicine.

HERBAL PREPARATIONS

Root or Seed Tea
Standard decoction
Drink 4–6 fluid ounces up to 4 times per day.

Root Tincture
1 part dried root
5 parts menstruum (65 percent alcohol, 35 percent distilled water)
Take 15–60 drops up to 5 times per day.

Seed Tincture
1 part dried seed
4 parts menstruum (75 percent alcohol, 25 percent distilled water)
Take 15–60 drops up to 5 times per day.

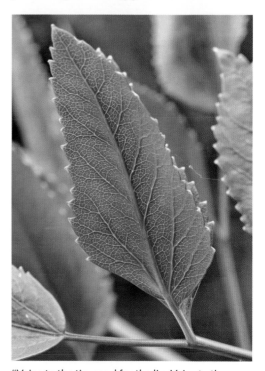

"Veins to the tip, good for the lip. Veins to the cut, bad for the gut." This couplet is helpful in distinguishing between angelicas and water hemlock, a deadly toxic plant, but not entirely reliable. Use other characteristics to make a positive identification.

sheep sorrel

Rumex acetosella
PARTS USED whole plant

Sour and cooling sheep sorrel increases urine output, stimulates the liver, and cleans the blood.

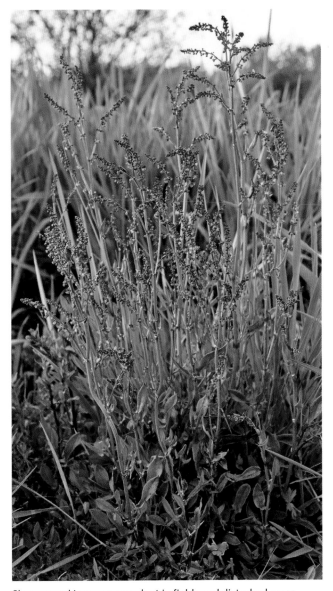

Sheep sorrel is a common plant in fields and disturbed areas.

How to Identify

Thin rhizomes spread to form sometimes dense colonies. Small, sour-tasting leaves, arrowhead-shaped with widely flaring lobes at the base, become less lobed and shorter-stalked as they climb the 4- to 18-inch tall stems. On separate plants, male and female flowers bloom yellowish to red in a series of small, branched clusters atop the stalks. Pollinated female flowers ripen into small, dry, triangular fruits. Thin sheaths wrap around the stem above each leaf.

Where, When, and How to Wildcraft

This introduced Eurasian perennial colonizes moist locales throughout temperate North America. Find it in disturbed areas, gardens, and along roadsides from low to middle elevations. Gather the whole plant from unpolluted sites while the plants are flowering from late spring to late summer.

Medicinal Uses

Sheep sorrel is a sour and cooling diuretic that stimulates

the liver and cleanses the blood. It is one of the ingredients in the Essiac formula that has been used to treat cancer. Adding the delightfully sour leaves to soups and salads also imparts a medicinal effect.

⚠ Caution

Sheep sorrel contains oxalic acids that can bind with and prevent the absorption of calcium and other minerals. There is some debate regarding the role of oxalate-containing foods in the formation of kidney stones. If you are prone to kidney stones, limit your ingestion of sheep sorrel and other foods high in oxalic acid, such as spinach, Swiss chard, rhubarb, beets, nuts, chocolate, wheat bran, strawberries, peanuts, and almonds.

Future Harvests

Like other weedy plants that prefer disturbed soils, sheep sorrel has no problem spreading itself far and wide.

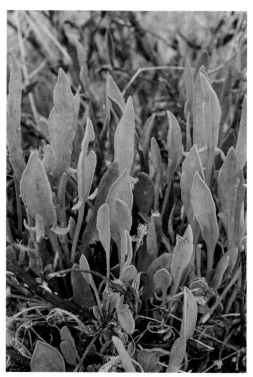

Distinctive, arrowhead-shaped leaves make sheep sorrel easy to identify.

HERBAL PREPARATIONS

Whole Plant Tea
Standard infusion
Drink 4–6 fluid ounces up to 5 times per day.

Whole Plant Tincture
1 part fresh whole plant
2 parts menstruum (50 percent alcohol, 50 percent distilled water)
Take 30–60 drops up to 5 times per day.

shepherd's purse

Capsella bursa-pastoris
PARTS USED whole plant

Best known as a remedy for postpartum hemorrhaging, this spicy and salty mustard stops nosebleeds, resolves edema, and lowers blood pressure.

How to Identify

From the crown of a small taproot, stalked basal leaves form a rosette of reverse-lance-shaped, 1- to 2-inch-long leaves that range from smooth edged to slightly toothed to lobed. Unstalked, alternately arranged, lance-shaped, and saw-toothed or smooth-edged leaves with ear-like lobes at the base clasp the 4- to 20-inch tall, simple or branched, erect stems. Small, white, 4-petalled flowers bloom continuously from early spring to mid summer in many-flowered clusters on thin, spreading stalks. Flattened, heart-shaped to triangular, 2-valved seed-pods, squared off or slightly notched at their broad tips, ripen from the bottom to the top of the stalk as the flowers continue to bloom upward. The lower part of the stem is generally covered in 3- to 5-rayed, star-like hairs.

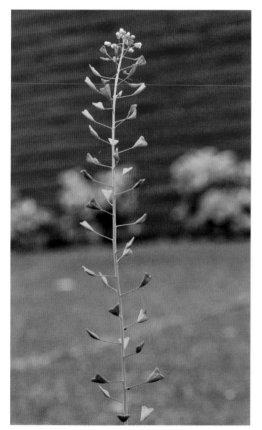

The heart-shaped to triangular seed pods look like the bags formerly used by European sheep herders.

Where, When, and How to Wildcraft

Introduced from Europe, this annual is found throughout North America and resides in dry-soiled, disturbed sites from low to high elevations. Find it in fields, gardens, waste places, and along roadsides. Harvest the whole plant with green seedpods present.

Medicinal Uses

Shepherd's purse whole plant tincture redistributes blood in the body to stop many types of bleeding. Take it for postpartum hemorrhaging, nosebleeds, blood in the urine or stool, or apply it externally to stanch bloody wounds. Take small doses all month to remedy excessive and heavy menstrual bleeding with sluggish, dark, and clotted blood.

As a diuretic, it stimulates the kidneys to resolve edema, clears bloody sediment from the urine, and removes uric acid buildup to relieve gout. It also lowers blood pressure, relieves diarrhea, and stimulates the flow of congested blood in the uterus to prevent uterine fibroids.

Caution

This medicine is not for use during pregnancy or for those with bradycardia, a slow heart rate of less than 60 beats per minute.

Future Harvests

Though this weedy mustard needs little assistance, you may choose to plant its seeds in dry, disturbed, nutrient-poor areas to increase the availability of its medicine and benefit the health of the soil.

HERBAL PREPARATIONS

Whole Plant Tincture

1 part fresh whole plant
2 parts menstruum (75 percent alcohol,
   25 percent distilled water)
or
1 part dried whole plant
5 parts menstruum (50 percent alcohol,
   50 percent distilled water)
Take 20–60 drops up to 5 times per day; for postpartum hemorrhaging take 30 drops every 15 minutes until the bleeding stops.

Sitka valerian

Valeriana sitchensis

PARTS USED root

*Sweet, bitter, and pungent roots calm the nerves, promote sleep,
relax cramping muscles, and invigorate the senses.*

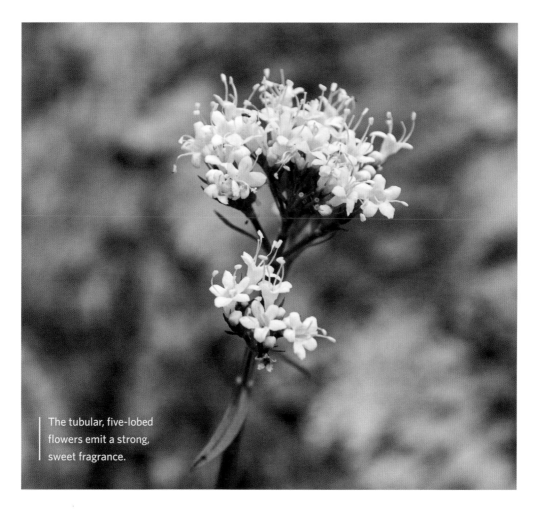

The tubular, five-lobed flowers emit a strong, sweet fragrance.

How to Identify

From small clumps connected by somewhat rigid, green rhizomes with thin, highly pungent, white side roots, unbranched stems rise 1–4 feet tall. Arranged opposite each other on the stalks, 2–5 pairs of deeply lobed to compound and often coarsely toothed leaves grow smaller and shorter-stalked as they ascend the stem. White to pink-tinged, tubular, and 5-lobed flowers bloom from early to late summer in compact heads atop the stems. Small egg-shaped seeds ripen from

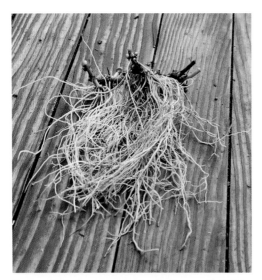

Some people have an aversion to the scent of Sitka valerian roots, comparing it to the smell of dirty socks. Others, like myself, enjoy the strong aroma.

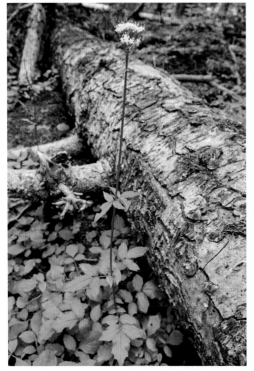

Sitka valerian is smaller than the European valerian (*Valeriana officinalis*), but its roots are no less potent.

late summer to early autumn. Basal leaves are smaller than the stem leaves, the terminal lobe or leaflet of the leaves is larger than the others, and the stamens of the sweet-scented flowers protrude past the corolla.

Where, When, and How to Wildcraft

Common throughout the northern portions of western North America, this herbaceous perennial forms large stands in wet, open-forested areas, in meadows, and along streams at middle to high elevations. Find it growing in this region from Alaska to northern California.

Gather the roots and rhizomes from late summer through mid autumn after the seeds mature and the plants begin to die back. When harvesting, be aware that Sitka valerian grows near toxic plants such as false hellebore (*Veratrum* species) and *Senecio* species whose roots may be entangled with those of Sitka valerian. Leave aboveground parts of the plants you harvest attached to aid in positive identification.

Medicinal Uses

Take the root tincture to relieve insomnia and promote sleep. Sitka valerian root has both relaxing and stimulating properties. It relaxes and sedates the nervous system, relieves muscle spasms and cramps, and improves vision and brain functioning while stimulating the cardiac, digestive, and respiratory systems. For those with strongly functioning or excess conditions of these organ systems, Sitka valerian might not work alone: the excitation may outweigh the relaxing effects. In these cases try combining Sitka valerian with red baneberry, which sedates the organs that Sitka valerian stimulates or work with other calming nervous system remedies such as California poppy, snapdragon skullcap, or western peony.

Sitka valerian root is one of the best adjunct therapies for healing tobacco addictions because it contains compounds that closely mimic the effects of nicotine, which also calms the nervous system and stimulates the cardiac, digestive, and respiratory systems. Whenever the impulse to reach for a cigarette comes, take some Sitka valerian root tincture instead. I've seen this work with many people, but I was truly sold when I saw it help an elderly Bulgarian woman who had been smoking several packs of dark, eastern European cigarettes daily since she was a young child. To aid the process, undertake a liver cleansing program 7–10 days after you've stopped smoking.

⚠ Caution

Do not use with sleeping medications, and use with caution at higher doses. Dependencies may develop with the stronger dry root preparations, and some people get nightmares from Sitka valerian. In my experience, a part of this plant's medicine is to teach us to how to work with our fears.

These nightmares may be a side effect of that process. If you would prefer not to engage in that dynamic, try something else.

Future Harvests

Harvest only part of each clump leaving roots and rhizomes to spread.

HERBAL PREPARATIONS

Root Tincture
1 part fresh root
2 parts menstruum (100 percent alcohol)
or
1 part dried root
5 parts menstruum (75 percent alcohol, 25 percent distilled water)
Take 5–30 drops as a restorative for the mind and senses; take 30–90 drops up to 4 times per day to relax the nerves and promote sleep. Because the dried root tincture is stronger than the fresh root preparations and may cause some agitation, cut the dosages in half.

smooth sumac

Rhus glabra

PARTS USED bark, leaf, berry

*Sour and astringent bark and leaves stanch watery discharges and bleeding,
relieve incontinence, and reduce inflammation in the mouth and throat.*

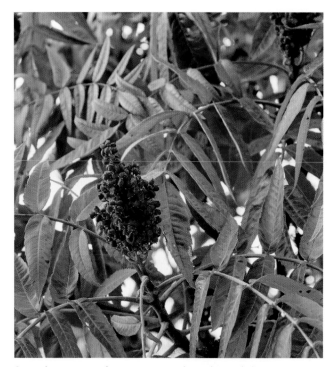

Smooth sumac produces attractive, fuzzy-berried clusters.

female flowers form on separate plants. Flattened berry-like fruits ripen reddish, hairy, and fleshy from early to mid autumn and may remain on the plant intact through winter. Birds and mammals eat the sour berries and distribute the seeds, and the plants spread via rhizomes.

How to Identify

Smooth-barked, brownish gray branches, sometimes slightly hairy near the flowering heads, exude a white, milky sap when cut. Compound leaves comprising 7–29 saw-toothed and broadly lance-shaped to elliptic leaflets spread outward like a bird's wings and turn a deep red or golden yellow in autumn. At the tops of the stems, dense pyramidal clusters of small yellowish flowers with 5 abruptly pointed petals bloom from mid spring to mid summer. Male and

Where, When, and How to Wildcraft

Growing throughout North America, this 3- to 10-foot-tall, thicket-forming shrub occupies dry rocky hillsides, open woodlands, and sunny river and stream banks in the eastern part of this region. Find smooth sumac growing at low to middle elevations from British Columbia southward. Harvest the bark in spring and summer after the leaves emerge, the leaves during flowering, and the bright red berries after they ripen in autumn.

Medicinal Uses

With their sour taste and astringency, the bark, leaves, and berries of sumac cool and tone tissues. The tea or tincture of the bark or leaves dries excessive mucus secretions in the lungs and upper respiratory tract, stops excessive sweating, and strengthens the kidneys to stop frequent urination and incontinence. Use either to stanch postpartum bleeding, to dry watery vaginal discharges or excessive and watery menstrual bleeding, or for prolonged cases of diarrhea.

Gargle the bark or leaf tea to soothe and cool inflammation of the mouth or throat or to speed the healing of mouth sores. The sour berries mixed with lemon balm make a cooling, relaxing, and refreshing summer beverage.

Recent research on Middle Eastern species of sumac shows that the traditional use of sumac berries for treating diabetes is well founded. Studies show that a daily dose of the powdered berries lowers blood sugar levels and decreases insulin resistance for those with Type 2 diabetes. It is possible that our native species may have similar properties, but further investigation is needed.

Future Harvests

When gathering bark, harvest no more than two stems per plant from healthy abundant stands. To make new plants, gather clusters of ripe berries, place them fully dried in a cloth sack, and beat the sack with a stick until the clusters break apart and the seeds are free of berry flesh. To aid germination, scar the hard seed coat with sand paper, nick it with a knife, or soak the seeds in water overnight. When stored well, the seeds remain viable for up to 10 years.

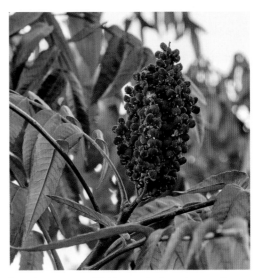

In autumn, pyramidal berry clusters ripen as the leaves turn a brilliant red.

HERBAL PREPARATIONS

Bark Tea
Standard decoction
Drink 6–8 fluid ounces 3 times per day.

Leaf or Berry Tea
Standard infusion
Drink 6–8 fluid ounces 3 times per day.

Leaf or Bark Tincture
1 part fresh leaf or bark
2 parts menstruum (75 percent alcohol,
    25 percent distilled water)
or
1 part dried leaf or bark
5 parts menstruum (50 percent alcohol,
    50 percent distilled water)
Take 15–30 drops up to 4 times per day.

Powdered Berries
*Place berries in a blender, blend for a short
    period to separate the flesh from the seeds,
    and strain to remove seeds and stems.
    Consume 3 grams per day.*

snapdragon skullcap

Scutellaria antirrhinoides
nose skullcap
PARTS USED leaf

Bitter leaves nourish the nerves to calm anxiety, soothe pain, and relax muscle spasms.

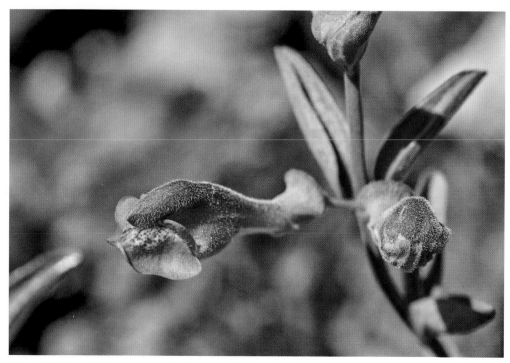

The reddish tinged ridge on the calyx gives the skullcaps their name.

How to Identify

Clusters of thin stems, 4–14 inches tall and covered with soft upturned hairs, stand erect from a branching base attached to slender, sometimes swollen-tipped rhizomes. Three to 5 prominent veins extend from near the base of short-stalked, oppositely arranged, egg-shaped to oblong, smooth-edged, and round-tipped leaves. Single, violet-blue, 2-lipped, softly hairy flowers bloom in the upper leaf axils from early to mid summer.

The side lobes of the spreading, 3-lobed lower lip attach to the hood-like upper lip, and blotches of violet-blue mottle the white-patched, wavy-edged, and widely spreading central lobe. After pollination 4 black nutlets mature enclosed in calyces with concave, prominently ridged tops.

Several other species of skullcap can be found in this region, including narrow-leaved skullcap (*Scutellaria angustifolia*), marsh skullcap (*S. galericulata*), and mad-dog or

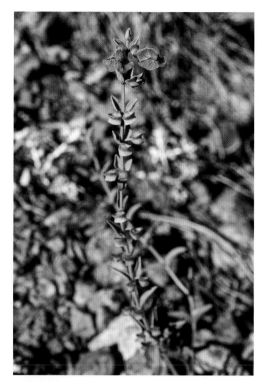

Unlike other species of skullcap, snapdragon skullcap prefers to reside in dry, rocky soils.

blue skullcap (*S. lateriflora*). Each can be used interchangeably for medicine.

Where, When, and How to Wildcraft

Scattered about in a few counties on both sides of the Cascades in Washington but fairly common in eastern Oregon and across a contiguous chunk of northern California and southwestern Oregon, this short-lived perennial mint, occasionally found on serpentine soils, prefers dry, rocky places. Find snapdragon skullcap growing in full sun at low to middle elevations on slopes and along ridges in oak woodlands and coniferous forests.

While flowering, clip stems near the base. Process fresh for tincture or dry in bags or on screens.

Medicinal Uses

Snapdragon skullcap leaf nourishes the nerves and increases blood flow to the brain. It is especially helpful for those affected by chronic stress and mental and physical exhaustion. Take the tea or tincture to relieve restlessness, agitation, fear, and worry that leads to anxiety and insomnia; to lift the spirit and calm feelings of overwhelm; to soothe overstimulated nerves; or to relieve nervous indigestion.

A specific remedy for the painful muscle spasms of tetanus or lockjaw, these same preparations relieve convulsions, uterine spasms, and twitching muscles and calm irritated nerves to reduce nerve, menstrual, tooth, and headache pain. They also help the nervous system recover from the effects of drug addiction and ease the withdrawal from benzodiazepine medications such as Valium, Xanax, and Ativan.

Future Harvests

Restrict your harvest to large healthy stands, and take only one or two stems from each plant. This will ensure that every plant has the opportunity to produce seed. Some species of skullcap are easily propagated by root division, and the seeds, sown in autumn or early spring, germinate readily.

HERBAL PREPARATIONS

Leaf Tea
Standard decoction
Drink 4-6 fluid ounces up to 3 times per day.

Leaf Tincture
1 part fresh leaf
2 parts menstruum (75 percent alcohol, 25 percent distilled water)
Take 15-45 drops up to 3 times per day.

spreading dogbane

Apocynum androsaemifolium
bitter root, dog's bane, werewolf root
PARTS USED root

Thin, bitter-tasting roots, used in the past to restore proper bile duct function, inspire great change that leads to psychological and emotional healing.

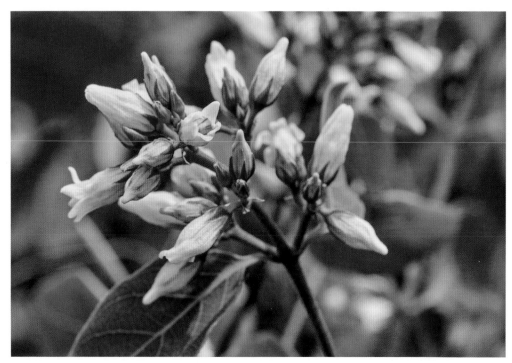

Like those of other members of the dogbane family, spreading dogbane's flowers twist open as they bloom.

How to Identify

Often reddish, many-branching stems with or without hair spread 7–18 inches from an interconnected, rhizomatous network of thin, woody, dark-barked roots. The upward-rising portions of the roots sometimes join the long, laterally running roots to form right angles. Smooth-edged, oval to egg-shaped, dark green leaves, 1½ to 3 inches long, arranged oppositely on the stem droop down with lighter-colored undersides. From early summer to early autumn at the ends of the stems or on stalks originating from the upper leaf axils, pink, bell-shaped, 5-lobed flowers form small clusters that bloom from top to bottom. The lobes of the flowers spread out or curve backward, and the flowers are sometimes a pale pinkish white marked with pink stripes. Pollinated flowers produce pairs of thin, 2- to 5-inch-long,

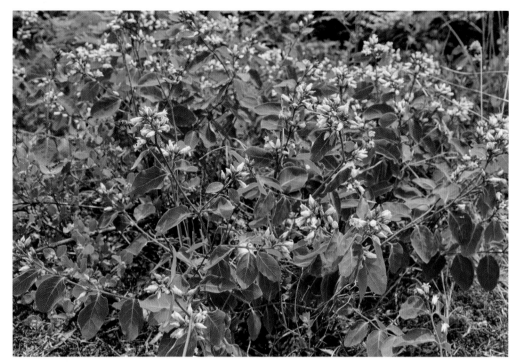

When blooming, spreading dogbane is unmistakable. During other times of the year look for the oppositely arranged, drooping leaves and reddish stems. Pinch off a bit of stem and check for milky sap to confirm the identification.

pincer-like pods with sometimes-touching tips. Numerous cotton-tufted seeds ripen in the arcing pods. The stems and leaves ooze a milky sap when cut.

Where, When, and How to Wildcraft

Often growing on south-facing road cuts, this low-growing perennial resides in dry, sunny locations throughout much of North America. In this region, find it at low to high elevations in dry meadows, rocky places, and forest openings from Alaska to California. Spreading dogbane is more frequently found at lower elevations and in hotter, drier locations with lower levels of annual precipitation.

Gather roots and rhizomes in autumn after the seeds have ripened and the tops have begun to die back. Dig straight down from the crown until you find the junction between the vertical and horizontally running rhizomes. Follow these running roots as far as you are able before removing them from the ground.

Medicinal Uses

Because it strengthens and tones the bile ducts, early American botanical doctors used spreading dogbane root to stimulate sluggish bile secretion. It was especially indicated for cases of jaundice, swelling of the liver, or for those with a sallow complexion, a damp, sticky, and yellow-coated tongue, or clay- or dark-colored stools, all of which are indicative of deficient bile duct function. By promoting the flow of bile, spreading dogbane was also said to be an efficient laxative.

Today, this often overlooked yet potent medicine is mostly used for psychological and emotional healing. Used in the proper context, spreading dogbane root has the ability to reconfigure and rewire connections in the brain to inspire profound change. Take small doses of the tincture to let go of addictions to substances, negative emotional states, or mental processes; to alter the way you unconsciously react to challenging situations or to people you perceive as difficult; or to break unhealthy habits and patterns that lead to depression, anxiety, or sorrow. After clearing away these impediments to health and happiness, spreading dogbane root will help you see your true self more clearly and allow you to establish positive relationships with others and more easily find your mission and purpose in life. To remove warts, apply the fresh milky sap directly on the affected area.

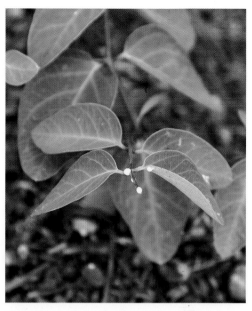

The milky sap oozes from cut stems and leaves and is used to remove warts.

 Caution

Do not use during pregnancy or with prescription medications. In larger doses, preparations of spreading dogbane may cause nausea or vomiting. Do not exceed recommended dosages or ingest the milky sap.

Future Harvests

Harvest conservatively from large healthy stands, and scatter ripe seeds in the areas where you are digging the roots.

HERBAL PREPARATIONS

Root Tincture
1 part fresh root
2 parts menstruum (75 percent alcohol, 25 percent distilled water)
or
1 part dried root
5 parts menstruum (50 percent alcohol, 50 percent distilled water)
Take 1–5 drops up to 3 times per day.

sweet gale

Myrica gale
bog myrtle, sweet bayberry
PARTS USED leaf

Astringent, bitter, and spicy leaves reduce inflammation, stimulate circulation, and clear the lungs of mucus.

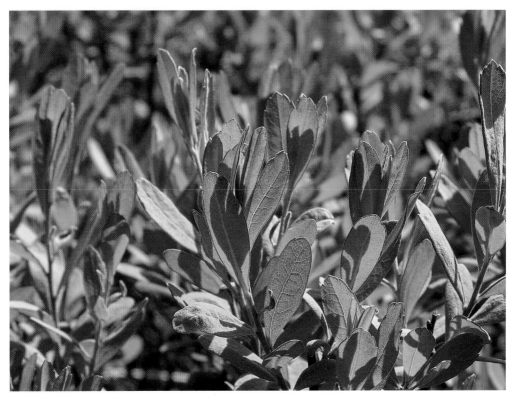

Sweet gale leaves may have rounded or few-toothed tips.

How to Identify

Finely hairy when young and becoming hairless as they mature, loosely branched stems with dark reddish bark extend 1½ to 6 feet. Alternately arranged, aromatic, reverse-lance-shaped leaves, 1¼ to 2½ inches long and hairy above and below, bear bright yellow wax glands and are smooth edged to few toothed nearer their rounded to blunt-edged tips. On separate plants from mid spring to early summer, male and female flowers form in stalkless catkins on the upper parts of the previous year's growth. Male catkins, ⅜ to ¾ inch long, crowd the branchlets housing flowers enfolded in broad, shiny brown to reddish bracts. A pair of spongy, wing-like bracts cradles each wind-pollinated female flower and remains attached as the fruits

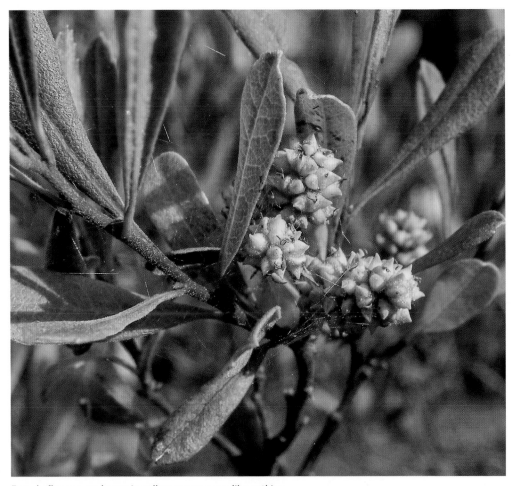
Female flowers are borne in yellow, waxy, cone-like catkins.

mature, allowing them to float upon the water for dispersal. These butterfly-like floral units organize into dense, waxy, yellow, cone-like catkins up to ⅜ inch long. Three-pointed, ovoid nutlets strewn with reddish yellow wax glands ripen in autumn. The deciduous leaves of this perennial, suckering shrub are sometimes hairless below.

Where, When, and How to Wildcraft

Considered somewhat rare in Oregon, where it is almost exclusively restricted to coastal counties, this shade-intolerant, nitrogen-fixing shrub occurs more frequently as its range extends northward into Alaska. Sweet gale can be found in temperate forests across North America and Europe inhabiting bogs, swamps, fens, and lake and stream margins at low to middle elevations. Harvest the leaves from mid spring through late summer.

Medicinal Uses

Not as potent but used similarly to the root bark of its cousin California bayberry (*Morella californica*), the astringent, bitter, and spicy leaves of sweet gale make a pleasant, stomach-settling beverage tea that reduces inflammation, stimulates circulation, and clears the lungs of mucus. The hot tea or tincture in hot water brings blood to the surface and opens the pores to dispel colds and flus and increases secretions to expel mucus from the lungs.

Swish the tea or diluted tincture to invigorate and tighten the gums, stop their bleeding, and/or reduce their inflammation. Apply a strong decoction simmered for 45 minutes in a covered pot externally to kill or repel lice and fleas.

For thousands of years in Europe, sweet gale has been made into a highly inebriating beer or has been added to other ales to increase their intoxicating effects.

⚠ Caution

Do not use during pregnancy. Because the strong decoction concentrates a potentially toxic oil (allowing it to kill fleas and lice), it should be used externally only. Taken internally, a strong decoction may cause nausea and vomiting.

Future Harvests

Be extra careful when harvesting sweet gale in Oregon, where it becomes increasingly rare at the southern limits of its range. That said, a respectful leaf harvest should pose little risk to the plants. Plant rooted cuttings or sprouted seedlings in boggy areas with moist, acidic soil to increase the size of native stands.

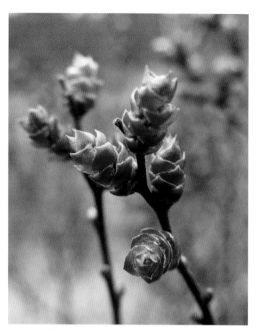

The male flowers are borne in bracted catkins at the branch ends.

HERBAL PREPARATIONS

Leaf Tea
Standard infusion
Drink 4–6 fluid ounces up to 3 times per day.

sweetroot

Osmorhiza occidentalis

western sweet-cicely, western sweetroot

PARTS USED root

Anise-scented roots harmonize digestion, reduce sugar cravings,
and help resolve fungal infections.

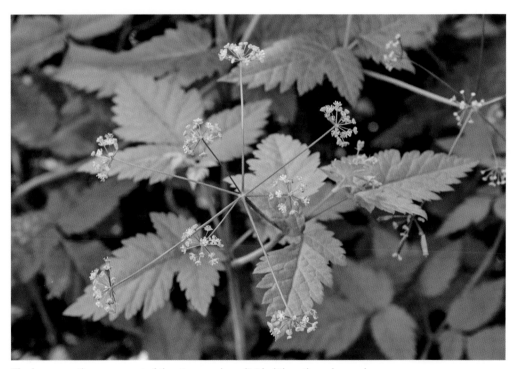

The leaves on the upper part of the stem are less divided than those lower down.

How to Identify

Erect, clustered stems, 1–4 feet tall, smooth to slightly hairy, hollow, and usually branched, arise from a mass of woody, dark-barked, oil-rich, and anise-scented roots. Compound leaves, 4–8 inches long, divide 1–3 times into lance- to egg-shaped, coarsely toothed, and irregularly lobed leaflets. Basal leaves attach to the root crown via long stalks and short-stalked leaves to the stem via compact sheaths. Both axillary and terminal compound umbels form from late spring to early summer bearing small yellow flowers that bloom in several loose, 5- to 12-rayed umbels lacking whorled bracts below. The short flower stalks elongate as hairless and barb-free, ½- to ¾-inch-long seeds mature. The green, sometimes anise-flavored, linear seeds flatten at the base, narrow to a beak-like tip, and as they dry turn dark brown to black and split lengthwise.

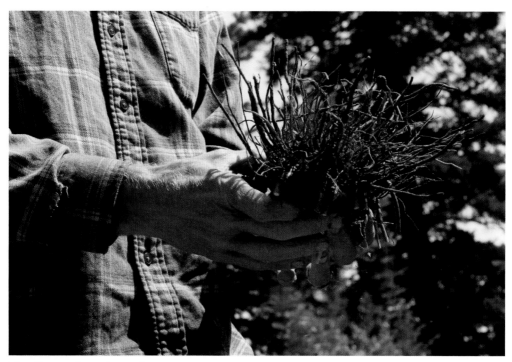
The oily roots form clumps that give rise to many stems.

Be absolutely sure of your identification before ingesting any part of this plant. Consult a botanical key to distinguish this plant from potentially deadly parsley family look-a-likes, and check the "Toxic Plants" section (page 32) for tips on identifying these poisonous umbels.

Where, When, and How to Wildcraft

Except for stands on the Olympic Peninsula, sweetroot mostly occupies lands east of the Cascades in Washington. From there its range extends westward to encompass much of Oregon and northern California. It reaches its southern limit in the east-central portion of California and can also be found in the extreme southern part of British Columbia. Find sweetroot growing in coniferous forests from low to high elevations in sunny, open areas with dry, rocky soil. Occasionally, it resides in somewhat moister, shady areas and along streams and creeks.

Start digging the roots in summer after the seeds mature and the leaves begin to die back. They grow fairly close to the surface. Use a digging fork or shovel to pop them out of the ground. Lightly beat them against the handle of your tool to remove dirt and rocks that get caught up in the intertwining mass of roots. Don't hit them too hard, because if you damage the roots you may lose some of their precious oil.

Medicinal Uses

The highly aromatic roots of sweetroot are warming, stimulating, and smell and taste like anise-flavored root beer. The tea or tincture stimulates the mucous membranes of the intestines to make the gut less hospitable to fungal infections such as candida. Apply the diluted tincture or the tea topically to speed the healing of ringworm, athlete's foot, jock itch, or other fungal outbreaks of the skin. Use the tea as a vaginal douche for yeast infections.

Take the tincture after eating foods that aggravate your gut. It relieves indigestion, gas, and upset stomach and is especially useful for those with gluten intolerance or other food sensitivities or allergies.

The tea or tincture reduces sugar cravings and regulates blood sugar imbalances for those tending toward diabetes. It is a mild laxative, eases the pain of sore throats, and works well in formulas because it improves the overall taste and harmonizes the action of combined herbs.

Future Harvests

Sweetroot generally grows in abundant patches. Harvest medium-sized plants from the outer edges or downhill portion of a stand, and replant chunks of root with the following year's growing buds intact. Gather mature seeds from the plants you harvest and sow them ¼ inch deep.

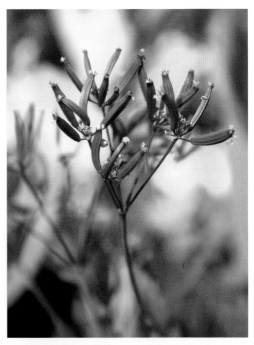

Finding flavorful seeds can be hit or miss. Sometimes they taste strongly of anise and other times like nothing at all.

HERBAL PREPARATIONS

Root Tea
Standard decoction
Drink 4–6 fluid ounces up to 4 times per day.

Root Tincture
1 part dried root
5 parts menstruum (70 percent alcohol, 30 percent distilled water)
or
1 part fresh root
2 parts menstruum (100 percent alcohol)
Take 30–60 drops up to 3 times per day.

thimbleberry

Rubus parviflorus

PARTS USED leaf, berry

*Astringent leaves tone and prepare the uterus for birth,
stem excessive menstrual bleeding, and relieve diarrhea.*

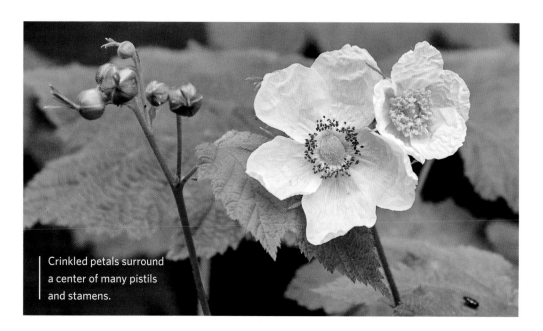

Crinkled petals surround
a center of many pistils
and stamens.

How to Identify

From an extensive network of rhizomes, thornless biennial stems with shredding gray bark stand erect, 1½ to 7 feet tall, bearing light green, 2- to 6-inch-long, 5-lobed leaves. Hairless or covered in fine glandular hairs, the alternately arranged and irregularly double saw-toothed leaves are slightly wider than long and emit a fruity aroma when rubbed. From late spring to early summer, 3–7 white flowers bloom in long-stemmed, flat-topped clusters at the end of second-year stems. Five glandular and densely hairy sepals with tail-like tips fuse together and with the 5 crinkled, egg-shaped petals cup a yellow center comprising numerous pistils and stamens.

Red, deliciously edible, raspberry-like fruits made up of many tiny drupelets in a velvety, thimble-like dome separate intact from the receptacle or floral base. A pair of stipules flare out lance shaped where the reddish leaf stalks meet the stem, and stalked oil glands cover the new-growth stems as well as the leaf and flower stalks. The leaf stalks are slightly shorter than the leaves, and the maple leaf–shaped leaves sometimes have 3–7 lobes.

Where, When, and How to Wildcraft

Common throughout western North America and the Great Lakes region, this shade-tolerant perennial shrub forms thickets in open areas, shrub lands, riparian areas, or in

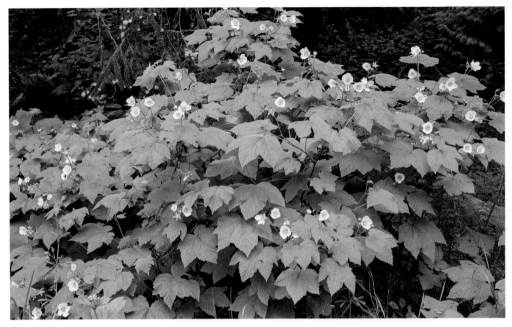
Thimbleberry forms large stands at the edges of mixed coniferous forests.

the understory of deciduous, coniferous, or mixed forests from sea level to subalpine elevations. In the Pacific Northwest, find thimbleberry growing in moist to relatively dry, nitrogen-rich soils from Alaska to California.

Pick the leaves individually or cut whole stems when the plant is in flower. To dry, lay the leaves out on screens; the stems can be bundled together in loose bunches and hung out of direct sunlight until dry.

Medicinal Uses

Gently astringent, thimbleberry leaf tea is a female reproductive tonic that tones and strengthens the uterine muscles and improves pelvic circulation. Drink it daily throughout pregnancy to prepare for birth or to support general reproductive health. After birth, take it to reduce inflammation and swelling in the uterus and to stop postpartum bleeding. It also decreases abnormally heavy or prolonged menstrual bleeding and relieves diarrhea.

The berries are high in antioxidant flavonoids. Eaten regularly, they promote cardiovascular health and may reduce the risk of cancer.

Future Harvests

Cut stems above an outward-facing bud to encourage bushier growth. Take no more than two stems from each plant, leaving many stalks to flower and produce berries that are an important food for wildlife and much sought after by humans. Dig the easily transplantable thimbleberry rhizomes in spring or autumn and plant them in appropriate locations to establish new colonies.

HERBAL PREPARATIONS

Leaf Tea
Standard infusion
Drink 6–8 fluid ounces 3 times per day to tonify the uterus or as needed for other uses.

thinleaf huckleberry

Vaccinium membranaceum
black huckleberry, tall huckleberry
PARTS USED leaf, berry

Astringent, sour leaves speed the healing of urinary tract infections and, along with the sweet and tart berries, moderate blood sugar, improve vision, and strengthen the integrity of blood vessels.

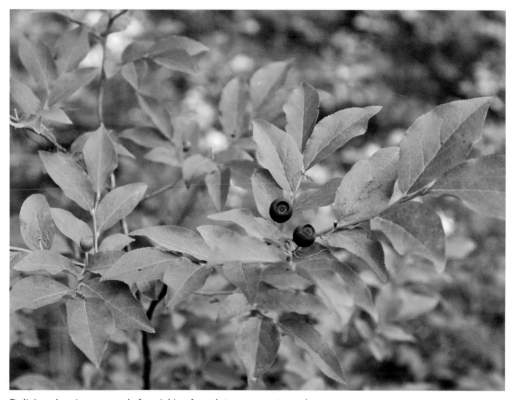

Delicious berries are ready for picking from late summer to early autumn.

How to Identify

Slightly squared, yellowish green, smooth to slightly hairy new-growth twigs emerge from erect to spreading, 2- to 6-foot long, densely branched stems with grayish, shredding bark. Thin, oval to egg-shaped, alternately arranged leaves with finely toothed edges and rounded bases taper to pointed tips and turn red before falling to the ground in autumn. Solitary, longer-than-wide, urn-shaped, and pale, yellowish pink flowers bloom on short stalks in the leaf axils from late spring to mid summer just as or slightly after the leaves unfurl. Sweet, globe-shaped, ¼- to ⅜-inch-wide berries without a whitish, powdery coating ripen blackish purple to dark purplish red.

The stems do not root in at the nodes, and the undersides of the ¾- to 2-inch-long, faintly-veined, dull-surfaced leaves are lighter in color and sparsely covered in glands.

Whortleberry (*Vaccinium myrtillus*), the main European *Vaccinium* species used for medicine, grows natively here, and other Pacific Northwest huckleberries such as evergreen huckleberry (*V. ovatum*), red huckleberry (*V. parvifolium*), grouseberry (*V. scoparium*), and bog blueberry (*V. uliginosum*) can all be used similarly for medicine.

Where, When, and How to Wildcraft

Found throughout the western parts of the United States and Canada with a range extending eastward to the Rocky Mountains and the Great Lakes region, this rhizomatous perennial inhabits mountain forests and sometimes forms dominant understory stands. In the Pacific Northwest, thinleaf huckleberry grows south from British Columbia through the Olympic and Cascade mountain ranges to California in acidic, well-drained, wet soils in partially closed or open-canopied, coniferous forests and wet meadows from middle to high elevations.

Collect green leaves from early summer to early autumn by cutting twig ends to an outward-facing bud. Dry in bundles or on screens. Once dried, remove leaves and discard the woody stems. Soil quality and ecological conditions affect medicinal activity. Seek out stands with somewhat fruity, sour-tasting leaves. Gather ripe berries from late summer through autumn and dry on screens or process fresh for tincture.

Medicinal Uses

Drink a tea of the leaves to reduce inflammation and pain in the bladder and urethra or to speed the healing of urinary tract infections. The leaf tea or tincture helps moderate elevated blood sugar levels, and for those with Type 1 diabetes, it may cut down the amount of insulin needed each day.

Antioxidant constituents and flavonoids in the leaves and berries strengthen and prevent damage to the capillaries of the eye and the retina. Take the leaf or berry tea or tincture alone or combined to improve night vision, to reduce retinal inflammation, to reduce the risk of age-related visual disorders, or to relieve eye strain from activities such as staring at a computer screen for prolonged periods. These same preparations may reduce the risk of cancer by protecting cells from free radical damage. They also strengthen the integrity of blood vessels to help prevent the buildup of plaque in the arteries thereby reducing the risk of stroke and lessening the effect of blood stagnation that leads to varicose veins and hemorrhoids.

Take the leaf tea or tincture for colitis or to soothe gastrointestinal inflammation and lessen the effects of diarrhea associated with the stomach flu. Swish the leaf tea or diluted tincture to mend damaged mouth tissue and to soothe swollen gums. The flavonoid-rich berries are high in vitamin C.

 Caution

If you plan on using huckleberry as a supportive therapy for diabetes, consult with a qualified health practitioner.

Future Harvests

Huckleberries respond well to pruning. Carefully cutting the twigs to an outward-facing bud will encourage bushier growth and increase berry production. To propagate huckleberries, carefully dig out and remove a small portion of the extensive rhizomatous root system in the early spring or autumn. Cut the rhizomes into pieces at least 4 inches long, making sure that each piece contains at least one bud. Plant in moist, acidic soil, keep them out of the sun, and water them frequently until they are well established.

In the past Native Americans periodically set fires in the autumn after harvesting berries to invigorate the soil, preserve clearings, and reduce resource competition from other plants. To this day many Native Americans still maintain and harvest from ancestral berry-picking patches. Please be respectful of this important cultural heritage. Do not harvest on tribal lands or in stands that look like they have been tended like gardens.

HERBAL PREPARATIONS

Leaf or Berry Tea
Standard infusion
Drink 3–4 fluid ounces up to 3 times per day.

Leaf or Berry Tincture
1 part fresh leaf or berries
2 parts menstruum (75 percent alcohol,
   25 percent distilled water)
*For a full-spectrum medicine, mix the leaf and
   berry tinctures in equal proportions.*
Take 20–30 drops up to 3 times per day.

Usnea species
beard lichen
PARTS USED thallus

Yellow-green strands or tufts of usnea decorate the forest and provide medicine that stimulates immunity and resolves bacterial and viral infections.

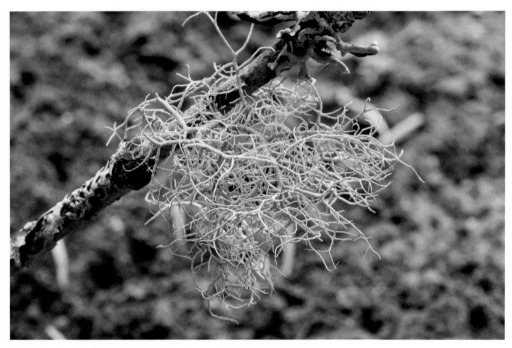

This tufted lichen species is growing on a western hemlock branch.

How to Identify

The Pacific Northwest is home to many species of usnea. These lichens come in two different forms: pendulous, hanging strands or stringy, short-stranded tufts. All usneas grow on the branches of trees and are yellow-green or gray-green with tough, elastic central cords. Gently pull on both ends of a wet or moistened usnea strand to reveal the often white or light-colored but sometimes brown or reddish central elastic core. If this cord is lacking, you most likely have a similar-looking but multi-branched *Alectoria* lichen, which has not traditionally been used as medicine.

The two most common species of usnea in the Northwest are Methuselah's beard (*Usnea longissima*), also known as beard lichen or old man's beard, and Wirth's beard lichen (*U. wirthii*), which is sometimes called blood-spattered beard. Methuselah's beard is a pendulous lichen with long, mostly unbranched, cylindrical central strands that grow 6–14 inches long. Short side branches, ⅛ to 1½ inches long, radiate out

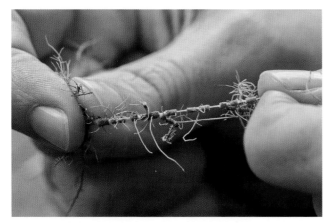

Polysaccharides in the central fungal core stimulate the immune system. Constituents in the outer cortex support a healthy inner ecology to speed the healing of bacterial and viral infections.

perpendicular from this central axis, and sometimes the external covering, known as the cortex, erodes to create a rough and patchy surface. Wirth's beard lichen forms tufts up to 2 ⅜ inches long and has a yellow central cord, an often red-spotted cortex, and branches divided into cigar-shaped segments.

Where, When, and How to Wildcraft

Methuselah's beard grows on hardwoods and conifers in old-growth and mature coniferous forests, hardwood forests, and along waterways west of the Cascades from Alaska to northern California. It prefers high-rainfall forests and foggy coastal areas. Its occurrence is limited throughout its range, but in the places it does inhabit, it is often found in abundance.

Wirth's beard lichen grows on both hardwood and coniferous trees. It thrives in wet, low-elevation forests from British Columbia to California and is very common west of the Cascades.

Gather vibrant and living usnea that have fallen to the ground throughout the wet growing season from early spring to mid summer. Discard discolored, dead portions of the thalli with dried out and cracked outer coverings.

Medicinal Uses

Cooling and drying usnea thallus speeds the healing of respiratory, urinary, and reproductive tract infections, and though it has an affinity for Gram-positive bacteria such as staph and strep, it is also helpful for resolving some Gram-negative bacterial infections. Take the tincture to resolve cases of pneumonia or strep throat as well as viral conditions such as herpes and Epstein-Barr. For vaginal infections, douche with ½ fluid ounce of the tincture diluted in 16 fluid ounces of water.

Externally the salve or powdered thallus not only prevents infection to cuts and scrapes but speeds the body's natural wound healing process. Apply tincture directly to the skin or diluted in a little water to speed the healing of staph infections.

Caution

Do not use internally during pregnancy.

Future Harvests

Usneas are slow growing and do not readily reproduce. Though you may find them locally abundant in some areas, they are becoming scarce in forests worldwide. They are also sensitive to air pollution (especially *Usnea longissima*), and the mature forest habitats they prefer are diminishing as humans expand their range and continue to cut down trees. With all of this in mind, limit your harvest to strands or tufts of usnea that have fallen to the ground, and don't harvest the ones growing attached to trees.

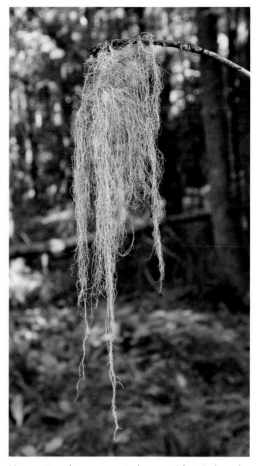

HERBAL PREPARATIONS

Thallus Tincture

1 part dried thallus

5 parts menstruum (50 percent alcohol, 50 percent distilled water)

Because some of its constituents are best extracted in alcohol and others are more water soluble, I recommend preparing usnea thallus as a tincture for internal use.

For urinary tract infections, add 90–120 drops to 32 fluid ounces of water and drink freely throughout the day; for acute lung or respiratory tract infections, take 15–20 drops every few hours up to 5 times per day.

Thallus Oil and Salve

For thallus oil, follow directions for Alternative Oil Method on page 64. For the salve, follow directions on page 65.

Powdered Thallus

Grind the dried thalli to remove the yellow-green or gray-green cortex from the mostly ungrindable white inner core. Apply liberally to wounded areas.

Usnea strands can grow to be over 1 foot in length.

Making Usnea Tincture

Tincturing usnea is a little different than making a standard tincture, as heat must be applied to get the full spectrum of healing constituents.

Use the standard dried herb ratio of 1 part of the herb by weight to 5 parts of liquid by volume. The menstruum should be 50 percent water and 50 percent alcohol.

1. Grind the thallus. The inner core is tough and generally resists grinding, but the long water decoction will extract its constituents.

2. Put the ground thallus in a crock pot with the measured distilled water. This will be half of your menstruum. The alcohol will be added later.

3. Cook on low heat for 48 hours.

4. While it's still warm, pour the thallus and the water into a jar and add alcohol.

5. Macerate for 2 weeks.

Some folks recommend macerating the thallus in hot alcohol, but applying heat to alcohol in the home is not without its dangers. I strongly recommend against it.

uva ursi

Arctostaphylos uva-ursi
bearberry, kinnikinnick
PARTS USED leaf

Astringent leaves help heal urinary tract infections, reduce postpartum inflammation and bleeding, stanch bleeding from cuts and scrapes, and add body to herbal smoking blends.

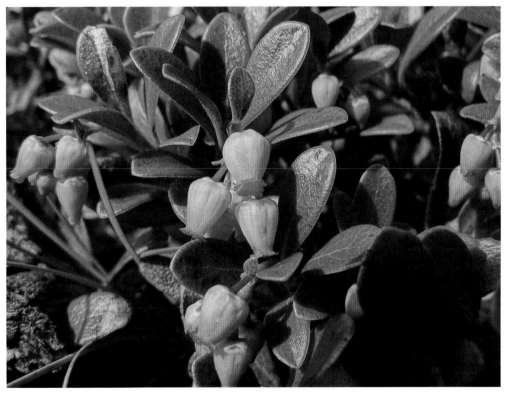

Urn- or bell-shaped flowers are characteristic of the heath family.

How to Identify

From peeling, reddish brown–barked mature branches, flexible, creeping stems with upward-curving tips crawl across the ground and root in at the nodes to form large mats. Alternately arranged, evergreen leaves, round at the tip and narrowing at the base, spread out along the stems on twisted stalks. The smooth-edged, oval- to spoon-shaped leaves, thick with a waxy coating and growing up to 1 inch long, are somewhat shiny and dark green above, lighter green below, and slightly hairy on the midrib and edges. From mid spring to early summer, pinkish, 5-lobed, and urn-shaped flowers bloom in hairy-bracted clusters at the ends of the stems. Shiny,

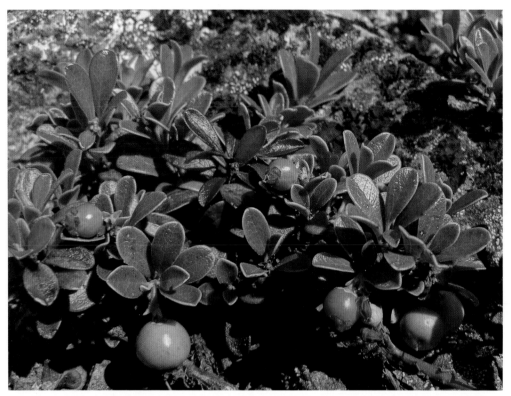

Round-tipped, glossy leaves, trailing stems with reddish brown peeling bark, and berries like miniature apples make uva ursi easy to identify.

bright red, apple-shaped berries, up to ½ inch wide, mature in summer and may remain on the plant through winter. These perennial shrubs rarely grow taller than 6 inches and secrete chemicals into the soil that inhibit the growth of other plants.

Pinemat manzanita (*Arctostaphylos nevadensis*), which can be used similarly for medicine, has a similar growth habit but produces pointy-tipped leaves and brownish red berries.

Where, When, and How to Wildcraft

Widely distributed throughout much of North America, uva ursi inhabits dry, rocky soils and exposed sites throughout this region. Find it growing on coastal bluffs at sea level and upward through open, mixed-coniferous and pine-dominant forests to dry, high-elevation and subalpine meadows.

Cut trailing stems from mid spring to mid autumn. After drying on screens or in bags, strip the leaves from the stem. Store the dried leaves in a glass jar and add a tablespoon of grain alcohol to soften the waxy coating and make the medicinal constituents more available.

Medicinal Uses

Astringent uva ursi leaves reduce inflammation, increase urine output, and make the urinary tract less hospitable to bacteria like *Escherichia coli*, the main cause of lower urinary tract infections. For acute urinary tract infections, drink the leaf tea along with 1 pint of unsweetened cranberry juice per day to alleviate pain and inflammation and prevent *E. coli* from adhering to the walls of the urethra. Avoid stimulants, sweets including fruit, and alcohol.

Use a douche of the leaf tea to reduce vaginal inflammation and speed the healing of yeast infections. Soaking the hips and groin area, known as a sitz bath, in tea-infused water reduces postpartum inflammation and bleeding, and as an external wash the leaf tea decreases redness and swelling, stops bleeding, and helps heal cuts, scrapes, and abrasions. Smoke the crushed leaves alone or use them to add body to herbal smoking blends containing mullein or other light fluffy herbs.

 Caution

Do not use during pregnancy. Because the astringent tannins can aggravate the gut, restrict internal use to 3–4 days.

Future Harvests

Transplant rooted sections of uva ursi into areas with dry, well-drained soil or scarify the difficult-to-germinate seeds before sowing them in summer. The overwintering seeds need a period of cold stratification, and if all goes well, they will sprout in spring. Scarification is a process that mechanically or sometimes chemically thins the seeds coat to encourage the seed to sprout. Nick with a knife, or rub with sandpaper to expose a small portion of the seed's white interior.

waxy coneflower

Rudbeckia glaucescens

PARTS USED root

Waxy coneflower roots stimulate the immune system and may strengthen the kidneys.

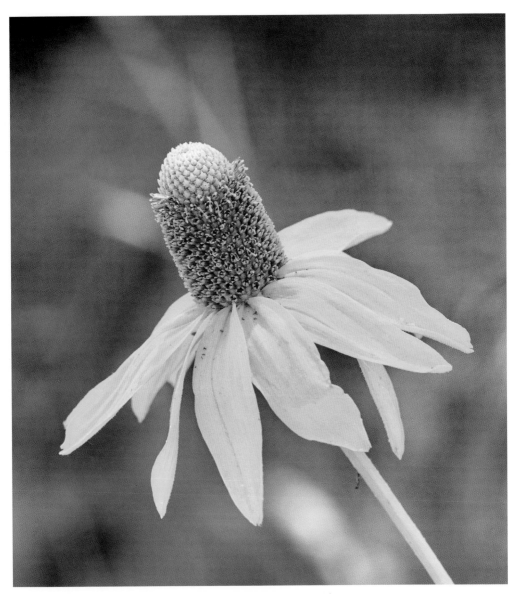

The blooming central cone of waxy coneflower is taller than it is wide.

How to Identify

Thin, usually unbranching stems stand 20–60 inches tall from thick rhizomes. Lance-shaped to elliptic blue-green leaves, basal and becoming stalkless and smaller as they alternately ascend the stem, spread 7¾ to 19½ inches long with smooth edges or a few shallow teeth. Single composite flower heads cupped by whorled bracts bloom from mid summer to early autumn at the tops of the stems. Semi-crinkled, sterile, often reflexed, yellow ray flowers radiate out from a central cone or column, taller than it is wide, of yellowish green disk flowers that ripen into seeds crowned with tiny, tooth-like scales. The stems and leaves are waxy-coated and without hairs.

The leaves of the related California coneflower (*Rudbeckia californica*), which doesn't grow on serpentine soils, lack a waxy coating, are occasionally lobed, and have hairy undersides. The root of this plant may be used interchangeably for medicine.

Where, When, and How to Wildcraft

Often growing on serpentine soils in the southern parts of this region, this perennial relative of black-eyed Susan inhabits meadows and seeps and grows at low to middle elevations along stream banks in the Siskiyou Mountains of southwestern Oregon. In northern California, find waxy coneflower (formerly *Rudbeckia californica* var. *glauca*) along the coast and in the Klamath Mountains. Dig the roots and rhizomes from late summer to mid autumn after the seeds have fully matured.

Medicinal Uses

Slightly diffusive—causing a tingly sensation on your tongue—in taste, waxy coneflower roots may be used in place of echinacea root, leaf, or seed to stimulate the immune system. Take the root tea or tincture to clear blood infections or to counteract the poisons of insect or snake bites.

Early American botanical doctors used the whole plant of a related species known as thimbleweed or coneflower (*Rudbeckia*

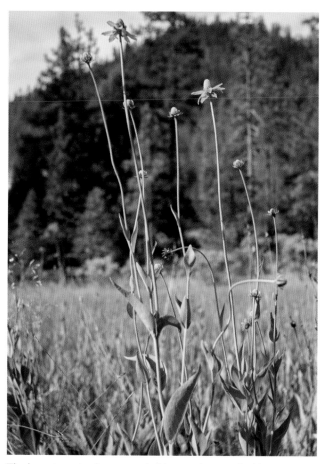

The long, tapering leaves are hairless and covered with a waxy coating.

laciniata) to relieve renal sluggishness to improve kidney function and as a treatment for Bright's disease, an inflammatory condition of the kidneys known today as nephritis. It was said to increase urine output, clear mucus discharges from the bladder, reduce urinary tract inflammation, and relieve blockages or soothe irritation in the bladder leading to painful or difficult urination.

 Caution

This plant is not for use during pregnancy. Do not consume large quantities of fresh plant material or teas from plants growing on serpentine soils, as they may uptake heavy metals such as nickel and chromium that can accumulate to toxic levels in the body.

Future Harvests

To expand a patch or establish a new colony, divide roots in autumn. Because plants growing on serpentine soils, which have lower levels of calcium and nitrogen than other soil types, generally grow more slowly, harvest only from large healthy stands growing on non-serpentine soils.

HERBAL PREPARATIONS

Root Tea
Standard decoction
Drink 3–4 fluid ounces up to 4 times per day.

Root Tincture
1 part fresh root
2 parts menstruum (75 percent alcohol, 25 percent distilled water)
Take 30–60 drops up to 4 times per day.

Aralia californica
California ginseng, California spikenard, elk clover
PARTS USED root, leaf, berry

Thick roots and large leaves reduce stress and support the lungs.
Purple berries relieve seasonal affective disorder and soothe sore throats.

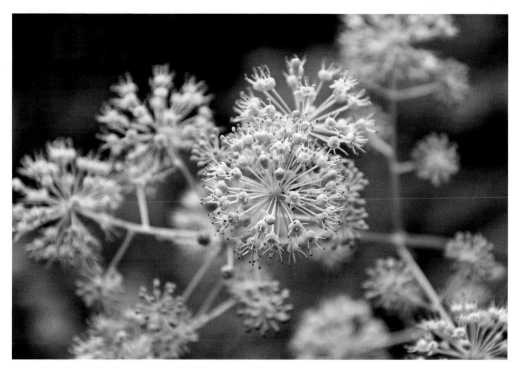

Globe-like flower clusters are typical of the ginseng family.

How to Identify

Large, chunky rhizomes anchored by thick side roots ooze a milky, resinous sap when cut. They rest just under the soil's surface, often in gravel or under rocks, bearing purple buds that will become the following year's growth. Spreading, graceful, 3-times-divided compound leaves reach 6 feet in length and clasp to thick, 6- to 10-foot-tall stalks. Wing-shaped, leaf-like appendages can be found at the base of the leaf stalks, and the surprisingly delicate, ovate to oblong leaflets are 6–12 inches long with serrated edges. Greenish white flowers radiate out from a central point to form spherical flower heads, several along a stem. Small, saponaceous, dark purple berries mature in late summer.

Where, When, and How to Wildcraft

This shrub-like herbaceous perennial occupies moist shaded canyons, forest edges, and the sides of streams, creeks, and rivers from Linn

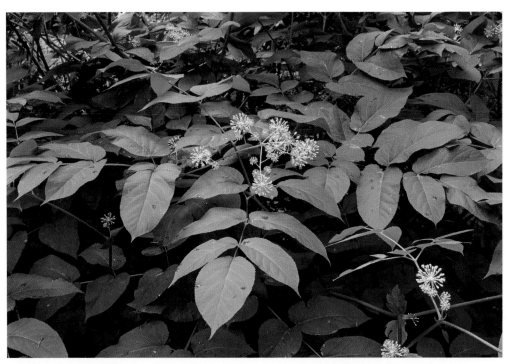

The large compound leaves and thick stems contain medicinally active oils and saponins.

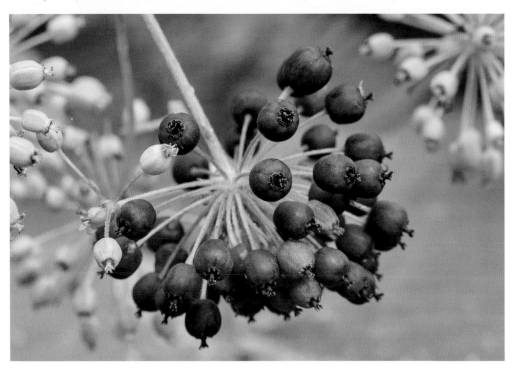

Juicy and saponaceous berries ripen to a dark purple.

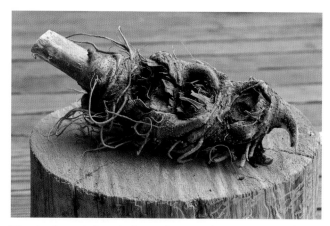

The chunky roots bear leaf scars from previous years' growth.

and joy to people suffering from seasonal affective disorder, and soothes sore throats. A syrup of the roots also soothes sore throats. Women who were raised by untrustworthy or mentally unstable mothers and who may suffer from womb pain caused by a distorted relationship to their own feminine nature can work with western aralia to restore trust in the strong and wild feminine within themselves.

County, Oregon, southward into California. Gather the leaves including the resin-exuding stalks from early to mid summer, the rhizomes along with their side roots from late summer to mid autumn, and the ripe berries from late summer to early autumn before the birds gobble them all up.

Medicinal Uses

The roots and leaves of western aralia, one of two Pacific Northwest native members of the ginseng family, have adaptogenic properties that moderate the body's reaction to stress. Take the root or leaf tincture during acute episodes of anxiety when the nerves are frazzled to bring calmness and peace of mind. For adrenal burnout and exhaustion caused by chronic stress associated with the pressures of everyday life, take the tea or tincture to restore balance to the neuroendocrine system and decrease the long-term effects of stress.

A tincture or tea of the roots clears mucus, reduces inflammation in the lungs, and supports the repair of tissue to aid those with lung damage from smoking or exposure to environmental pollution. A tincture of the berries elevates the mood, brings lightness

Future Harvests

Use the leaves rather than roots whenever possible. For a respectful root harvest that doesn't kill the plant, uncover the rhizome and remove a portion of the back end no greater than half its length. If the aerial parts are still present, cut them back to reduce stress on the root system. If you must dig a whole root up, replant a chunk from the bud-bearing front part of the rhizome. Leave plenty of berries for the birds and other creatures who eat them and distribute their seeds.

HERBAL PREPARATIONS

Root Tea
Standard decoction
Drink 4–6 fluid ounces up to 4 times per day.

Root, Leaf, or Berry Tincture
1 part fresh root, leaf, or berries
2 parts menstruum (75 percent alcohol, 25 percent distilled water)
Take 15–60 drops up to 4 times per day.

---

western bunchberry

Cornus unalaschkensis
Alaskan bunchberry, western cordilleran bunchberry
PARTS USED whole plant

Leaves, roots, and flowers relieve pain, lower fever, and reduce inflammation.

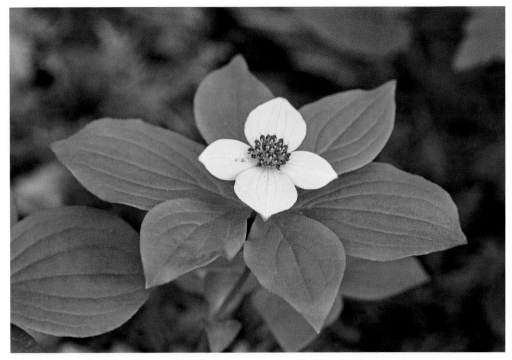

Purple-tipped petals distinguish western bunchberry from its close cousin Canada bunchberry
(*Cornus canadensis*).

How to Identify

Whorls of 4–6 oval, strongly parallel-veined, and overlapping leaves frame solitary flower heads that sit atop single, woody-bottomed stems. Surrounded by 4 pointy-tipped, whitish, petal-like bracts, 10–25 small, white, purple-tipped flowers make up compact flower heads that bloom from late spring to late summer. Clusters of edible, red, berry-like fruits, each containing 1 or 2 smooth-stoned seeds, ripen in late summer. This 2- to 8-inch-tall perennial spreads via rhizome to form sometimes dense patches and clumps. Occasionally a pair of opposite leaves grows on the stem below the whorl of leaves.

Canada bunchberry or bunchberry dogwood (*Cornus canadensis*) has the same medicinal properties as western bunchberry. It is occasionally found in the northern part of this region, has a much wider range than western bunchberry, and is distinguished by its white, but not purple-tipped, petals

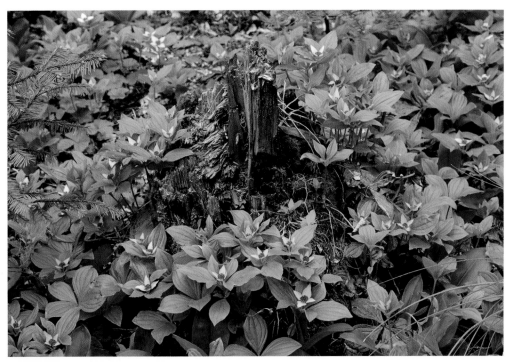

This small, spreading plant can grow in extensive patches that carpet the forest floor with interlocking leaves and white, eye-like flower heads.

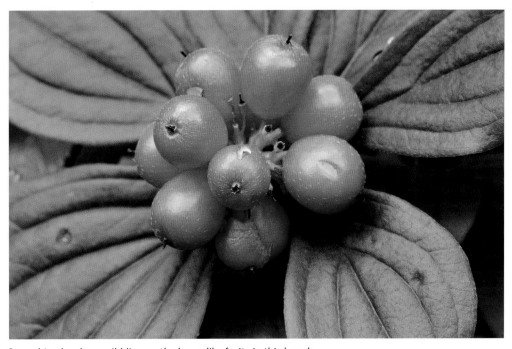

Something has been nibbling on the berry-like fruits in this bunch.

and bract-like stem leaves that are less than ⅜ inch long.

Where, When, and How to Wildcraft

Ranging from Alaska to California and commonly growing in thick forest duff or on rotted logs or the trunks of trees, western bunchberry prefers acidic soils in wet, shady forests from low to high elevations throughout the Pacific Northwest. Harvest the whole plant from early summer to early autumn.

Medicinal Uses

The bitter taste of western bunchberry, like that of its cousin Pacific dogwood (*Cornus nuttallii*), hints at the presence of aspirin-like salicylates and the alkaloid cornine. These constituents impart their medicinal activity when prepared as a whole plant tea or tincture. Take either preparation to relieve pain and inflammation from sprains, strains, or bruises or to reduce fevers.

The astringent tannins of the whole plant preparations, combined with the inflammation-reducing constituents, make the tea or tincture a particularly good remedy for diarrhea or inflammation of the digestive tract and bowels. Unlike other plants with aspirin-like effects, the milder bunchberries won't irritate the gut.

 Caution

Eating too many berries may cause diarrhea or other digestive upset.

Future Harvests

Because new growth is stimulated by disturbance, your harvest will encourage larger patches. However, gather only a few plants from each abundant patch. Rhizomes can also be transplanted during the wet season to other suitable sites in shady, moist forests with acidic soils topped by thick duff.

HERBAL PREPARATIONS

Whole Plant Tea
Standard decoction
Drink 6–8 fluid ounces up to 5 times per day.

Whole Plant Tincture
1 part fresh whole plant
2 parts menstruum (75 percent alcohol, 25 percent distilled water)
Take 30–60 drops up to 5 times per day.

---

western coltsfoot

Petasites frigidus var. *palmatus*
arctic sweet coltsfoot, butterbur
PARTS USED leaf, root

*Cooling, soothing, salty-tasting leaves relieve spasmodic coughing,
lessen pain between the ribs, and allay the effects of migraine headaches.*

How to Identify

From early to mid spring before large, round to kidney-shaped leaves emerge, 1- to 2-foot-tall flowering stalks burst forth from creeping rhizomes. The white to pink flowers bloom in rounded clusters of disk-like composite flower heads, and the long-stalked basal leaves, palmately lobed and cut almost to the base, extend 4–16 inches wide at the ends of thick, ridged leaf stalks. The coarsely toothed leaves, wider than they are long, are green and hairless above and white and wooly below. Sheathed, bract-like leaves line the flowering stalks, and each of the flower heads spreads out and droops as the flowers mature. Western coltsfoot is considered subdioecious: some plants produce only male flowers, some produce only female flowers, and others produce both.

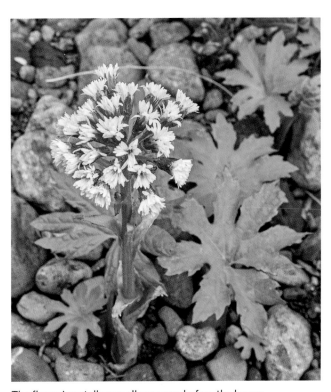

The flowering stalks usually emerge before the leaves.

Where, When, and How to Wildcraft

Western coltsfoot resides in the middle of slow-moving streams, in wetlands and bogs, below seeps, and along stream edges at low to middle elevations in the western portions of this region from Alaska to California. Gather the leaves along with the thick stems from early to late summer after the leaves have attained their maximum size. The roots are best harvested in spring.

Medicinal Uses

Western coltsfoot leaf relieves spasms and reduces inflammation. Take the leaf tea, tincture, or syrup to cool, soothe, and open

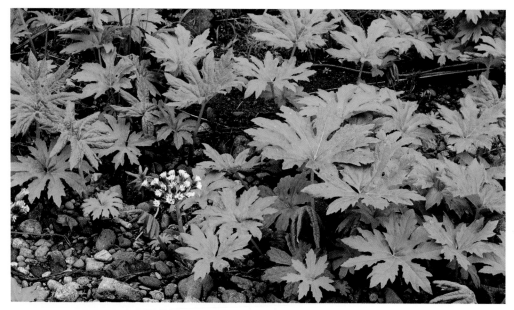

A western coltsfoot colony leafs out in spring.

the bronchial passages; to clear the lungs of mucus; or to relieve spasmodic coughs including those associated with allergies, asthma, emphysema, bronchitis, or whooping cough.

The leaf tea or tincture reduces pain between the ribs from too much coughing and relieves spasms in the digestive and urinary tracts. The tincture can be used to prevent and lessen the intensity of migraine headaches. Apply a poultice of the root or leaf externally to reduce pain and inflammation from bruises and sprains.

⚠ Caution

The young leaves contain very small amounts of pyrrolizidine alkaloids. The mature leaves and roots contain none. Because pyrrolizidine alkaloids are known to cause a severe and life-threatening disorder known as hepatic veno-occlusive disease, use with caution during pregnancy, when breastfeeding, or for those with impaired liver function.

Future Harvests

Take just a few leaves from each plant to avoid weakening the rhizomes. To establish new colonies, transplant chunks of rhizome to wet sites.

HERBAL PREPARATIONS

Leaf Tea
Standard infusion
Drink 2–4 fluid ounces up to 4 times per day.

Root Tea
Standard decoction
Drink 2–4 fluid ounces up to 3 times per day.

Leaf Tincture
1 part fresh leaf
2 parts menstruum (75 percent alcohol, 25 percent distilled water)
Take 30–60 drops up to 5 times per day; take 5–30 drops of the tincture up to 3 times per day to prevent and lessen the intensity of migraines.

western hemlock

Tsuga heterophylla
PARTS USED bark, leaf, pitch

Western hemlock is a safe and effective remedy for sore muscles, wounds, and chest congestion.

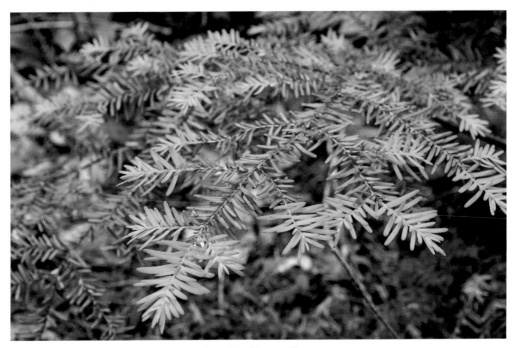

The new-growth leaves are lighter green than the older needles.

How to Identify

Smooth reddish brown bark roughens, darkens, and becomes deeply furrowed, thick, and scaly with age. Flat, blunt-tipped, and different-sized needles, ¼ to ¾ inch long and glossy-green above with 2 white bands running the length of the underside, attach randomly to the droopy-tipped branches via short leaf stalks. Yellow pollen-producing cones, about ⅛ inch long, form near the ends of branches, and green seed-bearing cones, ½ to 1 inch long, hang down at the branch tips. As the egg-shaped female seed cones mature, they turn light brown, and thin, papery bracts open to release tiny winged seeds that can travel up to a ½ mile from their parent tree. Pollination occurs between late spring and early summer, and open seed cones can be found in abundance on the ground below the trees. Topped by a distinctly drooping growing tip and clothed in foliage that appears feathery from a distance, this slow-growing, narrow-crowned tree, which grows up to 165 feet tall, is easily distinguished from the other conifers with which it shares habitat.

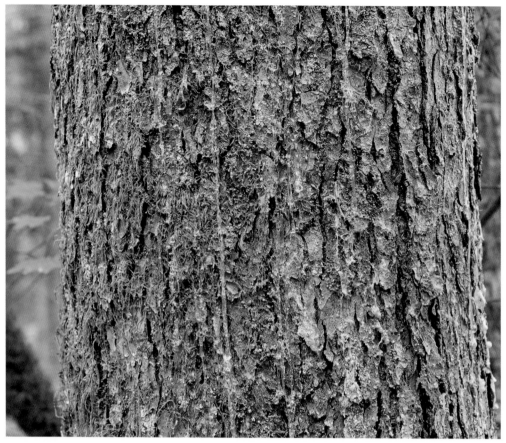

Pitch weeping from the bark of this young western hemlock is ready for collection.

Where, When, and How to Wildcraft

This shade-tolerant, evergreen tree can be found in deep, wet forests from sea level to middle elevations from Alaska to California. Young trees are often growing out of the stumps of dead trees or on fallen and decaying logs in the dense shade of other conifer species.

From mid to late spring, gather the fresh, light green growing tips from the ends of branches. This is also a good time to harvest branch bark. Remove thick lower branches, and strip the bark promptly to dry in bags or on screens. Throughout the year be on the lookout for pitch. The trees exude this resin, which varies in consistency from the thickness of honey when fresh to almost as solid as a rock when it dries, to protect and seal their wounds. Pry chunks off with a knife or scrape the ooze into a jar. Don't take too much from a large active wound or you will hinder the tree's natural mechanisms of healing and protection.

Medicinal Uses

A tea of the astringent bark stops internal bleeding, relieves diarrhea, and can be used externally as a wash to heal cuts, abrasions, or burns. Several Northwest native tribes also used the bark tea for tuberculosis. The warming and pungent pitch can be applied directly to wounds in the field to prevent

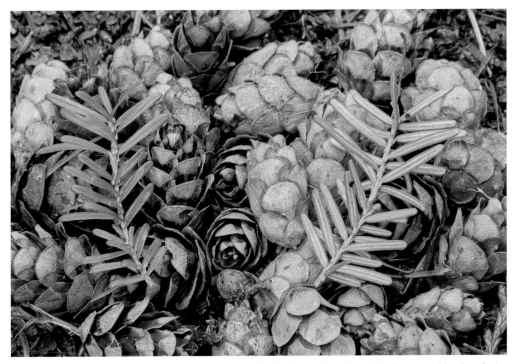

Bracts on the female cones flare open to release seeds. On the undersides of the leaves, a ridged midvein separates two white lines of stomata, pores that regulate gas exchange.

infection and speed healing. Apply pitch-infused oil to sore muscles; use the salve to speed the healing of wounds or as a chest rub to clear chest and sinus congestion during colds or flus. The spring tips, eaten fresh or brewed as a tea, are high in vitamin C.

Future Harvests

Respectfully remove only one or two branches from each tree when harvesting bark.

HERBAL PREPARATIONS

Bark Tea
Standard decoction
Drink 4–6 fluid ounces up to 3 times per day.

Leaf Tea
Standard infusion of the young tips
Drink 4–6 fluid ounces up to 3 times per day.

Pitch Oil and Salve
For pitch oil, follow directions for Dry Herb Infused Oil (page 64) but use 1 part pitch by weight to 10 parts oil by volume. For the salve, follow directions on page 65.

western juniper

Juniperus occidentalis
PARTS USED berry, leaf

Warm and pungent berries resolve chronic urinary tract infections, speed the healing of respiratory infections, and relieve joint pain.

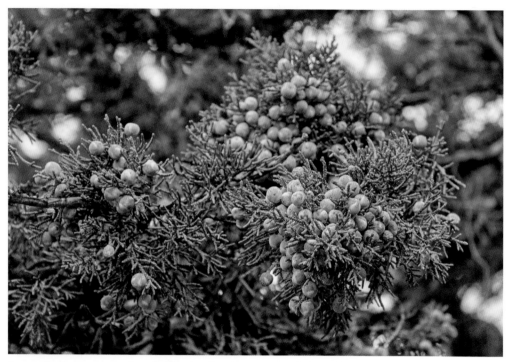

Juniper fruits are commonly called berries, but they are actually berry-like cones.

How to Identify

Fibrous, peeling, reddish gray to cinnamon-brown bark covers gnarled, twisting trunks and spreading branches that embody the stresses of the harsh environments where the trees live. Light green, scale-like leaves, arranged in whorls of three, form highly aromatic, resin-exuding, branch-like foliage. Woody, oval-shaped, pollen-producing male cones and fleshy, berry-like female cones form on separate trees from late spring to early summer. Covered with a white, powdery coating and containing 1–3 seeds, the green first-year berries ripen to a deep blue in their second year. These deeply rooted, dryland evergreen trees can grow as high as 65 feet tall with trunks up to 4 feet in diameter. On younger trees the awl-like leaves are sharply pointed and prickly. Some trees produce both male and female cones.

Where, When, and How to Wildcraft

Western juniper inhabits open forests and sagebrush steppe. It thrives in dry, rocky

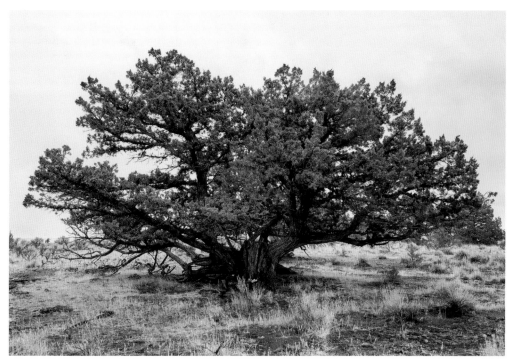

Older trees take on interesting shapes and tend to be more gnarled and twisted than younger individuals.

soils that receive as little as 8 inches of rain per year. The northernmost populations are in southeastern Washington. From there western juniper moves southward into eastern Oregon's high desert region. In the southern portion of Oregon, its range extends further westward before descending into California.

Harvest mature, second-year berries and dry for tea or tincture. The ripe fruit is sweet and juicy with a well-rounded pungency, but when consumed the oils can be irritating to the back of the throat. It can be difficult to tell if they are ripe by sight alone. Rub the berries to reveal the color beneath the white blush. If they are blue, they are ready. If they are green, they are still ripening. Usually all or most of the berries on an individual tree will be either green or blue.

Pick the ripe fruit one by one and dry on screens or on the lowest setting of a dehydrator. You also can clip berry-laden branch ends and remove the berries after they have dried. The leaves can be harvested any time of the year for smudges or steam inhalations. Snip off branch ends and hang in a bag or spread on a screen to dry.

Medicinal Uses

The diuretic berries stimulate, cleanse, and warm the genitourinary system and kidneys. Take the tincture in cold water to remedy chronic urinary tract infections resulting from cold, damp conditions. Inhale a steam of the leaves or take the berry tincture in hot water to clear mucus from the lungs or to speed the healing of respiratory tract infections.

Chew on a fresh or dried berry or take the berry tincture to relieve indigestion and gas. For creaky joint pain that is worse in the cold, take the berry tincture to warm the

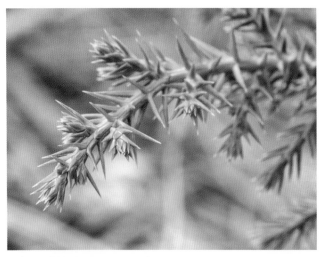
Spiky, awl-like leaves protect the young trees.

may be safely used for extended periods of time as a diuretic. Adulteration is common, so harvest the berries yourself to ensure that that the medicine you ingest only contains ripe berries. Caution is still advised in cases of acute kidney inflammation or for those with chronic kidney disease.

Future Harvests

Juniper berries are a valuable food source for birds. Harvest berries from lower branches that you can reach from the ground, and leave higher growing fruit for our avian friends who will distribute the seeds far and wide.

joints and to stimulate urine flow to flush out deposits that build up when energy stagnates in cold joints and limbs.

The oldest western junipers are more than 3000 years old, and the 2-year period of ripening for the berries is a signature for accumulated wisdom that ripens and sweetens with age. In the same way that western juniper's twisted, gnarled shape results from the stresses of its environment, the traumas that affect our lives mark our energetic and physical beings. Western juniper embodies the triumph of the human spirit and helps us to accept our history so we can align with and transform our traumas into gifts as we ripen into elders. A smudge of the leaves helps dispel heavy or dark energies from people and spaces.

Caution

Leaves, branches, or unripe berries all contain compounds known to irritate the urinary tract and kidneys and should not be used long term. Research published by herbalist Kerry Bone in 1995 suggests that preparations made with *ripe* juniper berries

---

HERBAL PREPARATIONS

Berry Tea
Standard decoction
Because resins are soluble in alcohol but not in water, western juniper berry medicine works best as a tincture. If you plan to make tea, use a dedicated pot or the resins will gunk up your everyday cooking vessels.
Drink 2–3 fluid ounces up to 3 times per day.

Berry Tincture
1 part dried berries
5 parts menstruum (75 percent alcohol, 25 percent distilled water)
Take 15–45 drops up to 3 times per day.

western mugwort

Artemisia ludoviciana
gray sagewort, silver wormwood, white sagebrush
PARTS USED leaf, flower

Leaves, long associated with the moon, enliven the dream life, support female reproductive health, and rid the body of worms. An oil of the flowers helps resolve fungal infections.

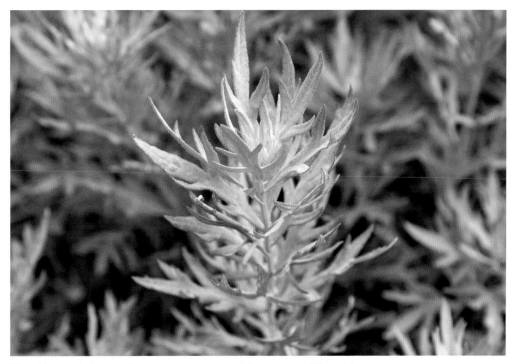

The white-wooly leaves of western mugwort can take on many different forms.

How to Identify

Fibrous roots from spreading rhizomes interweave just below the surface of the soil to form stands up to 10 feet in diameter. Matted, white to gray hairs cover 12- to 40-inch-tall stems that seldom branch below the inflorescence. Alternately arranged with wooly, white hairs on both sides or sometimes smooth to sparsely haired above, highly aromatic, smooth-edged to deeply lobed leaves, 1–4 inches long and lance-shaped, line the straight or slightly corkscrewed stems. Overlapping bracts encase disk-shaped composite flower heads of yellowish tubular flowers that form many-flowered, branching, spike-like clusters at the stem tips or upper leaf axils. Blooming from early summer to mid autumn, fertilized flowers produce smooth, dry, cylindrical seeds lacking a hairy crown.

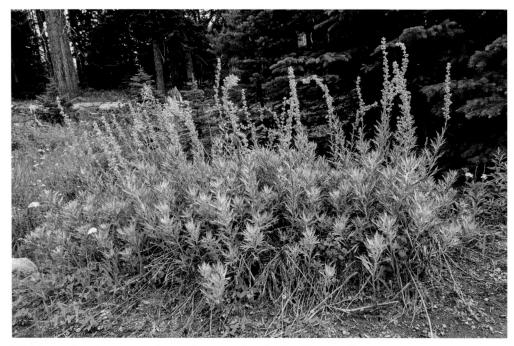

This clump of western mugwort is sending up stalks of yellow-blooming flowers.

Several forms of this highly variable species occur in this region, ranging from those with occasionally few-lobed, mostly smooth-edged leaves (*Artemisia ludoviciana* subsp. *ludoviciana*) to those with deeply cut, twice-divided leaves (*A. ludoviciana* subsp. *incompta*). They are all useful as medicine.

Where, When, and How to Wildcraft

Western mugwort is widely distributed throughout North America. It inhabits areas with dry, sandy or rocky soil from low to high elevations. In this region, it is mostly a mountain dweller ranging from southern British Columbia to California, growing on both sides of the Cascades in Washington and Oregon in open forests, sagebrush steppe, prairies, rangelands, and along year-round and seasonal streams.

While the plant is in flower, harvest four or five stalks per clump. Snip at the base and discard brown or damaged leaves. Bundle and hang to dry out of direct sunlight. After the herb is fully dried, remove the leaves and flowers separately. Reserve the flowers for oil, and use the leaves for tea or tincture.

Medicinal Uses

Like other medicinal *Artemisia* species, western mugwort is very bitter with a pungent, sagebrush-like taste and aroma. Drink the leaf tea hot to break a fever or to alleviate cold-induced menstrual cramping.

The cold infusion or the tincture calms an irritated stomach, promotes appetite, and rids the body of pinworms, the most common type of worm to infect humans. These thin, white, and ¼- to ½-inch-long worms live in the intestines and wriggle out at night to lay eggs in the folds of the anus. Wash your hands after using the toilet or scratching your anus to prevent the spread of eggs, and administer an enema of the body-temperature tea once a week for

6 weeks. Inhale a steam of the leaves to speed the healing of lung infections and to reduce respiratory inflammation.

Apply the flower oil or a wash of the leaves topically to red, itchy areas affected by athlete's foot, jock itch, ringworm, and other fungal infections of the skin.

The leaves in all forms—tea, tincture, smoke, or even hung above the bed or placed under the pillow—promote vivid dreams and help uncover, access, and transform areas of psychic unconsciousness. The flower oil rubbed on the middle of the forehead works the same.

The wadded leaves rubbed between the palms fluff up to make an excellent slow-burning smudge to clear negative energies from a space or can be used as a crude moxa. Add the dried leaves to smoking mixes for their mentally stimulating and sometimes giddiness-inducing effect.

⚠ Caution

Because of its uterine stimulating effect, do not ingest this plant in any form during pregnancy.

Future Harvests

To expand western mugwort populations, divide the vigorously spreading rhizomes. Dig up part of the root system, remove the top-growth, and break the roots into smaller chunks, each with new-growth buds, for replanting.

HERBAL PREPARATIONS

Leaf Tea
Cold or hot infusion
Drink 2–3 fluid ounces up to 3 times per day; for pinworm infections, drink 4 fluid ounces throughout the day.

Leaf Tincture
1 part dried leaf
5 parts menstruum (50 percent alcohol, 50 percent distilled water)
Take 20–45 drops up to 3 times per day.

Flower Oil
Follow directions for Dry Herb Infused Oil or Alternative Oil Method (page 64).

western pasqueflower

Anemone occidentalis

pulsatilla, white pasqueflower, wind flower

PARTS USED leaf

High-mountain leaves bring a breeze of tranquility to clear anxiety, harmonize thought, and stabilize mood swings accompanied by general nervous system overload.

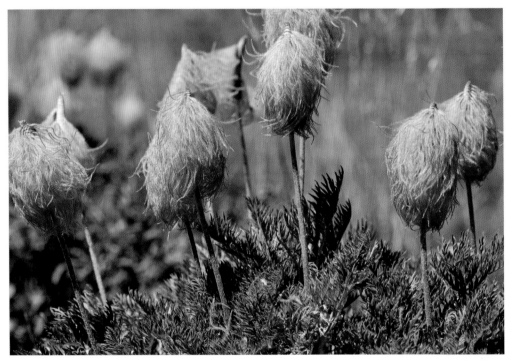

Heads of long-tailed, sperm-like seeds await dispersal on the wind.

How to Identify

This clumping, taprooted perennial with a woody-stemmed base grows 6–24 inches tall. In early summer as the mountain snows melt, hairy flowering stems rise upward. Atop each stem a single flower absent of petals blooms 1–2 inches wide. The center, filled with numerous yellow stamens, is cupped by 5–8 creamy white, petal-like sepals that are egg-shaped and hairy-backed with purple-tinged outer bases. Deeply dissected, 2–3 times divided, and long-stalked basal leaves spread out after the flowers bloom. Beneath the flower a whorl of 3 similarly shaped, stalkless leaves sits on the upper half of the stem. Many dry, elliptic seeds with long tails covered in feather-like hairs that aid their dispersal in the wind make up spherical seed heads resembling old, wild-haired humans.

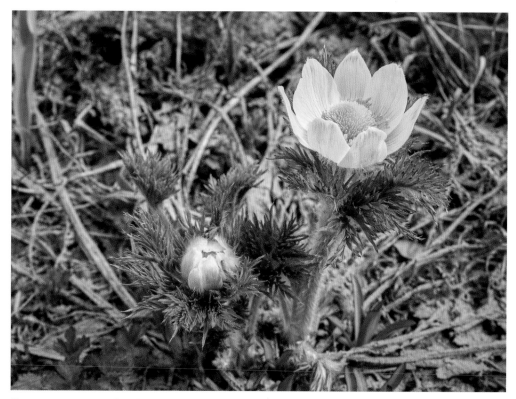

Flowers emerge just after the snow has melted away. Two weeks prior, there were several feet of snow in this area on Mount Rainier in Washington.

Some herbalists report that other *Anemone* species may be used the same as *Anemone occidentalis*. Taste a small piece of leaf to test for acridity, but be careful because the leaves of medicinally active anemones are so acrid they may burn your tongue. After nibbling on hundreds of leaves from other local species, I've only found a few that have the tell-tale bite, but you may have better luck.

Where, When, and How to Wildcraft

Western pasqueflower is found in alpine meadows and on open, rocky slopes at middle to high elevations from British Columbia to central California and spreading east as far as Idaho with isolated stands in Montana. It often grows at or above timberline in mountain ranges throughout the Pacific West. From the time they emerge until the seeds mature, conservatively gather vibrant green leaves from several different plants and process fresh for tincture.

Medicinal Uses

The leaves of western pasqueflower relieve anxiety and are best suited for people with nervousness characterized by rapidly changing moods, excessive thought, or an impending sense of doom. Take the leaf tincture to relieve panic attacks with a racing heart, to calm twitching overstimulated nerves, or to relieve insomnia caused by an overactive, worried mind.

Western pasqueflower leaf also harmonizes the mind and helps people prone to forgetfulness and scattered thought, who might be considered "airheads" by some, develop the positive gifts inherent to their constitution: swift, highly alert, relational thinking that connects widely varying ideas with the ability to quickly shift gears and stay emotionally unattached in situations where others may become mired in the muddy waters of the unconscious.

⚠ Caution

This is a low-dose plant. Exceeding the recommended dosage may significantly lower blood pressure and cause anxiety, nausea, and dizziness. This plant is not for use during pregnancy or for those with bradycardia, a slow heart rate of less than 60 beats per minute. If you notice any adverse effects from ingesting this medicine, stop taking it and try something else.

Future Harvests

Make a wish, and scatter the mature seeds into the wind.

HERBAL PREPARATIONS

Leaf Tincture

1 part fresh leaf

2 parts menstruum (75 percent alcohol, 25 percent distilled water)

The plant must be tinctured fresh to be effective, as the acrid taste of the medicinally active constituents is lost after drying. When stored well, the tincture is stable for about 2 years. As the medicine ages, you may need to use a slightly higher dosage to get the same effect.

Take 1–20 drops up to 5 times per day. Start with 1–5 drops, and continue with 1–5 drops every 15 minutes until you find the dosage that best suits your constitution.

Paeonia brownii
Brown's peony
PARTS USED root

Many-flavored roots relieve cramps, calm the nerves, and allow for the expression of suppressed feelings.

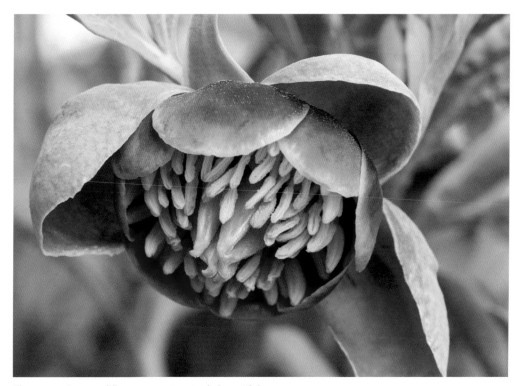

The many-stamened flowers are stunningly beautiful.

How to Identify

Fleshy, tuber-like roots grow in clumps with 5–8 fleshy, divided leaves per often-reddish stem. The leaves, coated with a whitish blue, waxy powder, are sometimes purple-tinged on the edges. Nodding buds bloom into exquisite, many-stamened flowers with 5–6 persistent, greenish to purplish sepals that bend backward as the flowers mature. The round, maroon to brownish petals, 5–10 per flower, are smaller than the sepals, have yellowish edges, and fall off after fertilization. A fleshy disc inside the flower exudes abundant insect-attracting nectar. A grouping of 3–5 stubby, pea-like pods, fused at the base, holds the light brown to purple-black, bean-like seeds, and the matured fruits rest on the ground. In full sunlight, these plants grow short and spread themselves wide; they grow taller, up to 20 inches, in shadier conditions.

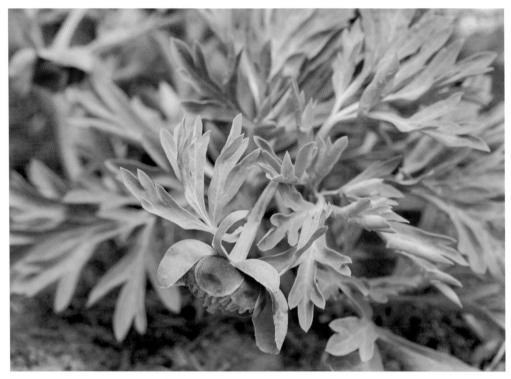

With its reddish stems, purple-tinged leaf edges, and nodding flowers, western peony looks like something out of a Dr. Seuss book.

Where, When, and How to Wildcraft

This long-lived perennial prefers open meadows, sagebrush steppe, dry forests, and bunchgrass prairies at middle to high elevations. Find western peony in central and southeastern Washington and through-out eastern Oregon. As it moves south, its range extends west of the Cascades into the Siskiyou Mountains of southwestern Oregon before descending into northern California.

Harvest the roots from mid summer to early autumn after the seeds have ripened. Excavate the soil along one edge of a large clump to expose some of the purplish- to brown-skinned, tuber-like roots. Gather a few roots from each clump and plant seeds in the loosened soil you use to refill the hole. Slice the roots in rounds to dry for tincturing. For teas, slice lengthwise so each dose contains the potentially different properties of the crown, middle, and tip of the root.

Medicinal Uses

The chalky, root beer–like taste of western peony root is a pleasant medley of sweet, bit-ter, pungent, and sour flavors. Take the root tea or tincture to relieve menstrual cramping with heavy bleeding, to initiate bleeding in slow-to-arrive periods, or to reduce the irrita-bility that can accompany either. These same preparations relieve testicular cramping and pain in the prostate and calm excessive and spasmodic coughing.

European peony (*Paeonia officinalis*), an old-time remedy for epilepsy, was known for its effect on the nervous system. West-ern peony root, with its watery and earthy nature, seems to have similar properties and cools and grounds overly excited nerves that bring twitching, shaking, and anxiety. To relieve anxiety from over-thinking, take the tea or tincture to ground and center yourself and get in touch with your feelings. For anxiety stemming from unexpressed emotions, especially grief, that may be at the root of your unease, take these same preparations to help you connect with and express your suppressed feelings.

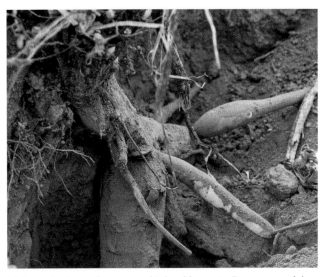

Mature plants produce several tuber-like roots. For a respectful harvest, remove only one or two from each plant.

 Caution

Eating or consuming preparations of the fresh root may cause nausea.

Future Harvests

Take only a few roots from each clump. I have successfully sprouted the seeds. To aid germination, scarify the thick-skinned seeds by thinning the seed coat with sandpaper or a file, nicking with a knife, or soaking in water overnight. Transplant seedlings to appropriate sites.

HERBAL PREPARATIONS

Root Tea
Standard decoction
Drink 3–4 fluid ounces up to 4 times per day.

Root Tincture
1 part dried root
5 parts menstruum (60 percent alcohol, 40 percent distilled water)
Take 15–30 drops up to 4 times per day.

western redcedar

Thuja plicata
canoe cedar
PARTS USED leaf

Aromatic and astringent leaves help speed the healing of respiratory, urinary, and fungal infections, relieve rashes, and remove warts.

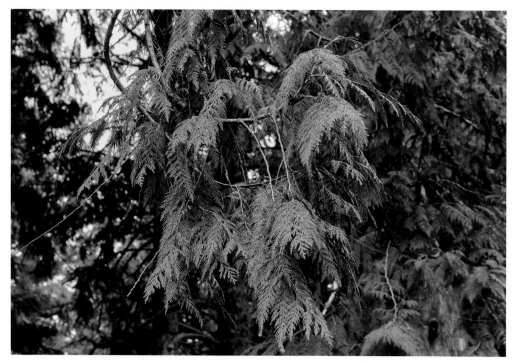

Graceful sprays of foliage hang down from upcurving branches.

How to Identify

Belts of thin, reddish brown bark, fibrous and easily peeling, run in vertical strips on tall, straight trunks that flare out at the base and become buttressed as the trees age. The growing tip or leader droops. Oppositely arranged pairs of small, overlapping leaves, glossy green and scale-like, press close to the stem in rows of 4 to form horizontally flattened sprays of aromatic, evergreen foliage that hang down gracefully from upcurving branches. The evergreen leaves turn brown and fall from the tree after 3 or 4 years. From mid to late spring, many tiny, yellowish to reddish, somewhat globe-shaped, pollen-producing cones form at the tips of the branchlets, and bluish green, egg-shaped, seed-bearing cones, about ⅜ inch long, emerge singly at the ends of branches and turn brown as they mature. Male and female cones form on the same tree. This long-lived tree can attain heights of up to 230 feet.

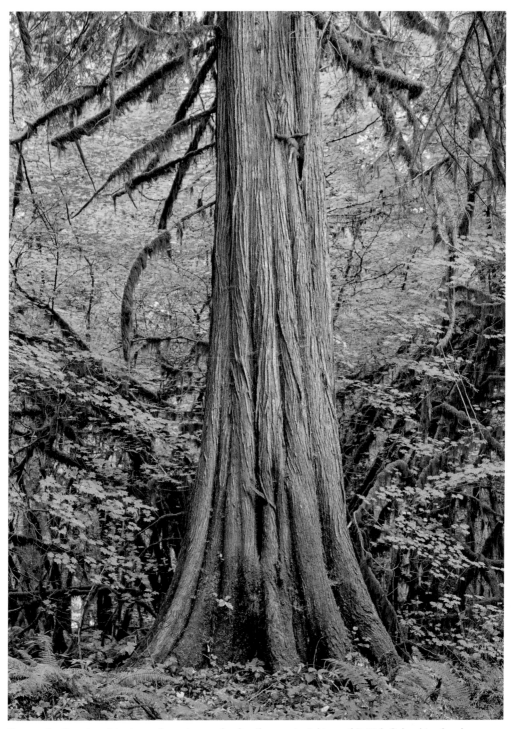

Famous for its rot-resistant wood, western redcedar, the provincial tree of British Columbia, develops a buttressed base as it matures.

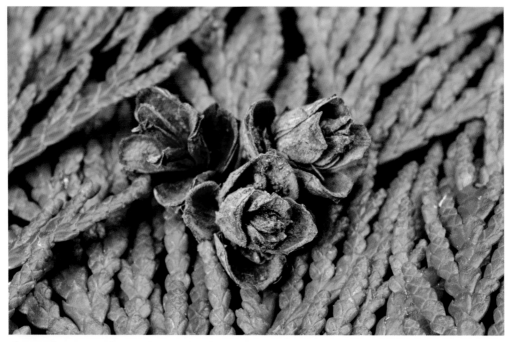

The woody cones are like small, many-petaled flowers, and the flattened aromatic foliage is made up of overlapping scale-like leaves.

Where, When, and How to Wildcraft

Restricted to coastal counties in northern California (the southernmost extent of its range), western redcedar, which also extends eastward into Idaho, Montana, and Alberta, mainly inhabits wet, mixed coniferous forests on the western side of the Cascade Mountains from Alaska to California. Find it growing in wet floodplains, in river and stream drainages, or near seeps and springs from sea level to middle elevations (about 4500 feet) in the mountains.

The leaves can be harvested throughout the year, but the best time is during the stormy season from autumn to spring, when you will often find fallen branches knocked to the ground by storms or vibrant, young growing tips scattered on the ground below the trees. If you find a downed branch or tree, taste the leaves to make sure they are still good for medicine. Even though the leaves

on fallen branches stay green for a long time, over time they lose their sweetness and their bitter taste predominates. Process the leaves along with green parts of the twig fresh for tincture or dry in a paper bag or on screens for smudge, tea, or infused oil.

Medicinal Uses

Western redcedar's cooling and drying leaves resolve hot, damp conditions in the body. Use the tea or tincture of the leaves to speed the healing of acute respiratory or urinary tract infections. The tea drunk hot, the tincture in hot water, or a steam of the leaves aids the lungs and upper respiratory tract; drinking the cooled leaf tea or the tincture diluted in cold water sends the aromatic oils to the kidneys and urinary tract.

Apply the infused oil, a wash of the leaf tea, or the simple lotion on red, oozy skin conditions like poison oak rashes or weeping eczemas to relieve irritation and speed their healing. Apply the salve or any of the above-mentioned preparations at the first sign of redness and itching from athlete's foot, jock itch, ringworm, or other fungal infections of the skin. When working with these types of imbalance, it is also important to address the internal ecology that gives rise to the condition. Consider avoiding sweets (even fruit) and stimulants that feed the fungus, and take cooling herbs like Oregon grape root or burdock root.

To get rid of warts, apply the leaf tincture directly on the affected area several times daily. The warts will usually fall off within a few days.

⚠ Caution

Because it contains thujone, a uterine stimulant, western redcedar is contraindicated during pregnancy. Do not take internally for long periods, as it can be damaging to the kidneys.

Future Harvests

While these trees are abundant, a respectful harvest would begin with a search for downed branches or leaf tips. Otherwise snip off a few fans of leaves from lower hanging branches.

HERBAL PREPARATIONS

Leaf Tea
Standard infusion
Infuse the leaves fresh or dried. Let the leaves infuse overnight to bring out the all of the subtle flavors.

Drink 3–4 fluid ounces up to 4 times per day.

Leaf Tincture
1 part fresh leaf
2 parts menstruum (100 percent alcohol)
Take 15–30 drops up to 4 times per day.

Leaf Oil and Salve
For leaf oil, follow directions for Dry Herb Infused Oil or Alternative Oil Method (page 64). For the salve, follow directions on page 65.

Leaf Simple Lotion
2 parts tincture
5 parts distilled water
1 part glycerin

Lysichiton americanus
American skunk cabbage, swamp lantern
PARTS USED root

In addition to its large leaves and distinctive yellow-bracted floral display, this beautiful bog dweller provides root medicine that expels mucus from the lungs and relieves spasmodic coughs.

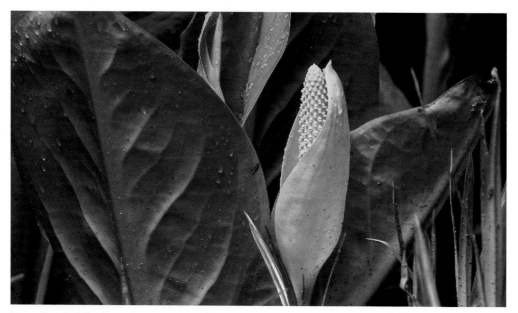

The yellow leaf-like bract, known as a spathe, surrounds the spadix, a dense, small-flowered spike on a thickened axis.

How to Identify
Sunk deep into the mucky earth and held fast by many fibrous side roots, a stout rhizome gives rise in spring to a thick, cylindrical spike of small, densely arranged, greenish yellow flowers on a 12- to 20-inch-long stalk. A bright yellow, leaf-like bract enfolds the spike of skunky-smelling flowers whose odor attracts pollinating insects. Short-stalked, fleshy, and waxy-coated basal leaves, broadly lance- to egg-shaped and 1–5 feet long, emerge after the flowers and emit a skunk-like odor when crushed. Egg-shaped, berry-like fruits, greenish to reddish in color and containing 1 or 2 seeds, remain embedded in the flower spike after maturing.

Where, When, and How to Wildcraft
Inhabiting swamps, bogs, ditches, marshes, stream edges, and wet forests from Alaska to northern California, this semi-aquatic perennial may live for 80 years. Find it from sea level at the coast to middle elevations on both sides of the Cascades.

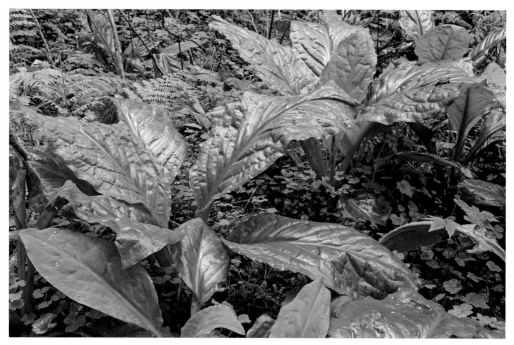

Being in the forest with this large-leaved plant transports me back to prehistoric times.

Harvest the difficult-to-remove rhizomes along with the side roots from late summer to mid autumn. It's a dirty, mucky job. Wash the roots well before drying.

Medicinal Uses

The root tincture clears mucus from the lungs and calms spasmodic coughing. It is especially indicated if the force of the coughing results in gagging or nausea. Consider it for cramps, spasms, or asthma brought on by stress or anxiety.

⚠ Caution

Do not consume the fresh plant or eat the cooked leaves. All parts of western skunk cabbage contain sharp, needle-like calcium oxalate crystals that mechanically injure the tissues of the digestive tract when ingested. Eating the raw plant may cause a burning sensation in the mouth and throat and/or a swelling of the tongue, lips, or throat.

In extreme cases the throat may even swell shut. In addition, consuming large quantities of the medicinal preparations may result in nausea or digestive upset.

Future Harvests

Respectfully harvest one or two plants from healthy, abundant patches. The roots can be divided and planted in boggy areas.

HERBAL PREPARATIONS

Root Tincture
1 part fresh root
2 parts menstruum (75 percent alcohol, 25 percent distilled water)
or
1 part dried root
5 parts menstruum (50 percent alcohol, 50 percent distilled water)
Take 15–45 drops up to 4 times per day.

Trillium ovatum

birth root, Pacific trillium, western wakerobin

PARTS USED leaf

Flowering western trilliums welcome spring and bring medicine that stops uterine bleeding and helps prepare the uterus for birth.

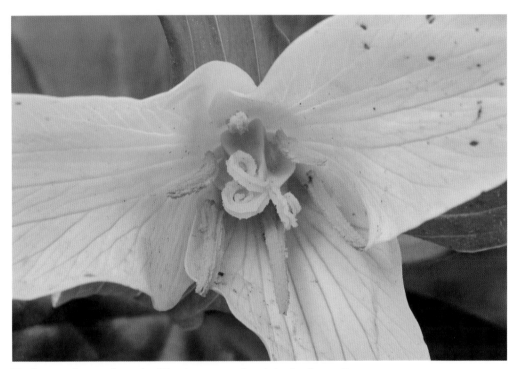

The large anthers at the ends of the stamens produce lots of yellow pollen.

How to Identify

From a stout, fleshy rhizome, a smooth, unbranched stem rises 4–12 inches in late winter. A whorl of 3 broadly triangular to oval, unmottled, unstalked, 2- to 8-inch-long, and pointy-tipped leaves unfurls to display a single showy flower atop an erect or slightly nodding stalk. Three white or slightly pinkish petals, ½ to 3 inches long, turn pink or purple as they age, and 3 green, lance-shaped sepals peek out from between the longer and wider petals. The reproductive parts of the flower are yellow. Fleshy, green to yellowish capsules with small, wing-like ridges split open to release their seeds. The egg-shaped seeds have fleshy appendages that entice ants to carry them back to their nests.

Where, When, and How to Wildcraft

Growing at low to middle elevations, this widely distributed perennial beautifies wet forested areas of this region from British

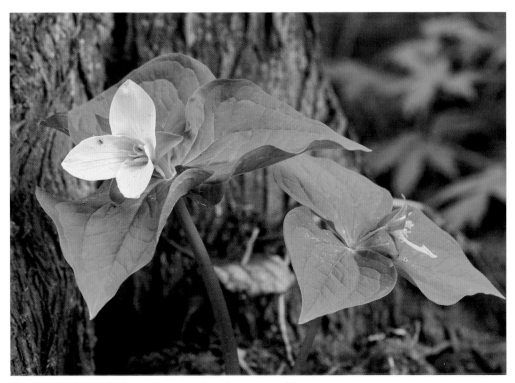

Showy flowers are framed by a whorl of three pointy-tipped leaves.

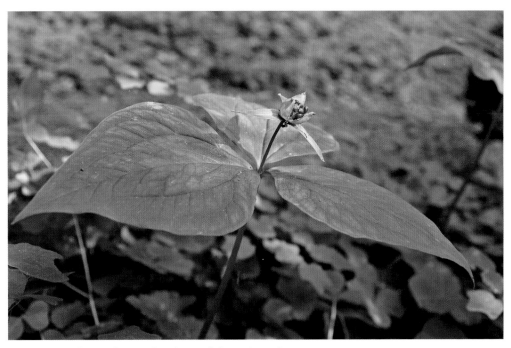

Harvest the still-green leaves after the seeds have ripened.

Columbia south to California. Harvest the leaves along with the stems in late summer just before the tops begin to turn brown and die back. The seed capsules will be just bursting open at this time. If you harvest them too early, the plant will not have enough time to store up food for next year's growth, and it might not make it through winter.

Medicinal Uses

Astringent tannins in western trillium leaves dry excessive discharges and stop bleeding. Take the leaf tincture to resolve damp, whitish or yellowish vaginal discharges known as leukorrhea or to stop postpartum hemorrhaging. You can also use it to stanch excessive bleeding after a miscarriage or bleeding from uterine fibroids. For the latter, use it for short-term, acute relief only.

To stimulate and tone the uterus in preparation for birth, take the tincture once a day for a week prior to the expected due date. The leaf tincture also stops bleeding in the lungs and reduces prostate inflammation with painful urination.

Caution

Do not use uterine-stimulating western trillium leaves or root during pregnancy except as noted above to prepare the uterus for birth. Use for the latter only under the supervision of a qualified health practitioner. Western trillium leaves and roots contain saponins that increase estrogen levels in the body. Because high levels of estrogen promote the growth of uterine tissue, long-term use is contraindicated for women with fibroids.

Future Harvests

Western trilliums are slow growing and long lived. Counting leaf scars on the rhizomes reveals their age. Only one true leaf may form in a plant's first 5–10 years of life, it may take 15 years for the plant to set its first flower, and a plant with a 3-inch-long rhizome may be over 70 years old. Do not harvest the roots of wild plants; only take the leaves and stems at the end of the growing season.

If you gather roots from cultivated plants, use half the recommended dosage because the roots are more potent than the leaves. Alternatively, consider yarrow leaf or shepherd's purse whole plant as alternatives to stop postpartum bleeding. For leukorrhea, substitute yellow pond-lily root or red root root bark.

If you would like to grow western trillium in your garden, be sure to add some soil from around a wild plant, because the plants, lacking root hairs, need specific soil mycorrhizae to facilitate the uptake of nutrients.

HERBAL PREPARATIONS

Leaf Tincture
1 part fresh leaf
2 parts menstruum (75 percent alcohol, 25 percent distilled water)
Take 20–40 drops up to 5 times per day.

western white clematis

Clematis ligusticifolia
white virgin's bower
PARTS USED leaf and stem

Leaves and stems, acrid and biting, reduce the severity and soothe the pain of migraine and cluster headaches, relieve uterine cramping, and calm anxiety.

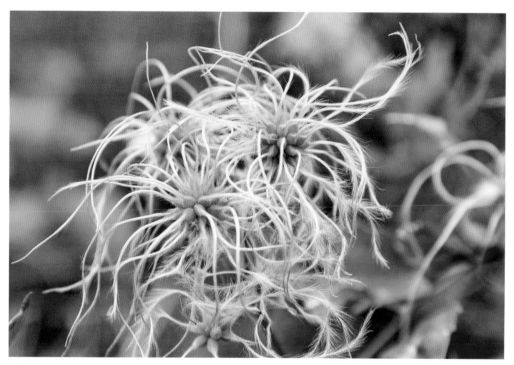

The feathery-tailed seeds are dispersed by the wind.

How to Identify

Tough, woody vines, up to 65 feet long, burst forth from stout, taprooted rhizomes to clamber on shrubs, climb trees, or trail along the ground. Pairs of smooth or slightly hairy compound leaves arranged opposite each other along the nearly smooth to softly hairy stems divide into 5–15 broadly egg- to lance-shaped, smooth, few-toothed, or irregularly lobed leaflets with persistent stalks that act as tendrils. Absent petals, 4 creamy white and hairy sepals grace both the male and female flowers, which bloom on separate vines from early summer to early autumn in bracted, several- to many-flowered clusters from the leaf axils of the current year's stems. Numerous non-pollen-producing, vestigial stamens surround the many pistils of the female flowers; the multi-stamened male flowers lack vestigial pistils. Pollinated flowers produce spherical tufts of several 1- to 2-inch-long, feathery-tailed, elliptic

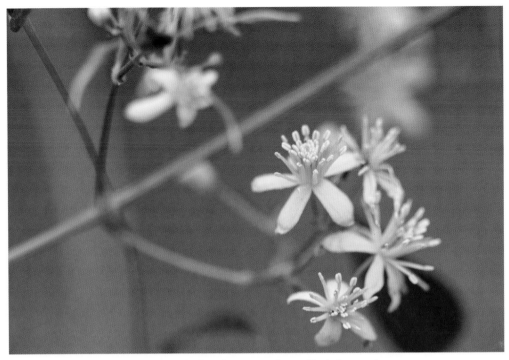

The reproductive parts of these petal-lacking flowers are framed by hairy sepals.

seeds that await dispersal by the wind. The leaves drop in late autumn, and though the first several feet of vine may live for a few years, the plants generally die back to the crown during winter.

Traveler's joy (*Clematis vitalba*), introduced from Europe and Africa, looks similar to western white clematis but has flowers with both male and female parts. It is mainly found west of the Cascades and is reported to have similar medicinal properties.

Where, When, and How to Wildcraft

Occupying most of the western half of North America, this long-lived native vine spreads by layering and makes its home along the banks of perennial or intermittent streams and in gullies, ditches, riparian thickets, and other wet places at low to middle elevations. It prefers full sun but tolerates some shade. In the Pacific Northwest, find western white clematis growing in southern British Columbia and mostly east of the Cascades in Washington. It is widely distributed throughout Oregon, and its range extends south into California.

Cut the ends of leaf-bearing vines during the spring and summer months and process them fresh or bundle them for drying. The medicinal strength of the vines varies depending on their age, climactic conditions, and the composition of the soil in which they grow. They are more potent earlier in the season. Chew a small piece of leaf; if it burns your tongue, it will make good medicine.

Medicinal Uses

The leaf and stem of western white clematis dilate blood vessels in the brain to relieve migraine and cluster headache pain resulting from weakness and lack of tone in the vasculature. For best results, take the tea or tincture

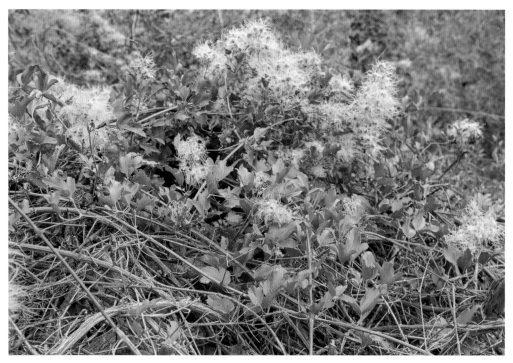

Burgeoning vines spread rapidly across trees, shrubs, and fences.

of the leaves and stems at the first sign of discomfort. These same preparations also relax dull, achy uterine and muscle spasms ameliorated by warmth and soothe arthritic joint pain aggravated by cold, damp weather.

The tea or tincture of the leaves and stems brings calmness, focus, and grounding to emotionally labile people while in states of anxiety, fear, or confusion. Early American botanical doctors used the related species *Clematis recta* for nervous insomnia, toothache, and swollen lymphatic glands in the groin.

⚠ Caution

This plant is not to be used during pregnancy, with pharmaceutical migraine medications, or with vasculitis, an inflammatory condition of the blood vessels. Do not exceed recommended dosages or use for extended periods of time.

Future Harvests

Carefully remove and transplant rooted nodes of this vigorously growing and drought-tolerant vine to appropriate locations, or sow seeds in autumn for spring germination.

HERBAL PREPARATIONS

Leaf and Stem Tea
Infuse 1 tablespoon of the recently dried herb in 8 fluid ounces of boiling water.
Drink 2–4 fluid ounces up to 2 times per day.

Leaf and Stem Tincture
1 part fresh leaf and stems
2 parts menstruum (75 percent alcohol, 25 percent distilled water)
Take 5–15 drops up to 3 times per day.

---

wild carrot

Daucus carota
Queen Anne's lace
PARTS USED seed, root

Pungent seeds, warming and stimulating, prevent conception, prepare the uterus for pregnancy, and aid digestion. Diuretic roots and seeds dissolve stones and rid the body of excess fluids.

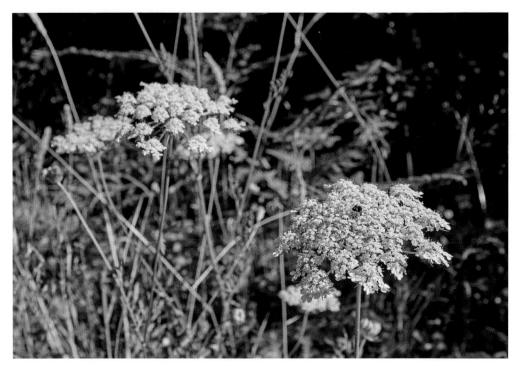

A single purple flower often blooms in the center of the flower head.

How to Identify

In its first year of growth, short-stalked, fern-like basal leaves emerge from a whitish, carrot-like taproot and divide many times into small linear segments. In the second year, the plant sends up a single, 1- to 4-foot-tall, branched flowering stalk covered in stiff hairs. A whorl of bracts divided into long, threadlike segments radiates outward from beneath 1½- to 4¾-inch-wide,

many-flowered, lacy flower heads made up of compact, white-flowered umbels borne on rays of unequal length. A single purple flower often dots the center of the flower head. As the early- to late-summer-blooming flowers ripen into egg-shaped, prickle-ribbed seeds, the outer rays of the flower head arch inward to form a bird's-nest-like seed head. The seeds are widest at the middle, and the root of this mostly hairy biennial smells like a garden

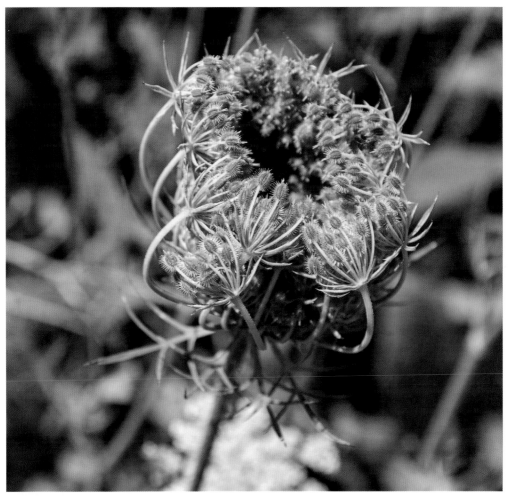

Harvest seeds as the seed head turns into a "bird's nest" and the seeds begin to turn from green to brown.

carrot for whom it is the wild ancestor.

This plant shares habitat and may be confused with poison hemlock (*Conium maculatum*), the deadly toxic plant that was supposedly used to kill Socrates. Be absolutely sure of your identification before ingesting any part of a wild carrot plant. Consult a botanical key to distinguish this plant from potentially deadly parsley family look-a-likes, and check the "Toxic Plants" section (page 32) for tips on identifying these poisonous umbels.

Where, When, and How to Wildcraft

Introduced from Eurasia, wild carrot makes its home in fields, waste places, and along roadsides throughout North America. In this region, it grows from British Columbia to California and from the coast to middle elevations in the mountains.

Collect seeds from mid to late summer as the seed bodies begin to turn from green to brown. Immature green seeds will be overly sharp and pungent, whereas brown dried out seeds will have lost most of their aromatic quality. When harvested at their peak, the flavor of the seeds is roundly pungent and feels expansive and opening. To kill insect eggs or larvae that will eat up your harvest when they mature, place well-contained seeds in the freezer for 2 weeks.

Harvest the roots of this biennial as they enter their second season of growth, between early autumn and early spring. After the flowering stalks emerge, the roots dry out and lose their medicinal virtue.

Medicinal Uses

The pungent seeds of wild carrot warm and stimulate the genitourinary and digestive systems. A tea or tincture of the diuretic seeds or roots improves urine flow to rid water-logged tissues of excess fluid and helps clear gravelly deposits from the bladder and kidneys. Take either for arthritic pain from water retention, to relax constriction in the urinary tract causing painful urination, to relieve gout, or to dissolve kidney stones. Aromatic oils in the seeds also aid digestion and reduce gas.

The seeds renew and refresh the womb by shedding old, stagnant blood. They can be used to promote conception by preparing a fertile ground for healthy embryo implantation. They can also be used as a form of birth control to prevent eggs from implanting by shedding the uterine lining during and after ovulation. To enhance fertility, take the tincture or 1 teaspoon of the seeds, chewed or crushed and mixed with water or juice, before ovulation. To prevent conception, take the same preparations during and after ovulation; and as an emergency contraceptive, take the seeds starting 8–12 hours after intercourse once daily for 3 days. Ingesting the seeds also harmonizes the menstrual cycle and helps clear placental tissue that remains adhered to the uterus after childbirth.

 Caution

Do not use during pregnancy. Before starting a wild carrot seed contraceptive program, do a careful and in-depth study of the available literature. Discontinue use if the timing of your menstrual cycle shifts or if you notice breast tenderness or other hormone-related issues.

Future Harvests

Although it is considered a noxious weed in many states, thank wild carrot for its beneficial medicine, and let it do its thing.

HERBAL PREPARATIONS

Seed Tea
Standard infusion of the crushed seeds
Drink 4–6 fluid ounces up to 4 times per day.

Seed Tincture
1 part fresh seed
3 parts menstruum (100 percent alcohol)
Take 15–30 drops up to 4 times per day; as a contraceptive, take 15–30 drops once per day for 3–7 days during and after ovulation.

Root Tea
Standard decoction
Drink 4–6 fluid ounces up to 4 times per day.

---

wild ginger

Asarum caudatum
British Columbia wild ginger
PARTS USED root

Spicy, warming roots promote sweating, relieve cramping, and bring on delayed menses.

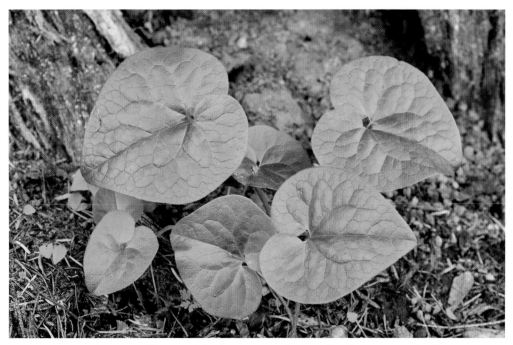

True to its name, the roots and leaves of this low-growing plant smell and taste somewhat like store-bought, tropical ginger.

How to Identify
Uniformly green, long-stalked, heart- to kidney-shaped leaves, 2 per node, attach directly to creeping rhizomes that spread near the soil surface to form loose mats. From the growing tips of the rhizomes, petal-less flowers made up of 3 maroon, 1- to 3-inch-long, tapering sepals emerge horizontally. The solitary flowers, blooming from mid spring to mid summer, are usually hidden under the leaf litter and ripen into fleshy capsules filled with seeds with fleshy appendages. The seed appendage contains an oil that attracts ants who carry the seeds back to their nests. When crushed all parts of this evergreen plant exude a strong, lemony-ginger smell. The prominently veined leaves and the stalks are lined with hairs.

Where, When, and How to Wildcraft
On both sides of the Cascades from British Columbia to California, wild ginger inhabits

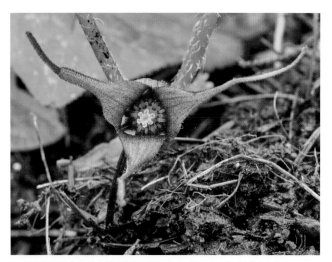

The striking maroon flowers are rarely seen because they usually lie hidden under fallen leaves.

Due to its uterine-stimulating effects, wild ginger should not be used during pregnancy. This plant should also not be used long term because it, as well as other members of the birthwort family (Aristolochiaceae), contains aristolochic acid which is reported to have kidney-damaging and cancer-causing effects. Despite its inviting, peppery-ginger flavor, it is best consumed infrequently and in small quantities as a wild food.

wet, shady forests at low to middle elevations. Gather roots and rhizomes from early to late autumn. Because the natural inclination of the plant is to grow outward, it is best to harvest from the edges of each mat-forming clump. The rhizomes grow right under the surface. Pull up on the end of a plant and gently pull it up out of the ground. You may need to dig under a little to help loosen the soil as you pry the plant from the ground. Cut the rhizome at a node.

Medicinal Uses

Wild ginger's pungent and stimulating roots warm the skin and promote sweating. Drink the root tea or the tincture in hot water to open the exterior and bring on sweating to clear and speed the healing of colds, flus, or acute respiratory infections. Either preparation relieves intestinal cramping with gas. For delayed menstruation accompanied by coldness and lower back pain, the tea or tincture lessens the pain and stimulates the uterus to encourage bleeding. In larger doses wild ginger root is reported to be emetic.

Future Harvests

Create new colonies of wild ginger by cutting small chunks of rhizome (make sure there are at least two nodes with attached rootlets) and planting them just under the surface of the soil with the tip barely exposed.

HERBAL PREPARATIONS

Root Tea
Standard decoction
Drink 3–4 fluid ounces up to 3 times per day.

Root Tincture
1 part fresh root
2 parts menstruum (100 percent alcohol)
Take 15–45 drops up to 3 times per day.

willow

Salix species

PARTS USED bark

Water-loving and ubiquitous, the willows provide bitter bark that reliably relieves pain and inflammation, reduces fevers, and clears urinary tract infections.

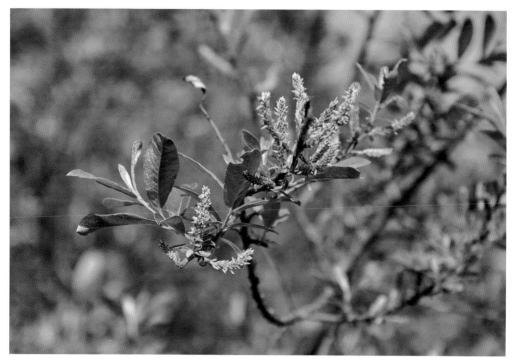

Capsules that contain ripening seeds arch upward on this willow found growing on the Washington side of the Columbia River Gorge.

How to Identify

In late winter fuzzy catkins, male and female on separate plants, emerge to stand upright from usually flexible yellow, orange, or red twigs. Soon after, leaves break free of single-scaled buds and unfurl linear to egg-shaped but always longer than they are broad. The leaves often have a pair of stipules growing at the bases of their stalks. Flowers of the female catkins produce capsules containing numerous tiny seeds, each with a hairy covering that carries them upon the wind. Willows often form extensive, shallow root systems that help stabilize stream banks.

Because the size and shape of leaves vary greatly within species and because they readily hybridize with other species to produce plants with mixed appearance, members of *Salix* can be quite difficult to positively

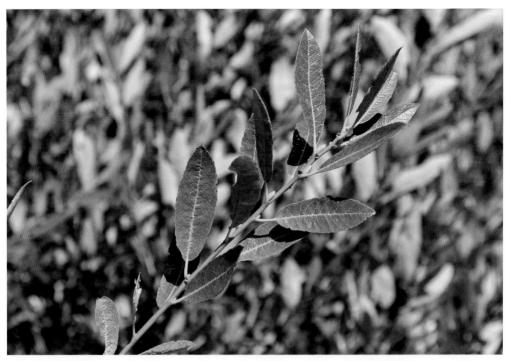

Notice the stipules growing at the bases of the leaf stalks.

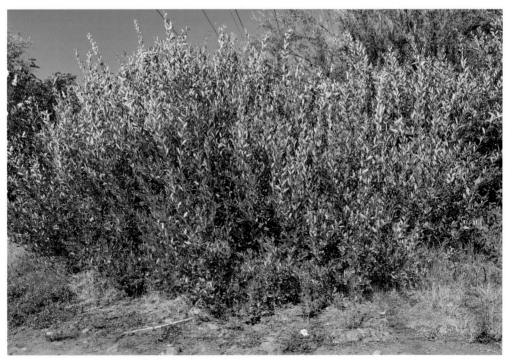

This willow grows on the banks of the Applegate River in southern Oregon.

identify and key out to species. For our purposes, what matters is the taste of the bark. If it is bitter like aspirin, you've got a medicinally active willow. The main species used by European herbalists, white willow (*S. alba*), can be found naturalized around urban areas in some parts of this region.

Where, When, and How to Wildcraft

There are more than thirty native species of willow in the Pacific Northwest, including trees, shrubs, and mat-forming, dwarf species. Throughout this region and at every elevation, willows grow where there is abundant water. Find them along streams, gullies, ditches, and swales and in swampy ground.

Finding suitable species for medicine takes some work. Not all species have high levels of the medicinally active salicin. In spring, cut little strips of bark from the branches and taste them to test for bitterness. When you find a suitable tree or shrub, remember where it is growing so you can return year after year for medicine.

From tree species remove thumb-sized or larger branches then strip the bark; from shrubs take a few stems from each clump. Gather in spring after the leaves emerge. As the season progresses the concentration of tannins rises and the amount of salicin decreases.

Medicinal Uses

Use bitter willow bark as you would aspirin. Take the tea or tincture internally for general pain, inflammation, fevers, headaches, or neuralgia. The bark tea relieves urinary tract pain and irritation, clears damp heat infections of the genitourinary system, and reduces genital discharges. Gargle the tea or tincture in water for mouth sores. Externally a wash soothes eczema or other red, itchy skin conditions; salicin reduces inflammation and the tannins tone the tissues.

Caution

Though it is gentler and can be used by those with aspirin sensitivity, take care with those prone to adverse salicylate reactions, and avoid use with pharmaceutical blood thinners.

Future Harvests

Because the tiny seeds are naked and without food stores, they must be sown immediately after collection. Propagate willows by planting the easily rooting stems in wet ground. You can also place twigs in a bucket or jar of water to root. Use this hormone-enriched water to stimulate the rooting of other plants.

HERBAL PREPARATIONS

Bark Tea
Standard decoction
Drink 3–4 fluid ounces up to 4 times per day.

Bark Tincture
1 part fresh bark
2 parts menstruum (75 percent alcohol,
    25 percent distilled water)
or
1 part dried bark
5 parts menstruum (50 percent alcohol,
    50 percent distilled water)
Take 15–30 drops up to 4 times per day.

---

woodland strawberry

Fragaria vesca

greenleaf strawberry, wild strawberry, woods strawberry

PARTS USED leaf, root

Astringent leaves support uterine health, relieve diarrhea and urinary tract infections, and soothe sore throats.

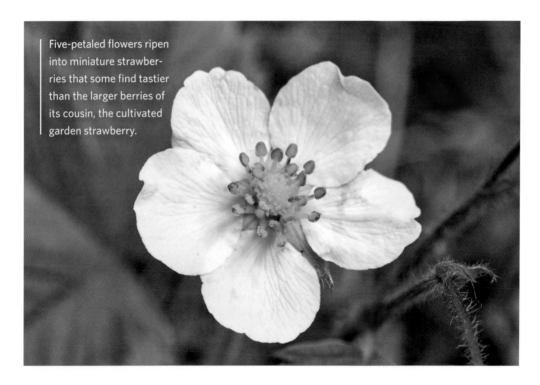

Five-petaled flowers ripen into miniature strawberries that some find tastier than the larger berries of its cousin, the cultivated garden strawberry.

How to Identify

From the crowns of short, scaly rhizomes, trailing stems (stolons) spread horizontally along the ground and root in at the nodes to form new plants. Prominently veined, bright green, 3-parted leaves unfold on hairy, 2- to 4-inch-long stalks connected to the crown. The thin, broadly oval to elliptic, stalkless leaflets, finely hairy below and nearly smooth above, fan out with strongly toothed edges. The tooth at the tip of each leaflet is larger than any of the others. Leafless stalks that attach directly to the rhizome rise above the leaves bearing diffuse clusters of 3–15 small, white flowers that bloom from mid spring to early summer. Five pointy-tipped lobes alternate with 5 small, narrowly oval bracts to form a persistent, green, silky-haired calyx that cups 5 egg-shaped petals. The thickened upper part of the stem that holds each flower, called the receptacle, swells to form a bright red, edible fruit. Many dry seeds are embedded evenly across the flesh of these ⅜-inch-wide strawberries.

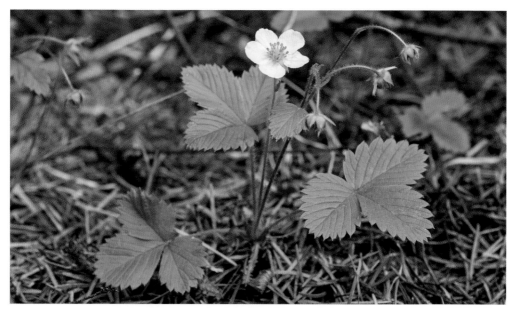
Tiny strawberries are ripening on this delightful little plant.

Where, When, and How to Wildcraft

With a range that extends the length of North America, this 4- to 12-inch tall perennial inhabits forest clearings and meadows, disturbed sites, and stream banks in moist to dry, semi-shaded forests throughout this region. Commonly found at low elevations, the occurrence of woodland strawberry steadily decreases as it rises toward the upper limit of its elevation range at 6500 feet above sea level. Collect green, intact leaves from mid spring to early autumn, and gather roots from late summer to mid autumn.

Medicinal Uses

A tea of astringent woodland strawberry leaves, like that made from the leaves of its rose family cousins, red raspberry and thimbleberry, tightens uterine tissue to prevent miscarriage and helps prepare the uterus for childbirth.

Drink the cooling root and/or leaf tea to relieve diarrhea, soothe urinary tract infections, or reduce stomach acidity. Gargle the tea for sore throats, inflamed gums, or mouth sores, or use it externally as a wash for wounds, eczema, or sunburn. The leaves are high in vitamin C.

Rub fresh berries onto the teeth to clean and whiten them. Leave the paste on for at least 5 minutes before brushing with baking soda.

Future Harvests

Conservatively harvest a few leaves per plant and gather rhizomes at the periphery of a patch to encourage outward growth. To establish new colonies, collect freshly rooted runners in spring and transplant in slightly acidic soil with the base of the root crown at ground level.

HERBAL PREPARATIONS

Leaf and/or Root Tea
Standard infusion
Drink 6–8 fluid ounces up to 4 times per day.

wormwood

Artemisia absinthium
absinthium
PARTS USED leaf and flower

Extremely bitter and stimulating leaves and flowers—the main ingredient in absinthe liqueur—improve appetite, relieve indigestion, strengthen the uterus, and act as a nervous system restorative.

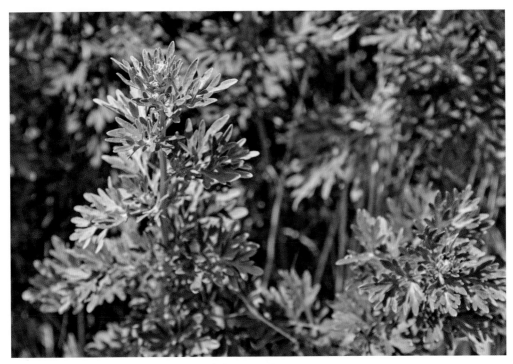

The lacy leaves smell sweet but are intensely bitter tasting.

How to Identify

Shallow lateral roots spread out from descending taproots. From a woody base many branching stems spread outward, slightly sprawling or standing erect 1–5 feet tall. Lacy, long-stalked leaves, grayish green, silky-haired and aromatic, deeply divide 2 or 3 times and terminate in oblong, blunt or round-tipped segments. The leaves become increasingly smaller, shorter-stalked, and less divided with more sharply pointed segments as they ascend the stem. Tubular, yellowish flowers, 30–50 in disk-like composite heads cradled by whorls of dry, papery bracts densely covered in long, silky hairs, bloom from mid summer to early autumn. Interspersed with small leaves, the many nodding flower heads, arranged in crowded, branching clusters, produce small, dry seeds lacking a hairy crown.

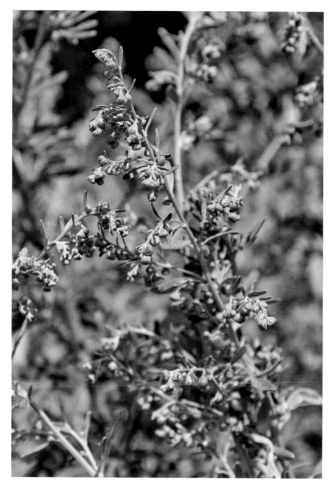

Many yellow tubular flowers make up each of the button-like, composite flower heads.

foliage, and strip the leaves and flowers from the stems for further processing.

Medicinal Uses

Small doses of the extremely bitter leaves and flowering tops stimulate digestion and relieve liver stagnation. Take the tea or tincture to encourage stomach acid secretion, improve appetite, and relieve indigestion, stomach inflammation, nausea, and heartburn. Take the leaves and flowering tops in either form to stimulate liver metabolism to clear liver congestion that leads to jaundice. For missed menstrual periods when the uterus is weak or lacks tone, the tea or tincture acts as a stimulant to bring on bleeding.

Long considered a tonic for the brain and mind, wormwood stimulates and restores energy to the nervous system to relieve nervous exhaustion from long-term stress or unhealed trauma leading to fatigue, anxiety, headache, heart palpitations, high blood pressure, depression, or despair.

Externally a warm compress or poultice of the leaves and flowers soothes sprains, contusions, and inflammations, and the infused oil or tea relieves fungal infections. In the past, wormwood was a popular remedy for the intermittent fevers of malaria and for expelling pinworms.

⚠ Caution

As a uterine stimulant, wormwood is contraindicated during pregnancy. Do not exceed recommended dosages or use while

Where, When, and How to Wildcraft

Introduced to North America from Europe in 1841, this woody perennial is widely naturalized throughout the northern part of the United States and across the southern Canadian latitudes. Find it growing in sunny, dry, disturbed sites such as abandoned fields and pastures and along roadsides at low to middle elevations throughout this region.

While in flower, harvest the upper green portion of branches. Cut to an outward-facing bud, and dry on screens or in upside-down hanging bundles. Discard brown or damaged

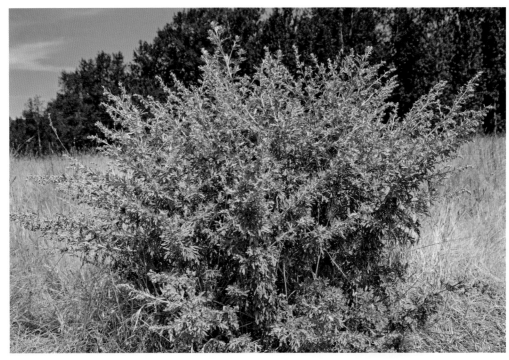

The branches sprawl, spread, or stand erect.

breastfeeding. Larger doses may irritate the stomach, increase blood pressure, or cause nausea, heart palpitations, and anxiety. Ingestion of the essential oil or long-term use of alcohol extracts is contraindicated due to high levels of thujone, a potential neurotoxin that may cause kidney damage, convulsions, tremors, or vertigo. While processing dried plant material, avoid inhaling large quantities of the leaf and flower dust, which may cause spaciness or delirium.

Future Harvests

To promote bushier growth, cut branches to an outward-facing bud while harvesting.

HERBAL PREPARATIONS

Leaf and Flower Tea
Standard infusion
Drink 2–3 fluid ounces up to 3 times per day.

Leaf and Flower Tincture
1 part dried leaf and flowers
5 parts menstruum (50 percent alcohol, 50 percent distilled water)
Take 5–15 drops up to 3 times per day.

Leaf and Flower Oil
Follow directions for Dry Herb Infused Oil or Alternative Oil Method (page 64).

yarrow

Achillea millefolium
common yarrow, milfoil
PARTS USED flower, leaf, root

Astringent leaves stanch bleeding; pungent, bitter flowers break fevers and speed the healing of colds and flus; and numbing roots soothe sore teeth and gums.

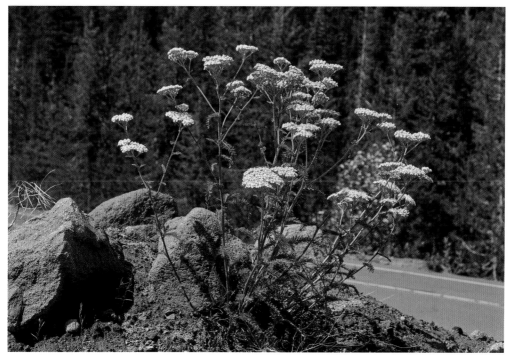

Common names from around the world reflect yarrow's use as a woundwort. The English name *yarrow* comes from the Old English *garwe*, which means "spear-well."

How to Identify

Spreading rhizomes form small clumps of erect-stemmed plants that stand 4–40 inches tall. Feathery, lance-shaped leaves, alternately arranged, aromatic, and finely dissected along the midrib, range in color from dark green to light grayish green and become smaller in size and shorter-stalked as they climb the stem. From mid spring to mid autumn, numerous composite flower heads bloom in flat- to round-topped clusters. Several whorls of dry, overlapping bracts cup each flower head, which is made up of 3–12 usually white but sometimes pinkish ray flowers and 10–75 pale yellow to cream-colored disk flowers. The tiny, flattened seeds lack crowns of feathery hairs. In wet places at lower elevations, yarrow grows lushly and up

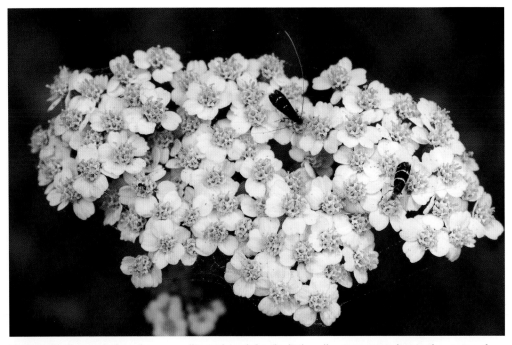

Harvest the flowers before they are pollinated. Look for the little yellow to orange dots in the center of each individual flower.

to 3½ feet tall. Sparsely leaved, high-elevation individuals growing in rocky soils may grow only a few inches tall.

Where, When, and How to Wildcraft

Yarrow's highly adaptable nature allows it to thrive in varied environments. It can be found just about anywhere: in the wildest or most domesticated places, in dry or wet places, and at all elevations from the seashore to timberline. Find it growing in open forests, grasslands, meadows, rocky hillsides, and disturbed areas all over the Pacific Northwest and throughout North America.

For the most potent medicine, harvest the aerial parts just before or as the individual flowers open and before the flowers have been pollinated. Pay close attention because the flowers are long lasting; even after the disk flowers turn brown, the ray flowers may remain white. If you see little, yellow to orange-colored, pollen-laden stamens in the center of the disk flowers, you will know that the flowers are in their prime. Flowers slightly past their prime may still make good medicine; taste and smell to be sure.

Snip the stalks near the base, one or two from each clump, and discard brown or wilting leaves. Process the leaves along with the flowers fresh for tincture. For teas or infused oils, place on screens or in bags or hang in bundles to dry. Harvest roots in autumn after the tops start to die back.

Medicinal Uses

Yarrow embodies opposites. It stops bleeding and moves stagnant blood, stimulates and relaxes, grounds and uplifts, and opens and enhances sensorial experience while providing energetic protection.

Yarrow leaves stop bleeding from the smallest cuts to the deepest wounds, prevent

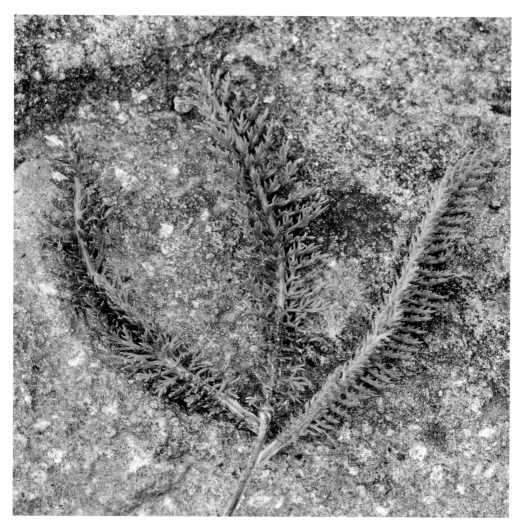

Cut to the midrib, yarrow's feathery, deeply cleft leaves are a signature for its ability to heal cuts to the bone.

infection, and relieve pain in wounded areas. Chew the leaves in the field to make a poultice or apply the tincture, oil, or salve to speed the healing of cuts and abrasions.

In the same way it closes physical wounds, yarrow also seals holes in the energetic body. If you feel overwhelmed when entering a room full of people, take small doses of yarrow leaf and flower tincture to strengthen and firm your energetic boundaries. Small doses of the tincture also open the senses

to enhance visual acuity and auditory perception.

Yarrow leaves move stagnant blood. To initiate a delayed or sluggish menses, especially when clotting is present, take the tincture or the tea. Apply the leaf oil or a wash of the leaves to clear stagnant blood from improperly healed bruises.

A tea of the aromatic flowers or the leaf and flower tincture in hot water, alone or combined in equal proportions with elderflower and field mint leaf, promotes sweating to drive out infection. At the onset of a cold or flu make a quart of the flower tea. Drink 3–4 fluid ounces, and pour the rest into a steaming hot bath. After bathing, bundle yourself up in a sleeping bag or a heavy blanket and allow your body to sweat out the infection. Chew the roots to alleviate tooth or gum pain.

Caution

Because of its blood-moving effect on the uterus, use yarrow sparingly during pregnancy.

Future Harvests

Even though yarrow grows abundantly in many places, take only one or two stalks from each clump so that individual plants will remain strong and healthy.

Rumex crispus
curly or sour dock
PARTS USED root

Bitter, astringent roots support healthy digestive function, relieve lymphatic congestion, and strengthen the bowels.

How to Identify

Stout, yellow- to orange-fleshed taproots, somewhat branching and 8–12 inches long or more, are crowned by oblong to lance-shaped, long-stalked basal leaves with round or wedge-shaped bases. Hairless, furrowed stems, unbranched below the inflorescence, often reddish, and with swollen nodes, stand 1½ to 4 feet tall. Alternately arranged stem leaves become smaller and shorter-stalked as they ascend. All leaves are wavy-edged, and a clasping sheath that becomes papery with age covers the base of each leaf's stalk. Dense, leafy-bracted clusters of numerous greenish to reddish brown flowers, arranged in whorls of 10–25 along the upper part of the stem and its branches, bloom from early summer to early autumn. Dry, reddish brown seeds, smooth and shiny, are 3-angled and enveloped by 3 papery, veined, heart-shaped bracts. The whole plant becomes reddish brown at the end of the season.

The roots of broad-leaved dock, *Rumex obtusifolius*, can be used in the same way as those of *R. crispus*. Its leaves are wider and less wavy, and the seed bracts have 1–3 spines on their edges.

A yellow dock with ripening seeds grows along the side of a road.

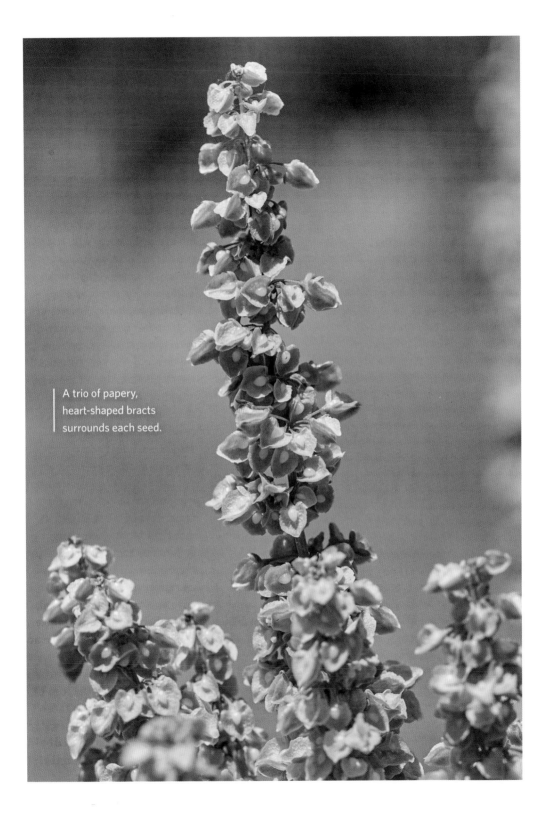

A trio of papery,
heart-shaped bracts
surrounds each seed.

Where, When, and How to Wildcraft

Introduced from Eurasia and now widespread throughout North America, yellow dock grows vigorously on a wide range of ground but prefers open sites with wet, nutrient-rich soil. Find it in wet meadows, gardens, waste areas, and along roadsides and ditches from low to middle elevations.

Dig the roots from early to late autumn. Thicker, darker-colored roots make the most potent medicine. Cut the roots width-wise into ¼-inch sections and dry on screens.

Medicinal Uses

Yellow dock root is bitter, sour, and astringent. It tones and cools the digestive tract and relieves sluggish digestion characterized by difficulty digesting fats, acid reflux, intestinal inflammation, and food allergies. It supports lymphatic circulation, purifies the blood, and relieves liver congestion to heal chronic cases of acne, eczema, or other skin eruptions. Use it to tone weak bowels that lead to diarrhea with loose but difficult to evacuate stools or in higher doses to relieve constipation. Take the tea or tincture for all of the above indications.

In cases of anemia, drink the tea to boost assimilation of iron. Like so many other high-tannin remedies, gargling yellow dock tea or the diluted tincture (30 drops in 4 fluid ounces of water) soothes sore throats, restores tone to lax and bleeding gums, and heals mouth sores. The tea or diluted tincture applied externally also reduces irritation from insect bites and speeds wound healing.

Future Harvests

This weedy species does just fine on its own.

HERBAL PREPARATIONS

Root Tea
Standard decoction
Drink 4–6 fluid ounces up to 3 times per day.

Root Tincture
1 part dried root
5 parts menstruum (50 percent alcohol, 40 percent distilled water, 10 percent glycerin)
Take 30–60 drops up to 3 times per day.

---

yellow pond-lily

Nuphar polysepala
Rocky Mountain pond-lily, spatterdock
PARTS USED root

*This cousin of the lotus has an affinity for the urogenital
and gastrointestinal systems.*

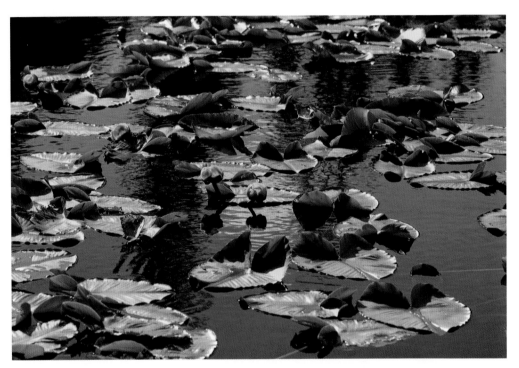

Mired in muck, very large rhizomes give rise to these beautiful flowers and leaves.

How to Identify

Large, scaled rhizomes with thick side roots cling to the bottoms of muddy ponds or slow-moving streams. Heart-shaped, thick-fleshed leaves emerge directly from the roots to unfurl on the surface, supported by thick, round, and fleshy stems up to 6½ feet long. Waxy, cup-shaped flowers made up of 6–9 thick sepals; 10–20 lance-shaped, yellow petals that are sometimes tinged green or red and smaller in size than the sepals; a disk-like, yellow stigma; and numerous yellow to reddish purple stamens sit atop stems similar to the leaf stalks, spread up to 4 inches wide, and bloom from late spring to late summer. Seeds suspended in a gooey mass mature within oval, many-chambered capsules crowned with round-tipped teeth. The greenish outer sepals are shorter than the inner, bright yellow sepals, and the usually floating leaves and flowers sometimes rise above the surface of the water.

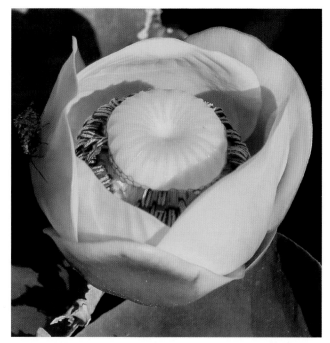

Fleshy sepals frame the flower's reproductive parts and petals.

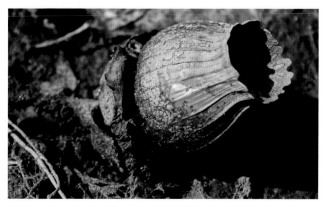

The seeds, separated from the gooey filling inside the capsule and dried, can be popped like popcorn.

Where, When, and How to Wildcraft

These aquatic plants are found at low to middle elevations in ponds, shallow lakes, and slow-moving streams throughout this region from Alaska to northern California. The massive rhizomes, sometimes the size of a baby, are challenging to extract because the roots tenaciously cling to the pond-bottom muck in which the plants reside. Look for places where yellow pond-lily grows in shallow water or where the water evaporates during summer to leave the rhizomes growing exposed or just beneath the surface at the edges of the pond. This mid summer to early autumn harvest is messy and best done as a group activity with a pre-arranged post-harvest cleanup plan. Have fun!

Medicinal Uses

Yellow pond-lily root is astringent and cooling and clears congestion in the pelvic area. It can be used, as a tea or tincture, for conditions presenting heat in the reproductive or urinary tracts, such as inflammation of the urethra, prostate, vagina, or ovaries. It is especially indicated when sharp pains and/or yellowish discharge are present. Take the tea or tincture to reduce inflammation of the stomach lining (gastritis) or of the colon (colitis), or to cool any other type of gastrointestinal inflammation.

Yellow pond-lily's affinity for the second chakra and reproductive organs makes it a useful ally in clearing the underlying disharmonies and traumas of our sexual lives. If left unattended, the energy in this area tends to stagnate, leading to chronic physical imbalances. Take a few drops of tincture or drink a cup of tea and imagine yourself sinking down into the lower chakra murk of your pelvic bowl. Use sound to express and move the stuck energies.

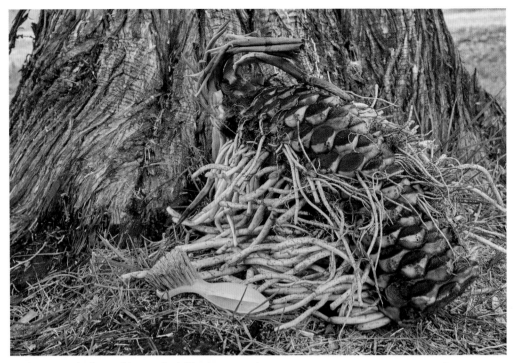
Leaf scars on the large rhizomes look like dragon scales.

Caution

Do not use yellow pond-lily for cold conditions with dull pain or when uterine fibroids are present.

Future Harvests

The interconnected rhizomes branch off to create new plants. One rhizome is enough to supply many individuals with medicine for a year and should suffice for most people's needs. If you find that you need a larger supply, take no more than a few rhizomes from each source.

yerba buena

Micromeria douglasii
PARTS USED leaf

Yerba buena, the "good herb," makes a tasty tea that soothes the digestive system and stimulates sweating to break fevers.

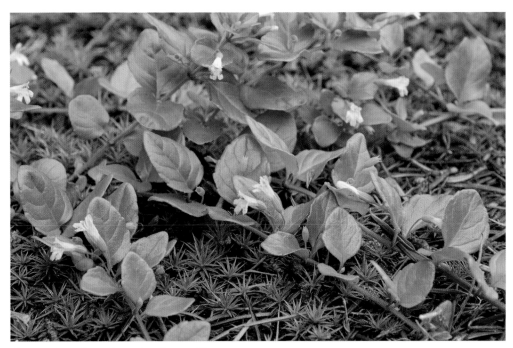

Flowers bloom from the nodes along trailing stems.

How to Identify

From woody rhizomes, ground-hugging stems with short, upward-reaching branches sprawl up to 3¼ feet and root in at the nodes to form new runners. Unevenly round-toothed and oppositely arranged, short-stalked leaves, ⅜ to 1⅜ inches long, attach to 4-sided stems. The deliciously minty-scented, egg-shaped to round, gland-dotted leaves unfurl bright green. Single, tubular, white and sometimes purple-tinged flowers emerge from the leaf axils on thin stalks to bloom from late spring to mid summer. The lower lip of the 2-lipped flowers spreads 3-lobed; the notched upper lip stands erect. Four shiny brown seeds form in the prominently ribbed, 5-toothed calyces. The stems and evergreen leaves are minutely hairy and often turn purplish in winter.

Where, When, and How to Wildcraft

Yerba buena (formerly *Satureja douglasii*) inhabits open, coniferous forests from sea level to middle elevations west of the Cascades. It grows abundantly in coastal regions from southwestern British Columbia, especially on the southern end of Vancouver Island, to southern California. It is occasionally found east of the Cascade Crest and rarely in Alaska.

All through summer but best when flowering, pull up trailing stems and cut them at a node. After drying the herb on screens or in bags, remove the leaves from the stem and store in an airtight jar or bag in a cool, dry place out of direct sunlight.

Medicinal Uses

Yerba buena leaf makes a pleasant beverage tea. Add it to formulas to improve the flavor of less palatable herbs. It stimulates sweating to break fevers during bouts of colds and flus, soothes the digestive membranes to calm an upset stomach, and relieves gas.

Future Harvests

Collect and plant seeds or carefully remove and transplant rooted sections to appropriate sites.

HERBAL PREPARATIONS

Leaf Tea
Standard infusion
Drink 6–8 fluid ounces up to 5 times per day.

Eriodictyon californicum

California yerba santa, consumptive's weed, mountain balm

PARTS USED leaf

The leaves of this "holy herb" clear mucus, relieve coughing, and speed the healing of urinary tract infections.

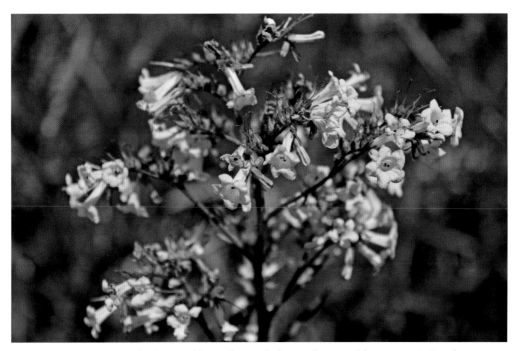

Tubular flowers, pollinated by bees and butterflies, unfurl on stalks resembling a scorpion's tail.

How to Identify

Woody lower branches with shredding bark stand erect. Sticky, yellow-green new-growth stems produce lance-shaped, 2- to 6-inch-long, usually hairless leaves. These toothed or smooth-edged leaves are dark green, sticky, and glossy above with hairs between the veins that form a net-like pattern on their lighter-colored undersides. Flowering stalks, lined with ⅓- to ⅔-inch-long tubular flowers that vary in color from white to pink to purple, unfurl like a scorpion's tail from late spring to early summer. Small seeds that can lie dormant for decades awaiting a fire or mechanical disturbance to stimulate their germination ripen in small capsules in late summer.

Where, When, and How to Wildcraft

This shallowly rooted, 2- to 8-foot-tall evergreen shrub forms stands in dry, sunny fields and open woodlands on south-facing, rocky slopes, and along roadsides at low to middle elevations. Its spreading roots help stabilize

Medicinal Uses

Yerba santa leaves warm and stimulate the respiratory system; reduce inflammation in the sinuses, throat, and lungs; and dry excessive secretions of the lungs or upper respiratory tract. Take the leaf tincture to relieve chronic asthma, bronchitis, or seasonal allergies accompanied by copious and easily expectorated mucus discharge, but keep in mind that yerba santa leaves can be very astringent. If taken in higher doses—more than about 45 drops—the drying effect may make your tongue feel like it's been wrung out, but if taken in smaller doses, you will find that yerba santa first gently dries and then remoistens and refreshes the mucous membranes.

The cooled tea or the tincture in room temperature water speeds the healing of urinary tract infections characterized by mucus discharge. The tea drunk hot or the tincture in hot water promotes sweating and increases circulation to the extremities and the surface of the skin.

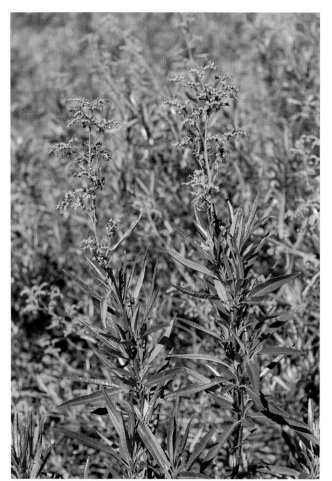

Glossy-topped, lance-shaped leaves line the stalks as the seeds ripen.

the soil on burn sites or in disturbed areas. From the northern limit of its range in Oregon's Josephine and Jackson Counties, yerba santa extends south into California.

Harvest the vibrant, new-growth leaves from early to late summer. Cut the twig ends just above an outward-facing bud to encourage bushier growth. Lay the stems with attached leaves flat to dry. Turn them regularly so the leaves don't stick together and turn brown. Remove the leaves from the stem for tincturing, teas, or smoking; leave them on the stems for smudge sticks.

Also known as consumptive's weed, yerba santa leaf has a history of use for treating tubercular cough and wasting away. Its high flavonoid content, represented by its sweet taste, points to its ability to nourish, build, and maintain the integrity of tissues.

Yerba santa has a very interesting taste characteristic—it starts out bitter and slowly gets sweeter. It teaches us how to find sweetness in the bitter experiences of life by bringing awareness to the initiatory

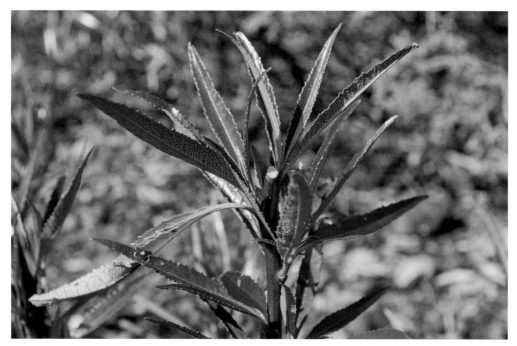

Cut the twig ends to an outward-facing bud to stimulate bushier growth. Note the distinct patterning on the undersides of the leaves.

power of trauma. In a similar way through its association with fire, yerba santa aligns us with the myth of the phoenix rising from the ashes. Burn the leaves as smudge to purify spaces and to clear heavy or dark energies from people. Crush the leaves and add them to herbal smoking mixes to help clear mucus from the lungs.

Future Harvests

Harvesting leaves stimulates new growth. The seeds will store for years if kept cool and dry. To fire treat the seeds to enhance germination, sow seeds in a wooden box (plastic pots will melt), cover the soil with small bits of bark and leaves and/or pine needles, and set aflame. Transplant seedlings to dry, rocky soil.

HERBAL PREPARATIONS

Leaf Tea
Standard infusion
Because resins are not soluble in water, yerba santa leaf is best prepared as a tincture for its mucus-clearing and respiratory-stimulating effects.
Drink 3–4 fluid ounces up to 5 times per day.

Leaf Tincture
1 part dried leaf
5 parts menstruum (65 percent alcohol, 35 percent distilled water)
I prefer making the tincture with dried leaves because the fresh leaves tend to clump up, making it more difficult to get a full extraction.
Take 10–30 drops up to 5 times per day

METRIC CONVERSIONS

INCHES	CENTIMETERS		FEET	METERS
¼	0.6		1	0.3
⅓	0.8		2	0.6
½	1.3		3	0.9
¾	1.9		4	1.2
1	2.5		5	1.5
2	5.1		6	1.8
3	7.6		7	2.1
4	10		8	2.4
5	13		9	2.7
6	15		10	3
7	18			
8	20			
9	23			
10	25			

TO CONVERT	MULTIPLY BY
feet to centimeters	30.5
inches to centimeters	2.54
inches to millimeters	25.4
pounds to kilograms	0.45
fluid ounces to milliliters	29.6
pint to milliliters	473
quart to milliliters	946

TEMPERATURES

degrees Celsius = 5/9 × (degrees Fahrenheit – 32)

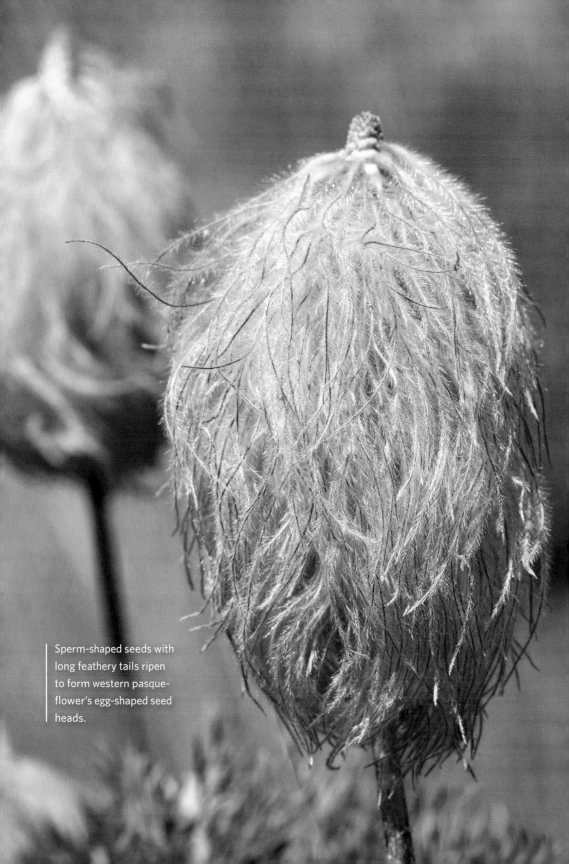

Sperm-shaped seeds with long feathery tails ripen to form western pasque-flower's egg-shaped seed heads.

REFERENCES

Arno, Stephen F., and Ramona P. Hammerly. 1977. *Northwest Trees: Identifying and Understanding the Region's Native Trees*. Seattle, WA: The Mountaineers.

Arora, David. 1986. *Mushrooms Demystified: A Comprehensive Guide to the Fleshy Fungi*. Berkeley, CA: Ten Speed Press.

Arora, David. 1991. *All That the Rain Promises and More: A Hip Pocket Guide to Western Mushrooms*. Berkeley, CA: Ten Speed Press.

Bennett, Robin Rose. 2014. *The Gift of Healing Herbs: Plant Medicines and Home Remedies for a Vibrantly Healthy Life*. Berkeley, CA: North Atlantic Books.

Bensky, Dan, and Andrew Gamble. 1993. *Chinese Herbal Medicine: Materia Medica*. Rev. ed. Seattle, WA: Eastland Press.

Bergner, Paul. *Symphytum: Comfrey, Coltsfoot, and Pyrrolizidine Alkaloids*. medherb.com/Materia_Medica/Symphytum_-_Comfrey,_Coltsfoot,_and_Pyrrolizidine_Alkaloids.htm. Retrieved May 13, 2015.

Bergner, Paul. *Symphytum: Hepatotoxicity of Pyrrolizidine Alkaloids*. medherb.com/Materia_Medica/Symphytum_-_Hepatotoxicity_of_pyrrolizidine_alkaloids_.htm. Retrieved May 13, 2015.

Buhner, Stephen Harrod. 2005. *Healing Lyme: Natural Healing and Prevention for Lyme Borreliosis and Its Coinfections*. Silver City, NM: Raven Press.

Buhner, Stephen Harrod. 2007. *The Natural Testosterone Plan: For Sexual Health and Energy*. Rochester, VT: Healing Arts Press.

Buhner, Stephen Harrod. 2012. *Herbal Antibiotics: Natural Alternatives for Treating Drug-Resistant Bacteria*. 2nd ed. North Adams, MA: Storey Publishing.

Buhner, Stephen Harrod. 2013. *Herbal Antivirals: Natural Remedies for Emerging and Resistant Viral Infections*. North Adams, MA: Storey Publishing.

Burke Museum of Natural History and Culture. WTU Image Collection: Plants of Washington, Lichens of Washington. biology.burke.washington.edu/herbarium/imagecollection.php. Retrieved March 29, 2016.

Cech, Richo. 2000. *Making Plant Medicine*. Williams, OR: Horizon Herbs, LLC.

Cech, Richo. 2009. *The Medicinal Herb Grower: A Guide for Cultivating Plants That Heal*. Vol. 1. Williams, OR: Horizon Herbs, LLC.

Cullina, William. 2000. *The New England Wild Flower Society Guide to Growing and Propagating Wildflowers of the United States and Canada*. New York: Houghton Mifflin.

Deur, Douglas, and Nancy Turner. 2005. *Keeping It Living: Traditions of Plant Use and Cultivation on the Northwest Coast of North America*. Seattle: University of Washington Press.

Donahue, Sean. *Ghost Pipe (Montotropa uniflora)*. greenmanramblings.blogspot.com/2010/07/ghost-pipe-monotropa-uniflora.html. Retrieved June 16, 2015.

Drum, Ryan. *Medicinal Uses of Seaweeds*. ryandrum.com/seaweeds.htm. Retrieved April 28, 2015.

Drum, Ryan. *Radiation Protection Using Seaweeds*. ryandrum.com/radiation protectionusingseaweeds.htm. Retrieved May 1, 2015.

Drum, Ryan. *Sea Vegetables for Food and Medicine*. ryandrum.com/seaxpan1.html. Retrieved April 28, 2015.

Ellingwood, Finley. 1915. *American Materia Medica, Therapeutics and Pharmacognosy*. Chicago: Ellingwood's Therapeutist.

Elpel, Thomas. 2008. *Botany in a Day: The Patterns Method of Plant Identification*. 5th ed. Pony, MT: HOPS Press.

Foster, Steven, and Christopher Hobbs. 2002. *A Field Guide to Western Medicinal Plants and Herbs*. New York: Houghton Mifflin.

Frances, Deborah. 2014. *Practical Wisdom in Natural Healing: Sage Advice for the Modern World*. Chandler, AZ: Polychrest Publishing.

Gilkey, Helen M., and La Rea J. Dennis. 2001. *Handbook of Northwestern Plants*. Rev. ed. Corvallis: Oregon State University Press.

Gladstar, Rosemary, and Pamela Hirsch, eds. *Planting the Future: Saving Our Medicinal Herbs*. Rochester, VT: Healing Arts Press.

Green, James. 2000. *The Herbal Medicine-Maker's Handbook: A Home Manual*. Freedom, CA: Crossing Press.

Gunther, Erna. 1973. *Ethnobotany of Western Washington: The Knowledge and Use of Indigenous Plants by Native Americans*. Seattle: University of Washington Press.

Hickman, James C., ed. 1993. *The Jepson Manual: Higher Plants of California*. Berkeley: University of California Press.

Hitchcock, Leo, and Arthur Cronquist. 1973. *Flora of the Pacific Northwest*. Seattle: University of Washington Press.

Hobbs, Christopher. 1986. *Medicinal Mushrooms: An Exploration of Tradition, Healing, and Culture*. Santa Cruz, CA: Botanica Press.

Holmes, Peter. 2006. *The Energetics of Western Herbs: A Materia Medica Integrating Western and Chinese Herbal Therapeutics*. 2 vols. 4th ed. Boulder, CO: Snow Lotus Press.

Jepson Flora Project, eds. 2013. *Jepson eFlora*, ucjeps.berkeley.edu/IJM.html. Retrieved March 29, 2016.

Jolley, Russ. 1988. *Wildflowers of the Columbia Gorge: A Comprehensive Field Guide*. Portland: Oregon Historical Society Press.

Klinkenberg, Brian, ed. 2014. *E-Flora BC: Electronic Atlas of the Plants of British Columbia*. ibis.geog.ubc.ca/biodiversity/eflora/. Retrieved March 29, 2016.

Kruckeburg, Arthur R. 1982. *Gardening with Native Plants of the Pacific Northwest*. 2nd ed. Seattle: University of Washington Press.

Lantz, Trevor C., Kristina Swerhun, and Nancy J. Turner, 2004. Devil's club (*Oplopanax horridus*): an ethnobotanical review. *HerbalGram* 62: 33–48.

Link, Russell. 1999. *Landscaping for Wildlife in the Pacific Northwest*. Seattle: University of Washington Press.

Masé, Guido. 2013. *The Wild Medicine Solution: Healing with Aromatic, Bitter, and Tonic Plants*. Rochester, VT: Healing Arts Press.

McDonald, Jim. *Mullein*. herbcraft.org/mullein.html. Retrieved June 23, 2015.

McGuffin, Michael, ed. *American Herbal Products Association's Botanical Safety Handbook*.

Boca Raton, FL: CRC Press.

Moore, Michael. 1993. *Medicinal Plants of the Pacific West*. Santa Fe, NM: Red Crane Books.

Moore, Michael. 2003. *Medicinal Plants of the Mountain West*. Santa Fe: Museum of New Mexico Press.

Parish, Roberta, Ray Coupé, and Dennis Lloyd, eds. 1996. *Plants of Southern Interior British Columbia and the Inland Northwest*. Vancouver, BC: Lone Pine Publishing.

Pojar, Jim, and Andy MacKinnon, eds. 1994. *Plants of the Pacific Northwest Coast*. Vancouver, BC: Lone Pine Publishing.

Rogers, Robert. 2011. *The Fungal Pharmacy: The Complete Guide to Medicinal Mushrooms and Lichens of North America*. Berkeley, CA: North Atlantic Books.

Rogers, Robert. 2014. Three under-utilized medicinal polypores. *Journal of the American Herbalists Guild* 12(2): 15–21.

Rose, Kiva. 2010. *Mending with the Devil's Darning Needles: The Pain Relieving Properties of Clematis*. bearmedicineherbals.com/clematis.html. Retrieved July 6, 2015.

Rose, Robin, Caryn E. C. Chachulski, and Diane L. Haase. 1998. *Propagation of Pacific Northwest Native Plants*. Corvallis: Oregon State University Press.

Schofield, Janice J. 1989. *Discovering Wild Plants: Alaska, Western Canada, the Northwest*. Portland, OR: Alaska Northwest Books.

7Song. *Herbalist's View: Anemone for Panic Attacks*. 7song.com/files/Herbalists%20 View-%20Anemone%20for%20Panic%20 Attacks.pdf. Retrieved March 8, 2015.

Storl, Wolf D. 2010. *Healing Lyme Disease Naturally: History, Analysis, and Treatments*. Berkeley, CA: North Atlantic Books.

Tilford, Gregory. 1997. *Edible and Medicinal Plants of the West*. Missoula, MT: Mountain Press.

Turner, Mark, and Phyllis Gustafson. 2006. *Wildflowers of the Pacific Northwest*. Portland, OR: Timber Press.

Turner, Mark, and Ellen Kuhlmann. 2014. *Trees and Shrubs of the Pacific Northwest*. Portland, OR: Timber Press.

U.S. Forest Service. *How to Identify and Control Dogwood Anthracnose*. http://na.fs.fed.us/spfo/pubs/howtos/ht_dogwd/ht_dog.htm. Retrieved February 17, 2015.

Vance, Nan. 2012. Finding Brown's peony a sweet attraction. *Kalmiopsis* 19: 1–6.

Weed, Susun. 1989. *Healing Wise: The Wise Woman Herbal*. Woodstock, NY: Ash Tree Publishing.

Weed, Susun. 2003. *Herbal Medicine Chest in Your Backyard*. susunweed.com/herbal_ezine/september03/herbalmedicine.htm. Retrieved May 14, 2015.

Weiss, Rudolf Fritz. 1988. *Herbal Medicine*. Beaconsfield, England: Beaconsfield Publishers.

Willard, Terry. 1992. *Edible and Medicinal Plants of the Rocky Mountains and Neighbouring Territories*. Calgary, Alberta: Wild Rose College of Natural Healing.

Winston, David, and Steven Maimes. 2007. *Adaptogens: Herbs for Strength, Stamina, and Stress Relief*. Rochester, VT: Healing Arts Press.

Wood, Matthew. 1997. *The Book of Herbal Wisdom*. Berkeley, CA: North Atlantic Books.

Wood, Matthew. 2004. *The Practice of Traditional Western Herbalism: Basic Doctrine, Energetics, and Classification*. Berkeley, CA: North Atlantic Books.

Wood, Matthew. 2008. *The Earthwise Herbal: A Complete Guide to Old World Medicinal Plants*. Berkeley, CA: North Atlantic Books.

Wood, Matthew. 2009. *The Earthwise Herbal: A Complete Guide to New World Medicinal Plants*. Berkeley, CA: North Atlantic Books.

ACKNOWLEDGMENTS

First and foremost, I'd like to extend my deepest gratitude to the plants who have given me hope and sustained me in this life and to all of the students with whom I've had the honor to share plant realm explorations. My appreciation for and experience of the majesty and magic of plants has been greatly enhanced by the work we've all done and continue to do together.

I would like to also thank my friend Bradford T. McLain, who showed up at just the right moment as I was trying to find out what all of these green things were out in the forest. He brought an understanding of botany out west just as I was trying to figure how these field guide and botanical key things worked. Many thanks to Dr. Deborah Frances for introducing me to the magic of plants; to Mark Disharoon for showing me how to harvest with speed, accuracy, and respect; to Christopher Hobbs for showing me how to balance science and wonder; to Cascade Anderson Geller for seeing something in me that at the time I was unable to see; and to Matthew Wood for affirming that I wasn't crazy to view the plants as more than physical beings.

Sincere thanks to my friends Cait, Nina, Sommer, Emily, and Lauren, who hung out with my boys while I was writing this book and showered them with love and tenderness; to my team, Jen Stickley, Kate Coulton, Amy Terepka, and Saliha Abrams, for holding down the fort and for being the pillars who hold a space for our community of plant medicine people to flourish; and to Elise Krohn, Gradey Proctor, Christopher Smaka, Erico Schleicher, Sean Donahue, and Howie Brounstein for their very important input: this book is much better for their involvement.

Eternal gratitude to Dr. J. J. Pursell for connecting me with this project, to Juree Sondker and Eve Goodman of Timber Press for their support and guidance through the process of writing my first book, to Lisa DiDonato Brousseau for her keen editing eye and her thoughtful and sensible suggestions, and to the whole Timber Press staff for making this life-long dream of writing a book possible.

Thanks to my family—Uni and Richard Sturt, Roeland Kloos (especially for helping me purchase a new camera lens), Joanne Dusseau, and Mark and Michelle Horton—for all of their support. Thanks also to Chiboola Malaambo for assisting me in procuring a lens.

Without the love of my beautiful wife, Kathryn, I wouldn't be where I am today. Thanks to her for putting up with my madness and for holding a space for me to prosper. Thanks to my boys, Finn and Joaquin, for filling my heart with more love than I thought possible and for inspiring me to do all that I can to make this world a better place. I am so proud to be a father of such wonderful children.

And finally, from the depths of my being I offer gratitude to the Queen of the Forest for guiding me to the hidden yet easily accessible wild places that exist inside my body and beyond the borders of my skin and for awakening me to all of the love, beauty, and knowledge that exists in this world. I will continue to walk proudly on the path she's laid before me, dedicated to serving her mission here on Earth.

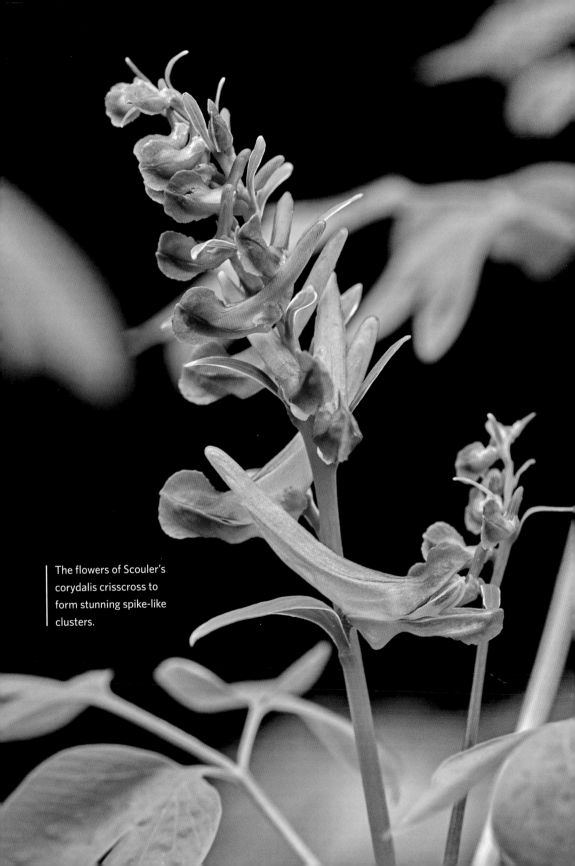

The flowers of Scouler's corydalis crisscross to form stunning spike-like clusters.

PHOTOGRAPHY CREDITS

*I am grateful to those who have made
their photos available for this book.*

Mackenzie Duffy, pages 37, 53, 317, 355,
   389 bottom
Robyn Klein, pages 33 top, 34
Sarah Milhollin, pages 3, 5, 6–7, 65

Flickr

Used under a Creative Commons
Attribution 2.0 Generic license
Andrey Zharkikh, pages 366, 388, 389 top
In Awe of God's Creation, page 206
Jason Hollinger, page 145
Mount Rainier National Park, page 360
Superior National Forest, page 207

Used under a Creative Commons
Attribution-ShareAlike 2.0 Generic license
Frank Mayfield, page 105
Matt Lavin, page 146
Ole Husby, page 315

Wikimedia

Used under a Creative Commons
Attribution 3.0 Unported license
Hajotthu, page 314

Used under a Creative Commons
Attribution-Share Alike 3.0 Unported license
Anneli Salo, page 275
Christian Fischer, page 110
Doug Murphy, page 93
Fritz Flohr Reynolds, page 106
Ivar Leidus, page 167
Qwert1234, page 232
Walter Siegmund, pages 327, 328

Public domain on Wikimedia Commons
George Chernilevsky, page 91
U.S. Army Corps of Engineers, page 313

All other photos are by the author.

INDEX

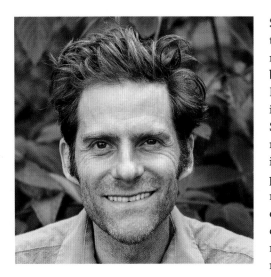

Scott Kloos is a plant medicine practitioner, ceremonialist, wildcrafter, medicine maker, and singer of plant songs. He has been working with the native plants of the Pacific Northwest since the late 1990s. He is the founder and managing director of The School of Forest Medicine (forestmedicine. net), which offers classes and courses that interweave direct spiritual experience with practical, hands-on participatory work and range from long-term initiatory journeys to evening Plant Teacher Circle meditations. He owns Cascadia Folk Medicine (cascadiafolk medicine.com), which supplies the community with high-quality, small-batch herbal extracts from the native plants of this region. In his healing practice, he works mainly with the psycho-spiritual aspects of plant medicine and was a founding member of the Elderberry School of Botanical Medicine (elder berryschool.com) in Portland, Oregon.